# BONE
# RADIOLOGY
# CASE
# STUDIES

# BONE RADIOLOGY CASE STUDIES

## Terrence C Demos MD

To

GINA
christine
terry

# CONTENTS

# FOREWORD

Physicians who care for patients suffering from diseases and injuries to the skeleton have always profited from a close relationship with the physical sciences. This was true in the Middle Ages when "state of the art" metallurgy was used to produce artificial hands for injured knights. Contemporary examples range from material science, which has produced artificial joints and ligaments, to signal analysis, which promises equal results in prosthetics and paraplegics.

However, none of the interactions between physical science and medicine has produced an equal to the application of the discovery of radiation to the development of bone imaging. With this, serious study of the skeleton was possible, and injuries and diseases were described and classified. This interaction between physics and medicine has continued, and with each improvement in imaging, additional information about skeletal disease becomes available.

The quality of the image is only one aspect of a plain roentgenogram, a tomogram, a CT scan, or a nuclide scan. Of equal importance is the extraction of information from the films and the application of this information to the patient. Missed information due to inadequate assessment is much more common than errors due to technical difficulties.

Learning to read roentgenograms accurately seems to be easy for some physicians but very difficult for others. One of the major hindrances to learning this process is hindsight bias. This mental trap allows the person who has equivocated in the interpretation of a roentgenogram to say, "Oh yes, that's what I thought." The only cure for this disease is a firm *a priori* commitment to an interpretation. The "surprise" of discovering that one might be wrong is a potent teaching tool.

Terrence Demos is an excellent teacher. He brings this technique into *Bone Radiology Case Studies* with the presentation of roentgenograms and a firm, clear question, "Your diagnosis?" The person with enough self-control to stop at this point and make a definite diagnosis will be rewarded. In the next few pages, the reader will find the correct answer and a great deal of information about the subject. This material will be better retained for having taken the time to form a diagnosis.

The case study method of learning a subject has long been a favorite way of teaching medicine and is still demonstrated each week in the *New England Journal of Medicine*. About the time that business schools discovered the case study method (and believed they invented it), medical editors began to prefer series data. Although averages and proportions are useful information, the random variation inherent in aggregates frequently obscures important details.

The debate between these two methods is best illustrated by an old medical-school story. It is Grand Rounds and a certain self-confident associate professor is pontificating, "Why, in my experience I've seen hundreds of these cases." At this point, the professor turns to him and answers, "But I have *studied* three." The title *Bone Radiology Case Studies* would seem to be on the side of the professor, but the book's content attempts to incorporate the best of both methods. The judgments are to be made about specific cases, but the series data is given to amplify and expand the reader's data base. For the more inquiring mind, the references provide additional information.

This book will be important reading for many classes of health professionals. Certainly orthopedists and radiologists (both puppies and old dogs) will find it most useful. Rheumatologists, oncologists, and others with an interest in the skeletal system will find sections of importance. Basic scientists involved in studies of the bony architecture should find the relation of form to function helpful.

Dr. Demos has taught us some important ideas about the skeletal system. He has taught us and made it fun.

**Wilton H. Bunch, MD PhD**
William M. Scholl Professor of Orthopaedics;
Chairman, Department of Orthopaedics and Rehabilitation
Loyola University Medical Center
Maywood, Illinois

# ACKNOWLEDGMENTS

The following physicians from the Loyola University Medical Center collaborated with the author on studies:

Manuel Alonso, M.D.

Mark Baker, M.D.

Michael Flisak, M.D.

David Gibson, M.D.

Philip Ludkowski, M.D.

John McCaffrey, M.D.

Richard Provus, MD

Sarcomatous Degeneration of an Enchondroma

Acute Lymphocytic Leukemia

Hemophilia

Sickle Cell Anemia

Computed Tomography

Fibrous Dysplasia

Osteosarcoma

Rheumatoid Arthritis

Vertebral Column Osteoid Osteoma

Partial Meniscectomy with Torn Remnant was written by Richard Cooper, M.D.

The text was typed by Joy Stella. The photographs were taken by Robert Vick and his staff. Ted Lewis and Harold Miller of Slack, Inc. were always available for advice. *TCD*

# INTRODUCTION

Most of the material in this volume first appeared in the journal *Orthopedics,* published by Slack, Inc. There are 39 studies, which have been supplemented with 100 new illustrations. The first study lists fundamental radiographic signs of bone and joint disease, and those that follow are arranged to emphasize these signs. Imaging with radionuclides, computed tomography, and arthrography is reviewed.

Radiographs and clinical information concerning a patient initiate each study and invite the reader to make a diagnosis. These patients have been selected because their radiographs are characteristic of a disease or emphasize a point concerning that disease. After the diagnosis is given, the salient features of the disease are reviewed, radiographic features are described and illustrated, and current references are listed.

There are several superb, comprehensive textbooks of bone and joint radiology. Most of these are not only large but have multiple volumes. This work is intended to give practicing physicians and residents a collection of concise, orderly, and well-illustrated reviews of a variety of diseases. It is hoped that the book's format and size will allow it to fit into the niches of busy schedules and provide a change of pace in the medical reading marathon.

# BONE RADIOLOGY CASE STUDIES

# RADIOGRAPHIC FEATURES OF BONE AND JOINT DISEASE

SIZE AND SHAPE          PERIOSTEUM

DENSITY                 SOFT TISSUE

CORTEX                  JOINTS

TRABECULAE

# Study 1

This 20-year-old woman is 4 feet 8 inches tall and has a horseshoe kidney. *Your diagnosis?*

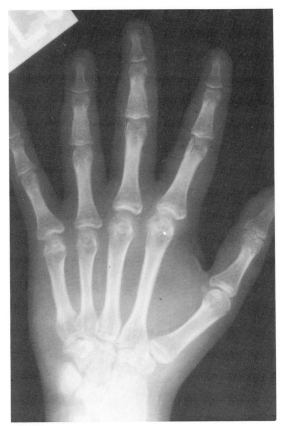

**Fig. 1A:** AP view hand.

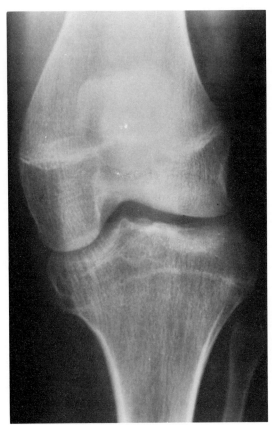

**Fig. 1B:** AP view knee.

# Diagnosis: Turner's Syndrome

In Fig. 1A there is decreased bone density, delayed skeletal maturation, a short ring metacarpal, and a decreased carpal angle with the proximal carpal row forming a V shape instead of gentle curve. In Fig. 1B there is overgrowth of the medial femoral condyle. These findings are characteristic of *Turner's Syndrome*.

I could not help laughing at the ease with which he explained his process of deduction. "When I hear you give your reasons," I remarked, "the thing always appears to me to be so ridiculously simple that I could easily do it myself, though at each successive instance of your reasoning I am baffled until you explain your process. And yet, I believe that my eyes are as good as yours."

"Quite so", he answered, "you see, but you do not observe. The distinction is clear . . . you did not know where to look, and so you missed all that was important."

*—Sherlock Holmes*

The Gestalt, or Aunt Minnie, approach to radiographs relies on instant recognition of the whole image. The diagnosis is then based on having seen the same image in the past, either in print or in another patient. Close attention to detail or thinking isn't required. This method works in "classic" cases and works more often for experienced interpreters. When lesions are atypical, however, errors are common. To make the proper diagnosis in these cases, Holmesean attention to detail is required.

Greenfield in his Textbook lists 31 features of bone lesions:

| | |
|---|---|
| loss of bone density | periosteum |
| altered bone texture | short bone |
| epiphysis | long bone |
| physis | overtubulation |
| zone of provisional calcification | undertubulation |
| metaphysis | contour change |
| medulla, spongiosa | expansion of bone |
| cortex | destruction of bone |
| endosteum | resorption of bone |
| erosion of bone | shape of lesion |
| bone sclerosis | margination |
| calcification | bone age |
| origin of solitary lesion | fracture |
| location of the lesion | soft tissue |
| invasion or lack of it | joints |
| size of lesion | |

This extensive list of radiographic features has been consolidated and organized as follows (features of growing bones and the solitary lesion are omitted):

4

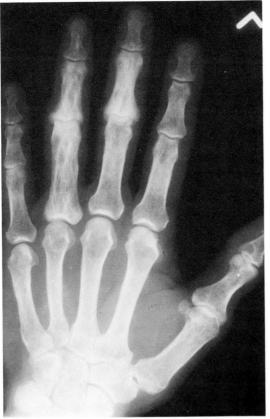

Figure 2

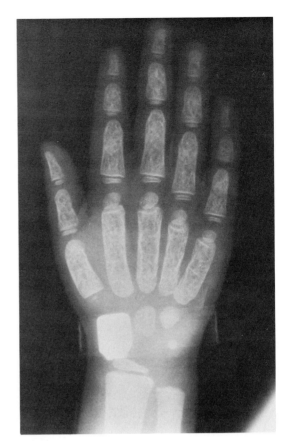

Figure 3

## Radiographic Features of Skeletal Disease

**Size**
Increased—General or local
Decreased—General or local

**Shape**
Overtubulated
Undertubulated
Deformed

**Density**
Increased—General or local
Decreased—General or local

**Cortex**
Thickened
Thinned
Discontinuous

**Trabeculae**
Destroyed
Thickened
Disrupted

**Periosteal New Bone**
Solid
Linear
Spiculated
Amorphous

**Soft Tissue**
Increased—General or local
Decreased—General or local

**Joints**
Wide
Narrow
Eroded
Calcified

**Fig. 2:** The enlarged phalanges have increased density, thickened cortex and widened trabeculae. *Paget's Disease.*

**Fig. 3:** All bones are rectangular (undertubulated) with decreased density, thin cortices, and fewer, but coarsened, trabeculae. *Thalassemia.*

These radiographic features of skeletal disease are illustrated by several congenital, traumatic, neoplastic, inflammatory, metabolic, and idiopathic bone lesions. The notes accompanying each feature mention a few entities which cause that feature.[2-6]

## Size

Endocrine problems and congenital short stature syndromes can cause generalized or local altered bone size (Fig. 1A). Size change in isolated bones can be related to diseases or trauma affecting the physis, fibrous dysplasia, or Paget's disease (Fig. 2).

## Shape

Diseases which decrease normal long bone modeling or expand bone result in a rectangular bone (Fig. 3) or a bulbous "Erlenmeyer Flask" bone end.

Diseases causing increased modeling or simple disuse can result in thin shafted, overtubulated long bones (Fig. 4).

A number of diseases and injuries result in abnormal shape and contour of bone (Fig. 1B).

## Density

The plain radiograph is very insensitive to bone loss. In a vertebra, for example, destruction is not seen until 40% of the bone is gone. In general, thin cortices, trabecular loss and prominent vertebral end plates indicate loss of bone density on plain films. Nuclear medicine transmission studies and computed tomography can accurately determine bone density. Generalized decreased bone density is not equated with osteoporosis since the decreased bone density found in hyperparathyroidism, osteomalacia, multiple myeloma, and other diseases looks identical to that found in osteoporosis; only specific findings such as subperiosteal resorption or pseudofractures (Fig. 5) allow a specific radiographic diagnosis of the etiology of decreased bone density. Bone destruction may consist of a single large hole (geographic) (Fig. 6), multiple coalescent medium sized holes (motheaten) (Fig. 7), or numerous tiny holes (permeative) (Fig. 8). Osteosclerosis can be general (Fig. 9) or local (Fig. 10). Avascular necrosis, infarcts, and metastasis are common causes of local sclerosis. Metastasis, hematologic disease, and Paget's can cause generalized increased density.

## Cortex

The most common cortical abnormalities are thin cortex in osteoporotic old people and discontinuous cortex due to fractures (Fig. 11). Cortical destruction indicates a process within the bone (Fig. 12) or adjacent soft tissue such as infection or neoplasm. Subperiosteal resorption is pathognomonic of hyperparathyroidism (Fig. 13).

## Trabeculae

Diseases which result in loss of small trabeculae (sickle cell disease, osteomalacia) are often associated with thickening of remaining trabeculae (Fig. 3) especially along lines of stress. Paget's disease is characterized by thickened trabeculae (Fig. 14). Infections and neoplasms result in destruction of trabeculae.

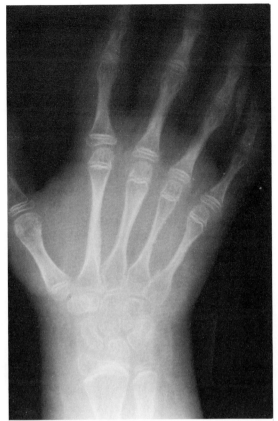

Figure 4

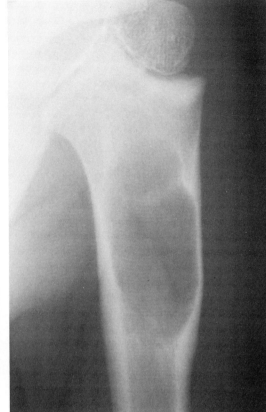

Figure 6

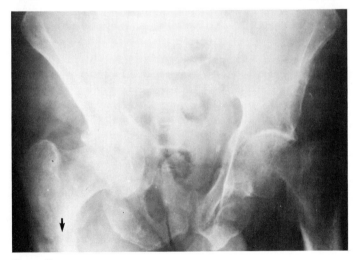

Figure 5

**Fig. 4:** Narrow (overtubulated) metacarpals with generalized decreased bone density. *Osteogenesis Imperfecta.*

**Fig. 5:** This patient has generalized decreased bone density, severe pelvic deformity, and a pseudofracture (arrow). *Osteomalacia.*

**Fig. 6:** Single sharply defined lucent lesion thinning the cortex and "expanding" the bone. Geographic bone destruction. *Bone Cyst.*

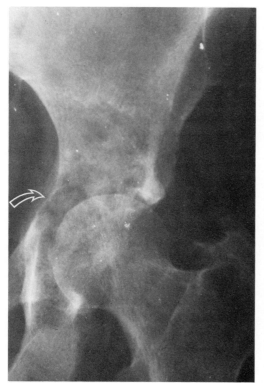

Figure 7

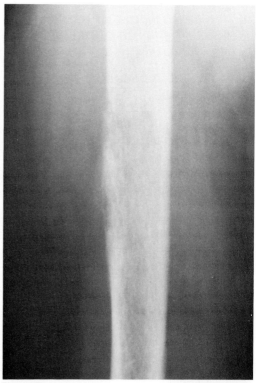

Figure 8

**Fig. 7:** Coalescent areas of bone destruction with loss of acetabular, pelvic rim cortex (arrow). Motheaten bone destruction. *Metastatic Adenocarcinoma.*

**Fig. 8:** Numerous tiny areas of bone destruction plus cortical destruction—permeative bone destruction. *Metastatic Lymphoma.*

**Fig. 9:** This patient has generalized increased bone density with "stripped" vertebra. Characteristic of *Secondary Hyperparathyroidism.* (Note central lucent stripes in vertebra.)

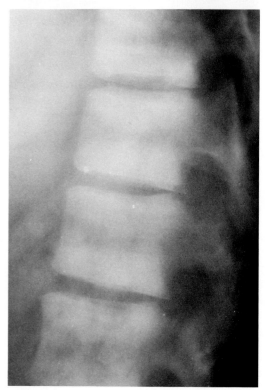

Figure 9

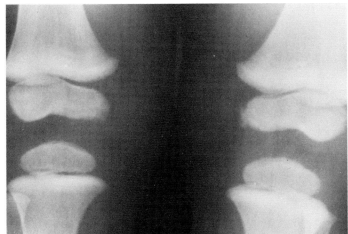

Figure 10

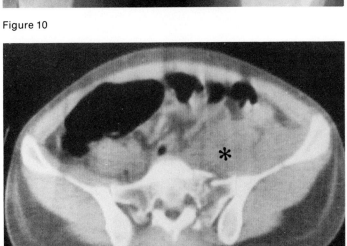

Figure 11

**Fig. 10:** Dense metaphyseal bands (zone of provisional calcification). *Lead Poisoning.*

**Fig. 11:** Discontinuous cortex left sacrum and pelvic hematoma (asterisk). The *Sacral Fracture* is obvious on this computed tomogram but was quite subtle on plain radiographs.

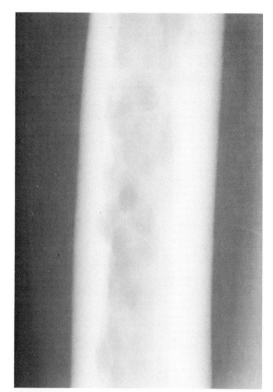

Figure 12

Figure 13

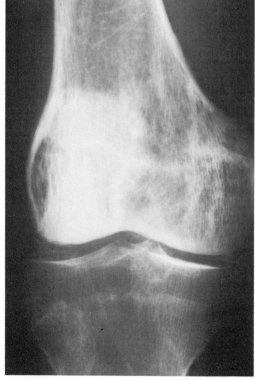

Figure 14

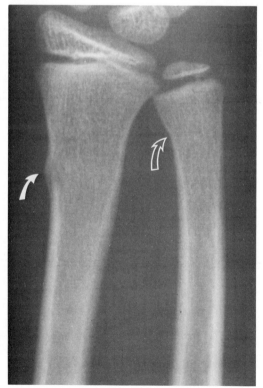

Figure 15

Bone Radiology Case Studies

Incomplete fractures, especially in children, or impacted fractures are marked by disordered trabeculae (Fig. 15).

## Periosteal New Bone

When the periosteum is elevated by pus, blood or neoplastic tissue, it may lay down new bone from its inner bone producing layer (Fig. 16). Multiple layers of periosteal new bone indicate multiple episodes of periosteal lifting. If a rapid process breaks through the central portion of lifted periosteum leaving the near and far edges of the lifted periosteum intact, the triangle formed by the cortex and intact periosteal remnant is called a Codman's triangle (Fig. 17). This triangle is a time honored sign of a rapidly moving process but is not pathognomonic of malignancy.

Very rapid progression of a bone lesion also results in parallel strands of periosteal new bone perpendicular to the cortex; the "hair on end" appearance (Fig. 17). If strands of periosteal reaction radiate from a point, a "sunburst" appearance is seen (Fig. 18). These latter types of periosteal new bone probably extend along Sharpey's fibers.

Amphorous periosteal reaction is seen with bone neoplasms and hypertrophic pulmonary osteoarthropathy (Fig. 19).

## Soft Tissue

Soft tissue may be calcified, ossified, enlarged, atrophic or the site of masses (Figs. 20, 21). Normal fat planes can be displaced or obliterated indicating abnormality in the underlying bone or joint (Fig. 22).

## Joints

Narrowing can be symmetric (rheumatoid arthritis) (Fig. 23) or asymmetric (osteoarthritis). Acromegaly causes widened joints (Fig. 24). Erosions of inflammatory arthritis occur earliest on intraarticular joints' surfaces unprotected by cartilage. Calcifications of cartilage due to calcium pyrophosphate dihydrate crystals may indicate the etiology of a patient's arthritis or lead to a diagnosis of hyperparathyroidism.

**Fig. 12:** Lytic lesions causing endosteal scalloping (arrows) and also seen as round lucencies. *Multiple Myeloma.*

**Fig. 13:** Extensive erosion of subperiosteal cortex (arrows) tuft erosion, and decreased bone density. *Hyperparathyroidism.*

**Fig. 14:** Diminished trabeculae and thin cortex of tibia—*Osteoporosis.* Thickened trabeculae and cortex of femur which is slightly enlarged—*Paget's Disease.* Incidental finding *Chondrocalcinosis.*

**Fig. 15:** Zone of disordered trabeculae medial to *Torus Fracture* (Closed arrow). Minimal angulation of ulnar cortex (Open arrow) indicates fracture also.

### References

1. Greenfield G: *Radiology of Bone Diseases.* Philadelphia, J.B. Lippincott, 1980.
2. Edeiken J, Hodes PJ: *Roentgen Diagnosis of Diseases of Bone.* Baltimore, Williams and Wilkins, 1981.
3. Aegerter E, Kirkpatrick JA: *Orthopedic Diseases: Physiology, Pathology, Radiology.* Philadelphia, W.B. Saunders, 1975.
4. Ozonoff MB: *Pediatric Orthopedic Radiology.* Philadelphia, W.B. Saunders, 1978.
5. Keats TE: *Normal Roentgen Variants.* Chicago, Year Book Medical Publishers, 1979.
6. Freiberger RM: *Bone Disease Syllabus* (Third Series). Chicago, American College of Radiology, 1980.

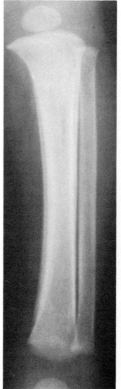

Figure 16

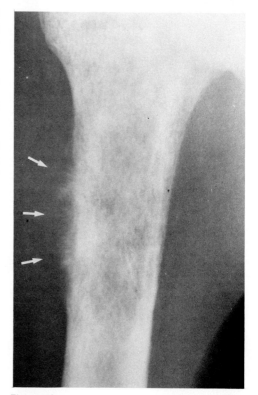

Figure 17

**Fig. 16:** Linear periosteal new bone of the tibia in a month old child with swelling in the mandible and leg— *Infantile Cortical Hyperostosis.*

**Fig. 17:** Spiculated periosteal new bone formation, Codman's triangle (arrows) and dense sclerosis of the distal femur—*Osteosarcoma.*

**Fig. 18:** Spiculated periosteal new bone (arrows), permeative bone destruction and cortical destruction. *Metastasis— Prostatic Carcinoma.*

Figure 18

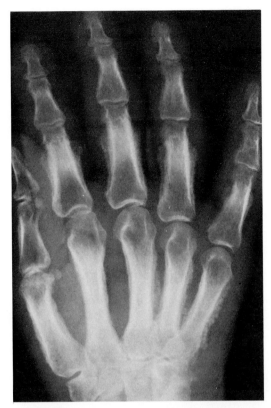

Figure 19

**Fig. 19:** Extensive amorphous periosteal new bone. *Pulmonary Osteoarthropathy* in a patient with bronchogenic carcinoma.

**Fig. 20:** Round soft tissue calcifications with lucent centers in a forearm mass. *Hemangioma* with phleboliths.

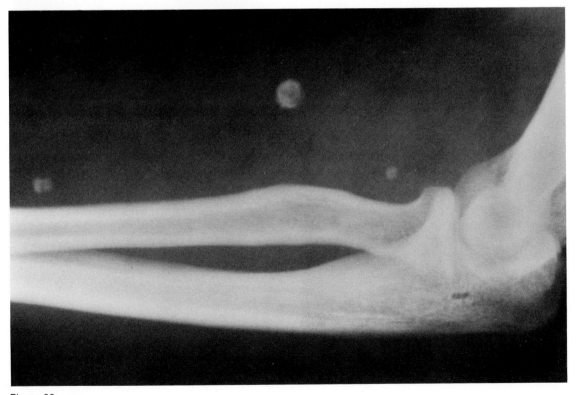

Figure 20

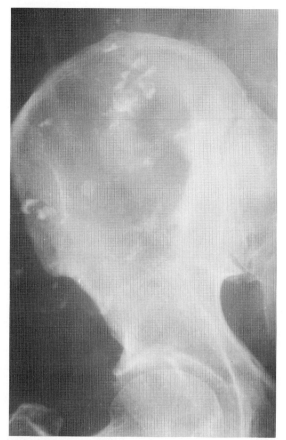

Fig. 21: Multiple irregular but sharply defined soft tissue calcifications and destruction of the iliac bone. *Chondrosarcoma.* Discrete calcifications are typical of a cartilage tumor.

Fig. 22: Displaced elbow fat pads (curved arrows) indicate a distended joint capsule. Subtle discontinuous cortex indicates radial neck fracture (straight arrow).

Figure 21

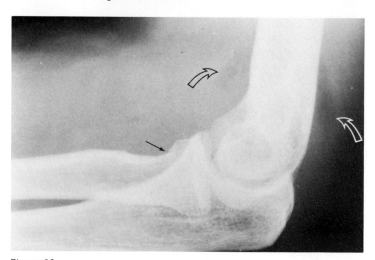

Figure 22

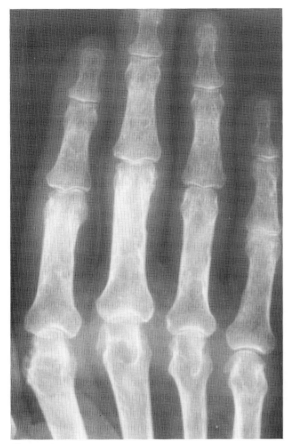

Figure 23

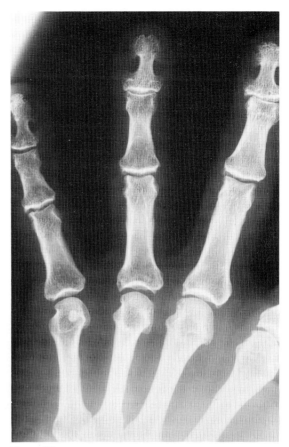

Figure 24

**Fig. 23:** Uniform narrowing of metacarpophalangeal joints and interphalangeal joints. Decreased bone
density. Multiple erosions of distal
metacarpals. *Rheumatoid Arthritis.*

**Fig. 24:** Widening of the metacarpophalangeal joints, tiny osteophytes,
and tuft overgrowth. *Acromegaly.*

# *SIZE AND SHAPE*

One or more bones may have altered size or shape, indicating the presence of disease or even a specific diagnosis. Changes may involve a whole bone or a segment of the bone. Endocrine disorders, genetic enzyme deficiencies, and short stature syndromes often cause such changes in mulitple bones. Change of size and shape in a single bone can be the result of disease or trauma affecting the growth plate, fibrous dysplasia, Paget's disease, neoplasm, and infection.

The shape of normal bone is the result of modeling by osteoclasts which form a collar around the metaphysis. Diseases involving the metaphysis can result in an overtubulated bone with a narrow diaphysis, an undertubulated bone with a wide diaphysis or an Erlenmeyer flask deformity when one end of the diaphysis is wide.

While increase in bone length by enchondral bone formation stops with epiphyseal fusion, increase in bone width by membranous bone formation is possible throughout life. Bone production and bone removal by osteoblasts and osteoclasts of the periosteum and endosteum are normally balanced, but indolent processes causing unbalanced activity can result in a bone with a focal "expanded" appearance.

# Study 2

This 43-year-old man gives a history of having been ill and confined to bed for one year when he was a child. Currently he says he has limitation of motion of the cervical spine but no other complaints. *Your diagnosis?*

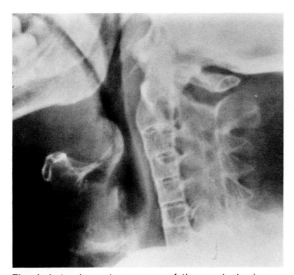

Fig. 1: Lateral roentgenogram of the cervical spine.

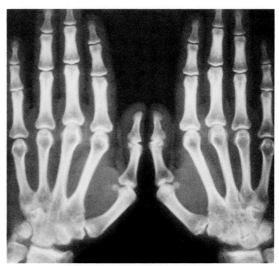

Fig. 2: Roentgenogram of both hands.

# Diagnosis: Juvenile Chronic Arthritis

In the U.S.A. chronic arthritis of childhood has been called juvenile rheumatoid arthritis. In England the term juvenile rheumatoid arthritis is reserved for the small minority of children who have chronic arthritis with positive rheumatoid factor, while Still's disease is the eponym applied to remaining cases of arthritis, which are seronegative. The chronic arthritis that occurs in childhood is not rheumatoid arthritis in a child. Most of these children have negative tests for rheumatoid factor and their arthritis and systemic findings differ from those associated with adult rheumatoid arthritis, so juvenile rheumatoid arthritis is a misnomer. Juvenile chronic arthritis (JCA) has been proposed as a general designation.[1,2] Rarely, seronegative juvenile type arthritis occurs in an adult.

A child under age 16 who has arthritis involving one or more joints and lasting for at least three months is considered to have JCA if other causes of arthritis have been excluded. Some feel that

**Fig. 3:** Lateral roentgenogram of the cervical spine, showing fusion of posterior elements of C1, 2, 3. Cervical ankylosis begins in and usually is limited to the upper cervical spine in juvenile chronic arthritis.

(The patient whose roentgenograms are shown in Figs. 1 and 2 had juvenile chronic arthritis with extensive cervical and carpal ankylosis. Cervical fusion involves the posterior elements and the vertebral bodies. The small vertebral bodies indicate that fusion took place at an early age.)

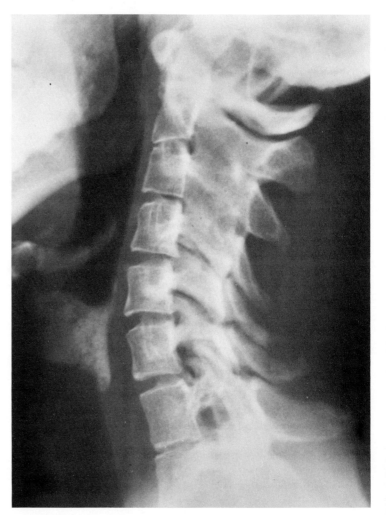

Figure 3

Bone Radiology Case Studies

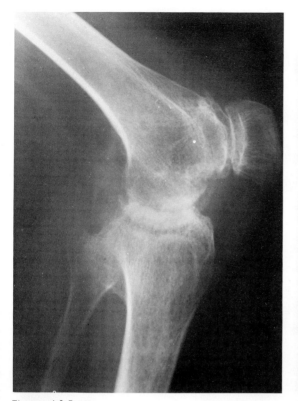
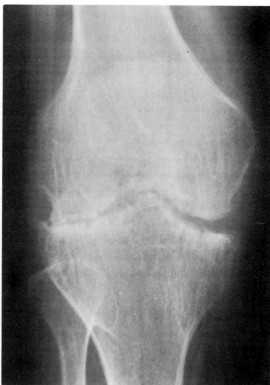

Figures 4 & 5

children with involvement of a single joint should have joint aspiration to rule out infection and synovial biopsy to establish the presence of synovitis.[3] The histology of the synovitis is nonspecific, however, and the diagnosis of JCA is a clinical diagnosis that follows exclusion of other causes of arthritis. When only one joint is affected trauma and infection present the most common problems in differential diagnosis.[4] Systemic lupus erythematosus and rheumatic fever may be very difficult to differentiate from polyarticular JCA with systemic onset.[5] A large number of diseases that cause joint signs and symptoms may mimic JCA. These include[1,4,5]:

Figs. 4, 5: Anteroposterior and lateral roentgenograms of the knee, showing narrowing of the knee joint with multiple erosions and enlargement of the patella. The knee is the joint affected most commonly in monarticular juvenile chronic arthritis.

| | |
|---|---|
| trauma | inflammatory bowel disease |
| infection | post-dysentery arthritis |
| tuberculosis | polyarteritis nodosa |
| joint hemangioma | systemic lupus erythematosus |
| nonspecific synovitis | dermatomyositis |
| Perthes' disease | Scheie's mucopolysaccharidosis |
| slipped femoral epiphysis | hypersensitivity angiitis |
| hemophilia | Behcet's syndrome |
| drug reaction | hypogammaglobulinemia |
| serum sickness | familial Mediterranean fever |
| psoriatic arthritis | leukemia |
| Reiter's syndrome | neuroblastoma |
| Henoch-Schonlein disease | |

Study 2

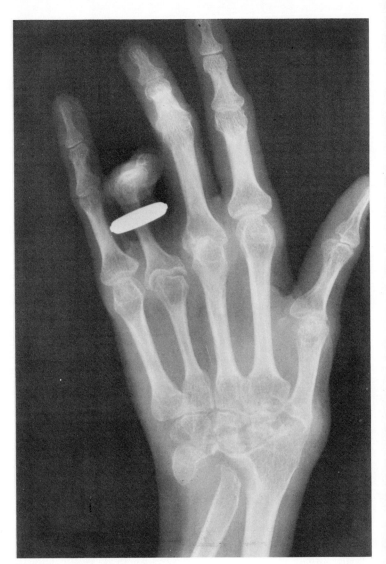

Figure 6

**Fig. 6:** Roentgenogram of the hand, showing extensive joint narrowing, erosions, carpal destruction, and a flexion contracture. This could be adult rheumatoid arthritis, but the short 4th metacarpal is due to early epiphyseal closure associated with juvenile chronic arthritis.

The incidence of JCA has been estimated to be one case per 1,500 schoolchildren, with three new cases per 100,000 general population per year.[4] Girls are affected twice as often as boys. The average age of onset is six years, but age at onset varies from less than one year to 15 years. The prognosis for JCA is good. Complete remission occurs in 50% of patients in less than 10 years, and 75% experience long remissions with no joint destruction.[2,6] Mortality, which occurs in fewer than 5%, is due most often to amyloidosis that affects the kidneys or heart, infection, or hepatic necrosis.

The disease is most often intermittent and may affect a single joint, a few joints asymmetrically, or may be polyarticular and symmetric. Subtypes of JCA, distinguished by differences in clinical presentation, laboratory findings, and prognosis include:[2]

1. System onset (20% of cases)
2. Polyarticular-seronegative (30%)

3. Polyarticular-seropositive (10%)
4. Pauciarticular-early onset (25%)
5. Pauciarticular-late onset (15%).

*Systemic onset* JCA, with acute onset and prominent systemic signs and symptoms, has been called the "classic" presentation. It occurs at any age. These patients have fever (>103 F), with wide temperature swings once or twice daily. Shaking chills are common. In up to 90% of cases there is a maculopapular rash with discrete, pale, salmon-colored lesions, often with central clearing. Usually the rash is on the trunk, but it may be found on the face and extremities, including the palms and soles (where the rash of rheumatic fever does not occur). Often the rash is evanescent and appears with fever spikes. There is pericarditis or pleuritis in 60% of cases. Most patients have hepatosplenomegaly or generalized lymphadenopathy. Almost all have leukocytosis with a leukocyte count of 15,000-25,000/cu mm; the count rarely exceeds 50,000/cu mm. Tests for rheumatoid factor and HLA-B27 are negative. Most of these patients have polyarthritis, but the systemic symptoms can precede the arthritis by weeks or months. Patients with delayed arthritis and those with arthritis that has been overlooked because of severe systemic problems may be considered to have a fever of unknown origin (FUO).[4] The acute systemic symptoms subside gradually, but often there is episodic recurrence. Polyarthritis persists in 50% of patients, and about 25% have severe arthritis with residual permanent deformity.[7]

*Polyarticular-seronegative* JCA is the most common subtype. It

**Fig. 7:** Lateral roentgenogram, showing micrognathia in addition to cervical spine abnormalities in a patient with JCA.

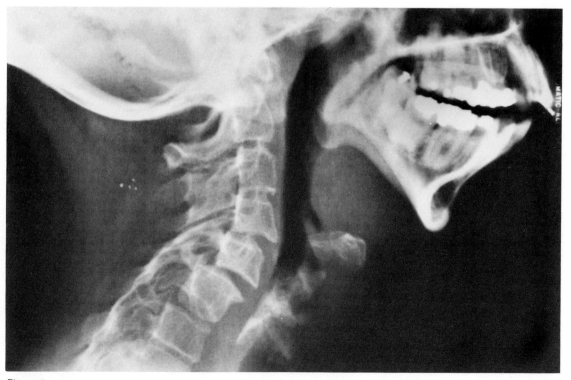

Figure 7

may occur at any age, but begins before five years of age in the majority of patients. There may be no systemic findings. The patients who do have these findings often have insidious onset of systemic problems, and the symptoms usually are mild in comparison with the "classic" presentation of JCA. Systemic findings include low-grade intermittent fever, lymphadenopathy, splenomegaly, mild anemia, rash, and moderate leukocytosis. Tests for rheumatoid factor and HLA-B27 are negative. The polyarthritis usually is symmetric and involves the hands and feet. A few large joints are involved in the majority of patients. Early cervical spine involvement is frequent. About 10% of patients have severe destructive arthritis; permanent deformity is found most often in the hips.

*Polyarticular-seropositive* JCA fortunately is the least common subtype, since it has the worst prognosis. It usually begins in late childhood. The disease in this group closely resembles adult rheumatoid arthritis. The rheumatoid factor test is positive and HLA-B27 is negative. The polyarthritis is symmetric and predominantly affects the hands and feet. Rheumatoid nodules are frequent. There are few systemic symptoms, but patients do develop vasculitis and rheumatoid lung. Roentgenographic changes of arthritis are found early, within one year. Most patients have persistent active arthritis with disabling joint destruction.[1]

*Pauciarticular-early onset* disease usually begins before five years of age. Less than six joints are involved. The large joints usually are involved asymmetrically. This subtype may affect a single joint. The knee is affected most commonly, followed by the ankle, hip, wrist and elbow. Initial shoulder involvement is unusual.[5] There are few systemic manifestations, and rheumatoid factor and HLA-B27 tests are negative. The most serious problem in this group is chronic iridocyclitis, which develops eventually in 50% of patients. The onset is insidious and without symptoms. Periodic slit-lamp examinations are necessary to ensure early diagnosis and treatment in order to prevent blindness due to this complication. Permanent bone and joint deformity is unusual.[2]

*Pauciarticular-late onset* JCA is the one subtype that is more common in boys. It usually begins after nine years of age. Rheumatoid factor test is negative; 90% of patients have positive tests for HLA-B27. Sacroiliac involvement is frequent, but may be delayed. Joint involvement is asymmetric, and more frequent in the lower extremities. Acute iridocyclitis is found in 25% of these patients, but they do not develop chronic iridocyclitis. Many of these patients will be identified as having ankylosing spondylitis later in life when characteristic sacroiliac and spine findings develop. Peripheral joint destruction is uncommon except for the hips and shoulders.[1,1]

Early roentgenographic findings in JCA are nonspecific periarticular osteoporosis and soft tissue swelling. Periosteal reaction occurs and is found most often in the phalanges and metatarsals. There may be striking changes related to the arthritis and synovitis that affect *growing* bones. There may be epiphyseal enlargement, especially in the knee (Figs. 4, 5). There may be

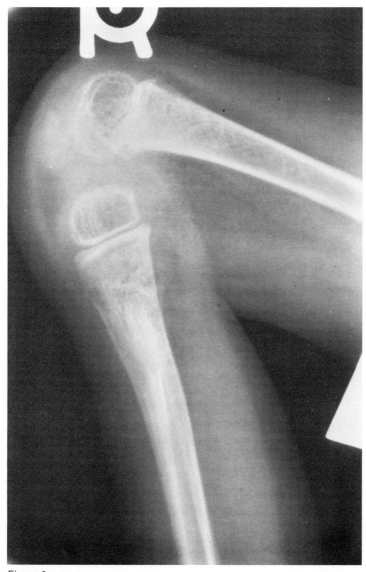

Figure 8

**Fig. 8:** Lateral roentgenogram of the knee, showing a flexion contracture and osteoporosis. Contractures are more frequent than ankylosis in *JCA*.

accelerated maturation. Early epiphyseal closure results in short bones, commonly the metacarpals (Fig. 6). Bones may also be abnormally long or thin. Micrognathia secondary to undergrowth of the mandible is seen in up to 20% of patients (Fig. 7).

Bone erosions similar to those found in adult rheumatoid arthritis are seen first on intra-articular bone surfaces unprotected by cartilage. Joint narrowing is a late finding (Figs. 4, 6). Fibrous and bony ankylosis (Fig. 2) are seen, but contractures (Fig. 8) due to fibrosis involving the joint capsule and periarticular tissue are more common problems that require orthopedic management.[3,5] Bony ankylosis most commonly involves the carpals and cervical spine. Cervical spine ankylosis begins in or is limited to the upper segments (Fig. 3), and involves the apophyseal joints and vertebral bodies. When roentgenograms are obtained later in life the small size of the fused vertebral bodies indicates the early date of fusion (Fig. 1). Odontoid erosions and atlantoaxial subluxation are also seen in JCA.[8]

It should be noted that distinctive radiographic findings in the knee, including decreased bone density, widening of the intracondylar notch, epiphyseal overgrowth, and "squaring" or shortening of the patella, are *not* specific for juvenile chronic arthritis and can also be seen in hemophilia, tuberculosis, and hemangioma of the knee joint with recurrent bleeding.

Orthopedic treatment frequently is needed to prevent contractures. Physical therapy, splints, casts, and traction usually are successful. A severe contracture, resistant to nonsurgical treatment, eventually will result in fibrous ankylosis. If roentgenograms do not show severe joint destruction, however, surgery of the soft tissue and tendon lengthening may salvage the joint.[3]

Synovectomy may prevent progressive bone destruction in selected patients. Arthroplasty is done most often for destroyed hips. Osteotomy is used when there is fixed deformity due to hip or knee ankylosis. Arthrodesis is used most often to correct finger or toe contractures.[3,9]

## References

1. Ansell BM: Chronic arthritis in childhood. *Ann Rheum Dis* 1978; 37:107.
2. Schaller JG: The seronegative spondyloarthopathies of childhood. *Clin Orthop* 1979; 143:76.
3. Bianco AJ, Peterson HA: Juvenile rheumatoid arthritis. *Orthop Clin North Am* 1971; 2:745.
4. Calabro JJ, Katz RM, Maltz BA: A critical reappraisal of juvenile rheumatoid arthritis. *Clin Orthop* 1971; 74:101.
5. Boone JE, Baldwin J, Levine C: Juvenile rheumatoid arthritis. *Pediatr Clin North Am* 1974; 21:885.
6. Goel KM, Shanks RA: Follow-up study of 100 cases of juvenile rheumatoid arthritis. *Ann Rheum Dis* 1974; 33:25.
7. Schaller J, Wedgewood RJ: Juvenile rheumatoid arthritis: A review. *Pediatrics* 1972; 50:940.
8. Martel W, Holt JF, Cassidy JT: Roentgenologic manifestations of juvenile rheumatoid arthritis. *Am J Roentgenol* 1962; 88:400.
9. Proceedings of the Conference on the Rheumatic Diseases of Children. *Arthritis Rheum* 20, Suppl, 1977.

# Study 3

This 30-year-old man fractured his femur in an automobile accident. At that time, he had swelling and tenderness of the left wrist. This was felt to be a sprain, and no roentgenograms were taken. The swelling subsided, but the wrist became painful with motion. There was a clicking sound with flexion, plus limitation of motion. These films were taken ten months following the accident. *Your diagnosis?*

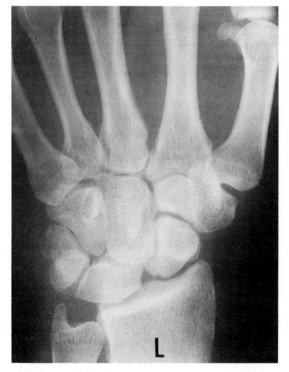

**Fig. 1:** Painful left wrist.

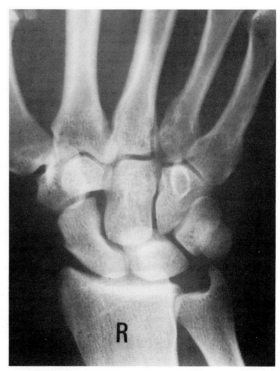

**Fig. 2:** Right wrist.

# Diagnosis: Rotational Subluxation of Navicular

In 59 patients with carpal dislocations and fracture dislocations there were:[1]

| | |
|---|---|
| Transnavicular perilunate fracture dislocations | 27 |
| Lunate dislocation | 14 |
| Dislocation lunate and half navicular | 6 |
| Perilunate dislocation | 3 |
| Dislocated navicular | 1 |
| Subluxation of navicular | 4 |

This uncommon problem, rotational subluxation of the navicular, is important since it may be missed unless actively considered as a diagnostic possibility. While the clinical presentation is nonspecific, the radiographic findings allow a definite diagnosis if proper films are obtained in subtle cases.

Rotational subluxation of the navicular refers to rotation so that there is dorsal movement of the proximal pole and volar movement of the distal pole, with the navicular assuming a more vertical position. This movement is allowed to occur when there is disruption of the ligaments between the navicular, lunate and capitate, plus tearing of the dorsal radiocarpal ligment overlying the navicular-lunate joint.[2] Etiology includes:

1. Trauma with rotatory subluxed navicular accompanying a lunate or perilunate dislocation (the subluxed navicular may persist following satisfactory reduction of the other carpals).[3]
2. Trauma with isolated rotatory subluxation of navicular.
3. Rheumatoid arthritis (the ligaments are destroyed by granulomatous process).
4. Rotational subluxation with no history of significant trauma.

There is a great range of disability in these patients. Symptoms may be insignificant or require only external support.[4] In others, symptoms are severe and require open reduction and one of several surgical procedures which have been used.[5]

Patients may complain of pain and weakness. There may be limitation of motion and a clicking sound with wrist flexion.

The radiographic findings are often clearcut. They are (Fig. 2 and 3):

1. *Widened space between the navicular and lunate.* To assure that widened space isn't obscured by rotation, insist on an AP film with little or no overlap of the distal radius and ulna.[4] Compare to the opposite hand. Two millimeters is top normal.
2. *Ring appearance of distal navicular* looks like a large hamate hook (due to volar movement causing distal pole of navicular to be seen on end).[6]
3. *Foreshortened navicular* in AP view (due to rotation).
4. *Increased vertical angulation of navicular* on lateral view. Varying radial-navicular angles are given in the literature as indicating abnormal position, but this sign is of little value. It

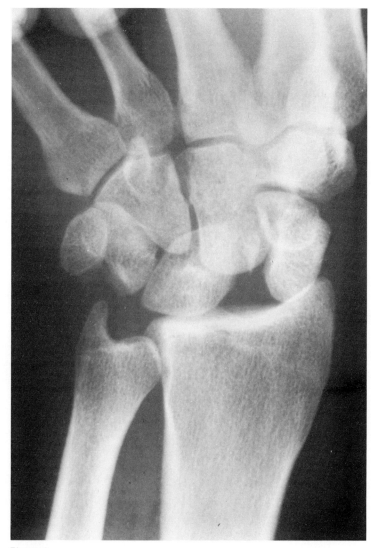

Figure 3

**Fig. 3:** Left wrist in ulnar deviation with further increase in widened space between navicular and lunate. Navicular foreshortened and "ring" appearance of distal navicular also are present. (Incidentally noted is ununited bone fragment from lunate.)

is usually difficult to get a true lateral view, and in this position the navicular is often difficult to identify.[4]

It isn't always so easy. In a patient with doubtful findings, other views may be necessary. Several different views and hand positions have been claimed as being superior in demonstrating subluxation. None have proven to be consistently superior. If AP, lateral and oblique views are not definitive, films should be obtained with radial and ulnar deviation and in pronation and supination (Fig. 3).

Occasionally a patient may have a navicular which is intermittently subluxed.[5] In these cases and in cases unresolved with plain films, cineradiography is of value.[7]

### References

1. Russell TB: Intra-carpal dislocations and fracture dislocations. *J Bone Joint Surg* 1949; 31B:524.

2. England JP: Subluxation of the carpal scaphoid. *Proc Roy Soc Med* 1970; 63:581.
3. Thompson T, Campbell RD, Arnold WD: Primary and secondary dislocation of the scaphoid bone. *J Bone Joint Surg* 1964; 46B:73.
4. Hudson TM, Caragol WJ, Kaye JJ: Isolated rotatory subluxation of carpal navicular. *Am J Roentgenol* 1976; 126:601.
5. Howard FM, Fahey T, Wojik E: Rotatory subluxation of the navicular. *Clin Orthop* 1974; 104:134.
6. Crittenden J, Jones D, Santarelli A: Bilateral rotational dislocation of the carpal navicular. *Radiology* 1970; 94:629.
7. Arkless R: Cineradiography in normal and abnormal wrists. *Am J Roentgenol* 1966; 96:837.

# Study 4

This 4-year-old boy fell on his outstreched left arm. He was brought to the emergency room soon after the injury because of pain, swelling, and deformity, and the roentgenograms shown above were taken. *Your diagnosis?*

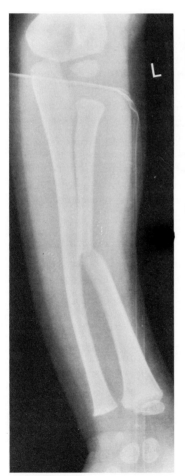

**Fig. 1A:** *AP* view of left forearm.

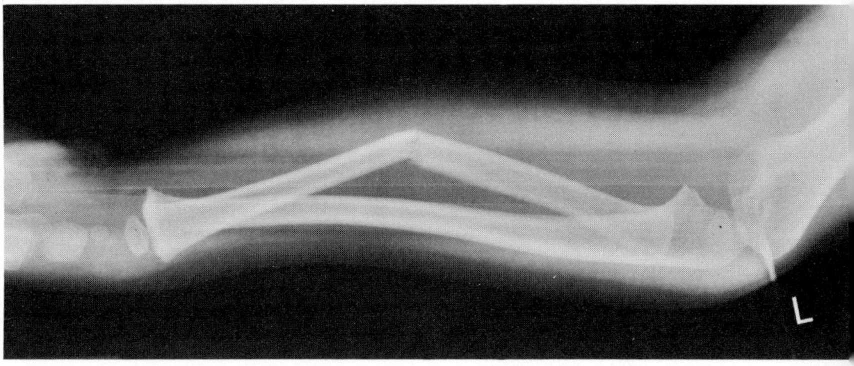

**Fig. 1B:** Lateral view of left forearm.

# Diagnosis: Traumatic (Plastic) Bowing Fracture

Fractures of the shaft of a bone in children may be classified as complete or incomplete. A complete fracture crosses the bone shaft; an incomplete fracture does not cross the entire shaft. Types of incomplete fracture include:

*Torus Fracture:* localized projection of the cortex, which has a buckled appearance.

*Greenstick Fracture:* fracture line crosses only one cortex, with opposite cortex intact. The fracture line may extend up and down the shaft.

*Stress Fracture:* fracture line or a zone of reparative sclerosis resulting from the effect of repeated stress below the magnitude required to fracture a normal bone.

*Bowing Fracture:* fixed bowing deformity of a bone with no gross fracture of the bone.

Bowing fractures are rare and were described first in the literature in 1974.[1] These fractures were produced in the dog ulna in 1972 and the relationship of applied stress to bone deformity has been described, along with the histology of plastic bowing.[2,3]

When a longitudinal compressive force is applied to a naturally curved bone, tensile stress is produced at the convex surface while compressive stress is produced at the concave surface, and the bone bends. Figure 3 shows a curve representing deformities caused by single stresses of increasing magnitude. Low level stresses, up to magnitude P, cause bending proportional to applied stress, but the bone reverts to normal when the stress is removed. This is called an elastic response. Stress that exceeds the elastic limit (E) causes fixed bending that does not change when the stress is removed. This fixed bending is not associated with a gross fracture and is called a plastic response. Further increase in applied stress finally reaches a level causing gross fracture, which is the limit of the plastic zone of response. (Between points P and E on the curve, stress and deformity are no longer proportional. Plastic bowing does not occur when a single stress is applied. If this same stress is applied *multiple* times, however, the curve shifts from the elastic to the plastic zone of response and fixed deformity does occur. This segment of the curve between P and E is called the fatigue zone.)

While the bone with plastic bowing is grossly intact, multiple oblique fractures can be seen microscopically. These microfractures are located mainly in the compressed concave cortex of the bent bone. Minimal periosteal new bone formation on the concave side may result finally in cortical thickening, but in dogs periosteal reaction has not been seen roentgenographically.[3]

In reference to stress-deformity curves, microfractures do occur in the plastic response zone but do not occur in the elastic response zone when a single stress is applied. (In the fatigue zone, which is located at the end of the elastic response zone, the summation of the effect of repeated stresses will cause microfractures).

Plastic bowing fractures almost always occur in children. This is

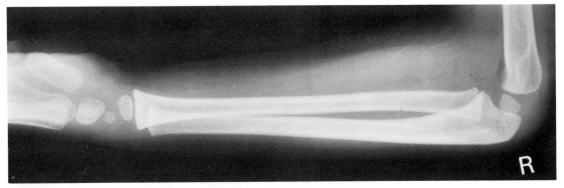

Figure 2

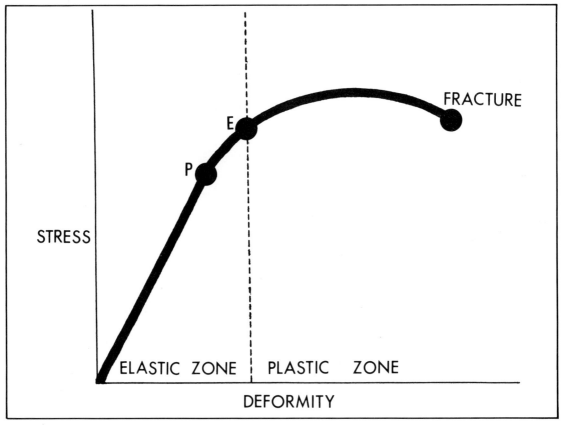

Figure 3

**Fig. 2:** Lateral view of the patient's normal right forearm for comparison with Fig. 1B. Figs. 1A and 1B show an angulated fracture of the radius plus lateral (Fig. 1A) and anterior (Fig. 1B) bowing of the ulna.

**Fig. 3:** Stress/deformity curve (modified from Chamay and Tschantz.[1]) P = proportional limit. E = elastic limit. Vertical axis = Compressive force applied to longitudinal axis of bone. Horizontal axis = Bending deformity of bone.

**Figs. 4A, 4B:** Patient 2 (14-year-old boy). AP view of injured right forearm (4A) shows greenstick fracture of the midshaft of the ulna, plus medial bowing of the radius. Comparison AP view (4B) shows normal left forearm.

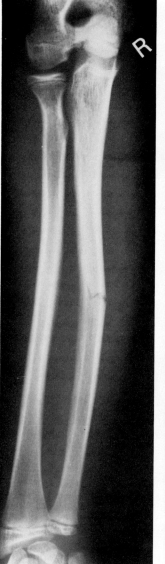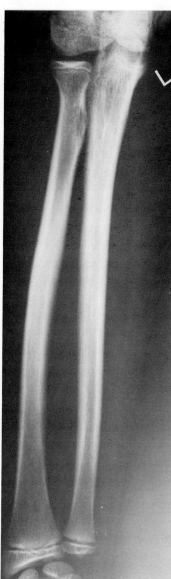

Figures 4A & 4B

Bone Radiology Case Studies

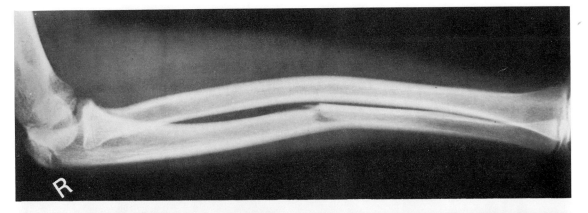

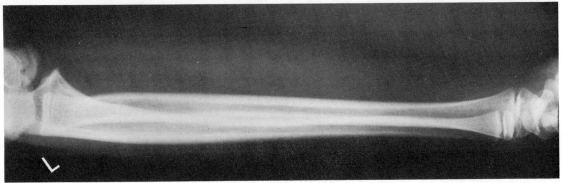

due to the wide zone of plastic response of bones in children when compared with those of adults.

In reviewing 74 cases of plastic bowing, the bones affected were:[1,4-11]

| | |
|---|---|
| Forearm | 58 (78%) |
|   Ulna | 26 (35%) (Figs. 1, 6) |
|   Radius | 15 (20%) (Figs. 4, 5) |
|   Unspecified | 6 (8%) |
|   Both Bones | 11 (15%) |
| Fibula | 14 (19%) (Fig. 7) |
| Femur | 1 (1%) |
| Tibia | 1 (1%) |

**Figs. 5A, 5B:** Patient 2. Lateral view of injured right forearm (5A) shows angulated greenstick fracture of the mid-ulna, with anterior bowing of the radius. Comparison lateral view (5B) shows normal left forearm.

The forearm is the most common site of plastic bowing. The applied force is almost always longitudinal, because a non-longitudinal force is a shearing force that will result in metaphyseal or epiphseal fractures. (A single case of plastic bowing of the forearm produced by a wringer injury indicates that tangential trauma can produce plastic bowing, however.[10]) The most common mechanism of injury is a fall on the outstretched hand. Most often a portion of the traumatic force is in the zone of plastic response for the other bone and results in fixed bending. There may be bowing of both bones, but this is less frequent than the combination of a fracture of one bone and bowing of the other. Three cases of dislocation of the radial head with bowing of the ulna (Monteggia

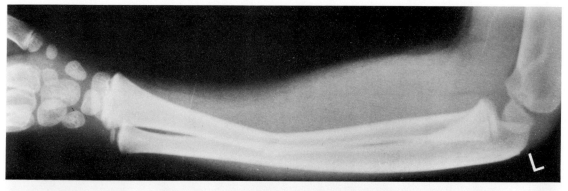

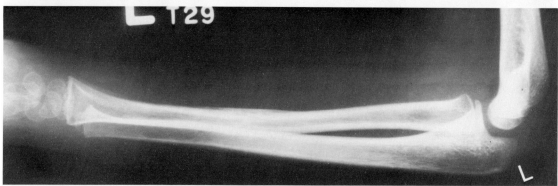

**Figs. 6A, 6B:** Patient 3 (8-year-old boy). Lateral view of injured left forearm (6A) shows posterior angulation of greenstick fracture of the radius plus posterior bowing of the ulna. Lateral view of injured left forearm 6 weeks later (6B), following removal of cast, shows that the ulna is no longer bowed.

equivalent) have been reported.[4,5] The deformed bone usually, but not always, forms a single broad curve.

Plastic bowing of the fibula usually results from a direct blow.[6] In this situation an oblique direct blow is translated into sheer and compressive vectors.[7] Most bowing is associated with tibial fractures. The only adult with plastic bowing in the 74 cases reviewed was a 21-year-old man.[8]

There was one report of three children who had posttraumatic posterior displacement of the capitellum in relation to the distal humerus without other evidence of fracture; these cases were interpreted as plastic bowing of the humerus.[12] These cases were not included in the 74 cases compiled.

Children with bowing fractures are seen because of pain, tenderness, deformity, and limited motion. On roentgenogram a fracture (or dislocation) usually can be identified easily in one bone of the forearm. Often the fracture is angulated. Sometimes the bowed bone is detected in only one view. If the bowing is subtle it may be necessary to obtain views of the opposite extremity for comparison. Followup roentgenograms seldom demonstrate periosteal reaction of the bowed bone, but a thickened cortex on the concave surface of the curved bone may develop.[1,5]

The bowed bone may make it difficult to reduce the grossly fractured bone. If straightening of the curved bone is attempted it may require a great deal of force. Preferred treatment is not well-defined but, in general, children less than 10 years of age do not have functional loss even if the curvature of the bowed bone is not reduced. Subsequent remodeling is greater the younger the child.

Older children may have residual reduction of supination and pronation if plastic bowing is not reduced.[1,5]

## References

1. Borden S: Traumatic bowing of the forearm in children. *J Bone Joint Surg* 1974; 56A:611.
2. Chamay A: Mechanical and morphological aspects of experimental overload and fatigue in bone. *J Biomech* 1970; 3:263.
3. Chamay A, Tschantz P: Mechanical influences in bone remodeling, experimental research on Wolff's law. *J Biomech* 1972; 5:173.
4. Crowe JE, Swischuk LE: Acute bowing fractures of the forearm in children: A frequently missed injury. *Am J Roentgenol* 1977; 128:98.
5. Borden S: Roentgen recognition of acute plastic bowing of the forearm in children. *Am J Roentgenol* 1975; 125:524.
6. Martin W, Riddervold MO: Acute plastic bowing fractures of the fibula. *Radiology* 1979; 131:639.
7. Manoli A: Traumatic fibular bowing with tibial fracture. *Orthopedics* 1978; 1:145.
8. Cook GC, Bjellan JC: Acute bowing of the fibula in an adult. *Radiology* 1979; 131:637.
9. Cail WS, Keats TE, Sussman MD: Plastic bowing fracture of the femur in a child. *Am J Roentgenol* 1978; 130:780.
10. Rydholm U, Nilsson JE: Traumatic bowing of the forearm. *Clin Orthop* 1979; 139:121.
11. Stenstrom R, Gripenberg L, Bergius A: Traumatic bowing of the forearm and lower leg in children. *Acta Radiologica* 1978; 19:243.
12. Rogers LF, Malave S, White M: Plastic bowing, torus, and greenstick supracondylar fractures of the humerus. *Radiology* 1978; 128:145.

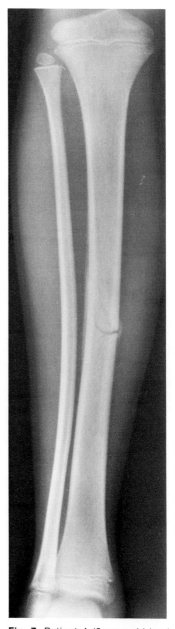

**Fig. 7:** Patient 4 (8-year-old boy). AP view of lower leg shows greenstick fracture of tibia and medially bowed fibula.

# Study 5

This 13-year-old boy has limited range of motion of both wrists. He is healthy and has no symptoms. There is a fixed nontender protuberance over the left sixth costochondral junction and another over the proximal right tibia. *Your diagnosis?*

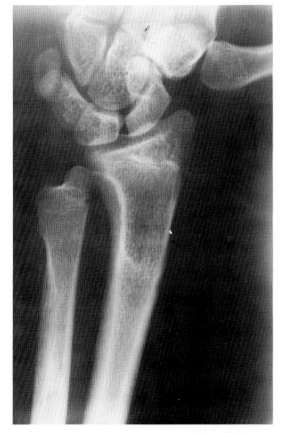

**Fig. 1:** AP right wrist.

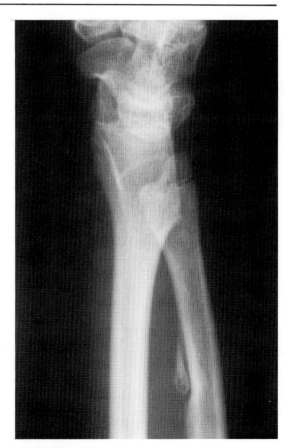

**Fig. 2:** Lateral right wrist.

# Diagnosis: Multiple Hereditary Exostosis With Madelung Deformity

Madelung's deformity is the end product of asymmetric growth of the distal radial epiphysis. Retarded growth of its medial aspect results in a triangular shape of the epiphysis with ulnar tilting of the articular surface (normal angle 25°). Usually there is increased volar tilt of the radial articular surface (normal angle 5°) with resultant prominence of the normally positioned ulnar styloid. The radius is shortened and bowed. The carpal angle formed by intersecting lines across the proximal ends of the navicular-lunate and triangular-lunate is decreased (normal angle greater than 117°).

The carpals have a triangular configuration as they are wedged into the widened space between the deformed radius and ulna. The most constant findings are radial shortening, triangular shape of the distal radial epiphysis and decreased carpal angle.[1]

### Bilateral Madelung-Type Deformity
Isolated anomaly
Dyschondrosteosis
Multiple hereditary exostosis
Multiple enchondromatosis
Multiple epiphyseal dysplasia
Turner's syndrome
Morquio's disease
Hurler's disease
Thalidomide embryopathy

### Unilateral Madelung-Type Deformity
Trauma
Infection
Rickets
Rheumatoid arthritis

Most commonly, Madelung's deformity is an isolated problem or is associated with the congenital mesomelic bone dysplasia, dyschondrosteosis. Some think that the isolated anomaly is actually a mild expression of the mesomelic bone dysplasia.[2] In multiple hereditary exostosis the wrist deformity is further distinguished by a short ulna, as in this patient (Fig. 1 and 2).

Multiple hereditary exostosis is transmitted as a dominant with more cases reported in males. Lesions may occur in any enchondral bone and usually number 10 to 20, although hundreds may be present. Osteochondromas are rare before age 2. They are frequently palpated as asymptomatic soft tissue lumps. Uncommonly, symptoms occur because of pressure on adjacent nerves, vessels, tendons or joints.[3] Many patients have fibula and ulna shortening with Madelung-type deformities. Short metacarpals and phalanges occasionally occur.

Growth of osteochondromas ceases with epiphyseal

closure. Sudden growth, growth after adolescence or pain may indicate sarcomatous degeneration. The reported incidence of malignancy varies from 2 to 20%.[4] The lower figure is more generally accepted. An individual lesion may not have any greater potential for malignancy than an isolated osteochondroma. Patients with numerous lesions have a higher incidence of malignant degeneration, possibly related to chance.

### References

1. Felman A, Kirkpatrick J: Madelung's deformity: Observations in 17 patients. *Radiology* 1969; 93:1037.
2. Langer L: Dyschondrosteosis, A hereditable bone dysplasia with characteristic roentgenographic features. *Am J Roentgenol* 1965; 95:178.
3. Solomon L: Hereditary multiple exostosis. *J Bone Joint Surg* 1963; 45-B:292.
4. Jaffe HL: *Tumors and Tumerous Conditions of the Bones and Joints.* Philadelphia. Lea & Febiger, 1958.

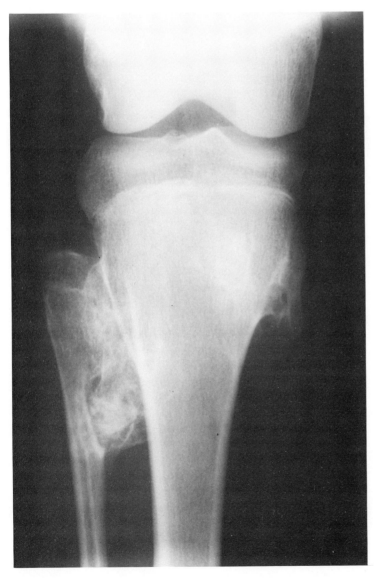

**Fig. 3:** AP right knee. There is under-tubulation of the proximal tibia with osteochondroma. The wrist in Figure 1 and 2 has a Madelung-type deformity with a short ulna—commonly seen in multiple hereditary exostosis. There is an osteochondroma of the ulna and under-tubulation of the distal radius in Figure 2.

# Study 6

This 23-year-old man has a paraspinal mass in the thorax (arrows) and papillary necrosis of the kidneys (Fig. 1). *Your diagnosis?*

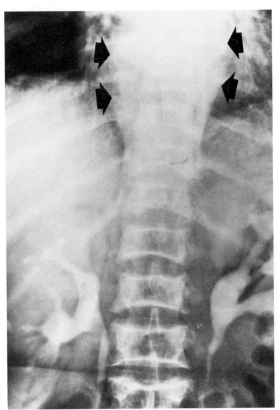

**Fig. 1A:** AP film of excretory urogram.

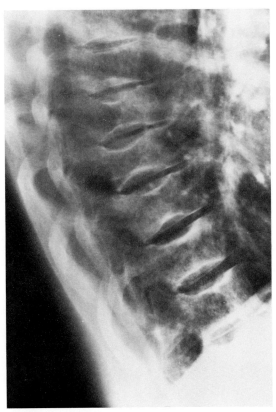

**Fig. 1B:** Lateral radiograph of thoraco-lumbar spine.

# Diagnosis: Sickle Cell Anemia

The thoracic paraspinal mass represents extramedullary hematopoiesis. Papillary necrosis is common in sickle cell disease. There is decreased bone density and focal central depressions of the vertebral end plates, which are characteristic for this disease.

**TABLE 1**

## CLASSIFICATION OF HEMATOLOGIC DISORDERS AFFECTING BONE
### (Modified from Williams)

*I. ERYTHROCYTE DISORDERS (ANEMIA)*
    *A. Anemia predominantly due to decreased red cell production*
        *1. Stem cell disturbance*
            *a. Aplastic anemia*
            *b. Thrombocytopenia with absent radii syndrome (TAR)*
            *c. Congenital hypoplastic anemia*
        *2. Hemoglobin synthesis disturbance*
            *a. Iron deficiency*
            *b. Thalassemias*
    *B. Anemia predominantly due to increased red cell destruction*
        *1. Increased destruction secondary to abnormal shape*
            *a. Hereditary spherocytosis*
        *2. Increased destruction secondary to enzyme deficiency*
            *a. Pyruvate kinase deficiency*
        *3. Increased destruction secondary to antibodies*
            *a. Isoimmune hemolytic disease of the newborn (erythroblastosis fetalis)*
        *4. Paroxysmal nocturnal hemoglobinuria*
        *5. Abnormal globin*
            *a. Sickling diseases*
*II. MYELOPROLIFERATIVE DISORDERS*
    *A. Myelofibrosis*
    *B. Acute myelogenous leukemia*
    *C. Chronic myelogenous (granulocytic) leukemia*
    *D. Mastocytosis*
*III. LYMPHORETICULAR DISORDERS*
    *A. Acute lymphocytic leukemia*
    *B. Lymphoma (Hodgkins and non-Hodgkins)*
    *C. Plasma cell dyscrasias*
*IV. BLEEDING DISORDERS*
    *A. Hemophilias*

## Skeletal Manifestations of Anemias

In order to better understand bone changes secondary to blood

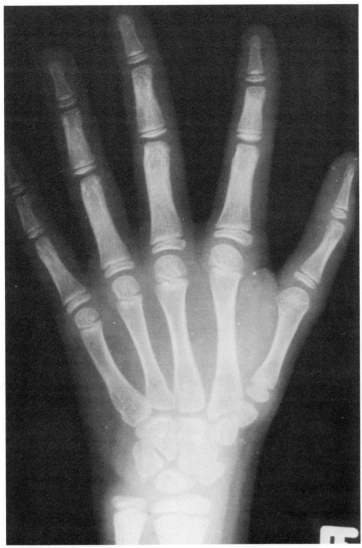

Figure 2

**Fig. 2:** Hypoplastic thumb and scaphoid. These findings occur in Fanconi's anemia, but they are also associated with several other inherited syndromes and other isolated anomalies.

disorders, an organized patho-physiologic-morphologic approach is necessary. These disorders have been organized according to the blood component affected. A chart after the approach in Williams' textbook is provided (Table 1).[1] Many of these disorders affect bone in a nonspecific fashion, while others cause characteristic, almost pathognomonic changes.

### Anemia

The blood disorders most often recognized as causing bone changes are the anemias. Anemia is best defined as an abnormally low hemoglobin concentration. The anemias causing bone changes are secondary to hemoglobin synthesis abnormalities, hemolysis secondary to abnormal shape, membrane or enzyme deficiency, and abnormal globin synthesis. The unifying concept behind the bone changes is the body's response to anemia. As the hemoglobin

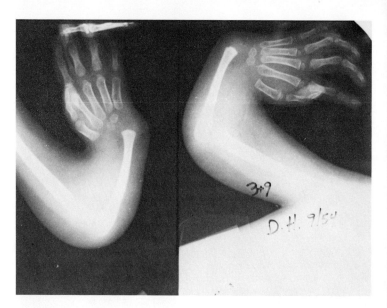

**Fig. 3:** Characteristic radial aplasia in a patient with *TAR* (thrombocytopenia absent radius) syndrome.
(Courtesy of Arnold Cohn, M.D., Northfield, Illinois)

concentration decreases, tissue hypoxia initiates a complex response resulting in red cell precursor proliferation in the bone marrow. The severity of the anemia often dictates the marrow response. The primary pathologic and radiographic findings result from marrow expansion. These findings are trabecular resorption, cortical thinning and decreased bone density leading to bone deformity and pathologic fractures if severe enough. Secondary changes in specific cases include delayed maturation, thrombotic propensity and increased susceptibility to infection.

Aplastic disorders result from an abnormality in the production or maturation of one or more stem cell precursors.[1] The etiology is multifactorial, but only the congenital disorders cause bone changes.

*Fanconi's aplastic anemia* is characterized by pancytopenia, brown skin pigmentation, hypoplasia of the kidneys and spleen, microcephaly, genital abnormalities, mental retardation and bone changes.[2] The onset of pancytopenia is insidious and delayed, often appearing after seven to eight years. Unfortunately, most die within two to three years of onset. The most prominent skeletal changes are radial element hypoplasia or aplasia (Fig. 2). Abnormalities of the thumb, radius, first metacarpal, greater multangular and navicular bones commonly occur.[3] The thumb anomalies are nonspecific and can be found in a number of other syndromes including Holt-Oram, thrombocytopenia-absent radius, ectodermal dysplasia, craniosynostosis, and trisomy 18. Thumb anomalies can also be a part of the "VATER" complex (vertebral, anal, tracheal, esophageal and radial abnormalities) or associated with malformations such as cleft palate and renal anomalies. Other skeletal abnormalities include congenital hip dislocation, webbing of the second and third toes, flat feet, Klippel-Feil deformity, club feet, extra terminal phalanges of the third and fourth toes and Sprengel's deformity.[4]

Bone Radiology Case Studies

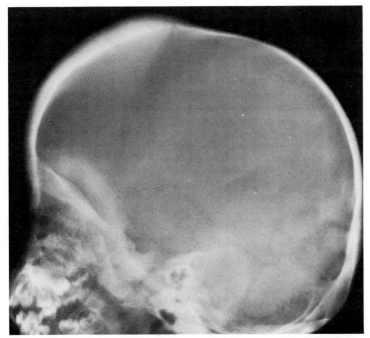

Figure 4

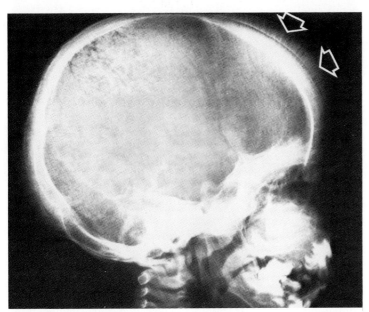

Figure 5

**Fig. 4:** Thickened frontal bone in a child with iron deficiency anemia.

**Fig. 5:** Thalassemia major. Calvarial thickening spares the inferior occiput. There is a striated appearance over the frontal bone where the outer table has been penetrated by hyperplastic marrow (arrows). The dense obliterated maxillary sinuses are characteristic of thalassemia but rare in sickle cell disease.

A distinct yet similar entity is the *thrombocytopenia with absent radii* syndrome (TAR).[5] The important characteristics are bilateral radial absence in 100% of the patients (compared to approximately 50% in Fanconi's anemia), presence of a thumb, and congenital hypomegakaryocytic thrombocytopenia present at birth (Fig. 3). Other bones are deformed, especially the ulna, humerus, shoulder girdle and feet; and cardiac anomalies are found in one third of cases. These children often improve spontaneously.

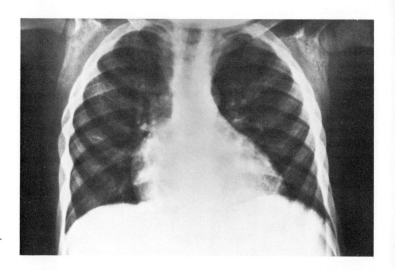

**Fig. 6:** Thalassemia major. Characteristic widened ribs.

*Congenital hypoplastic anemia* (pure red cell aplasia) is characterized by an isolated anemia with reticulocytopenia. Skeletal changes are unusual and nondiagnostic, and consist primarily of growth retardation and either an extra digit or phalangeal hypoplasia.[4,5] The triphalangeal thumb hypoplastic anemia syndrome is considered by Moseley as part of CHA.[6]

*Iron deficiency anemia* results from inadequate iron intake, malabsorption, chronic blood loss, hemoglobinuria, dialysis and pregnancy. Symptoms are nonspecific unless the anemia is severe. Classically the anemia is microcytic and hypochromic with decreased iron stores.[7] Skeletal changes are mild, nonspecific, and generally found in infants and children. Changes result from marrow hyperplasia. Osteoporosis can occur. The diploic space in the skull may widen and the outer table may be thinned (Fig. 4).[8,9] Skeletal changes do not correlate with the severity of the anemia.

The *thalassemias* are a group of inherited disorders of globin synthesis. Anemia results from alteration in the rate of globin synthesis causing ineffective erythropoiesis and decreased peripheral survival (hemolysis) secondary to a cell membrane abnormality The beta-thalassemias are the best known and occur in heterozygous (minor), homozygous (major), and intermediate forms.[10] Thalassemia minor is a relatively asymptomatic disorder (except under extreme stress) characterized by a mild microcytic, hypochromic anemia, a normal to increased red cell count, elevated hemoglobin $A_2$ and a minimally elevated fetal hemoglobin. Thalassemia major is a fatal disorder characterized by failure to thrive, stunted growth, frequent infections, massive splenomegaly, a severe anemia with elevated fetal hemoglobin and characteristic bone changes. Patients rarely survive the first few years of life. The intermediate form occurs in patients with either homozygous or heterozygous states but whose clinical course goes contrary to the expected.

The bone changes in the homozygous form are severe and directly related to exuberant marrow hyperplasia.[11] In the skull, there is osteoporosis, diploic space widening and outer table thinning. The classic "hair-on-end" appearance results from breakthrough of the outer table by marrow with subsequent bone deposition (Fig. 5). The paranasal sinuses are obliterated by bone expansion (Fig. 5). Overgrowth of the maxilla and mandible may lead to the almost pathognomonic "rodent facies." The occipital squama inferior to the occipital protuberance is spared as no marrow exists in this bone (Fig. 5). Changes in the spine result primarily from osteoporosis. The trabecular pattern is accentuated and softening may lead to

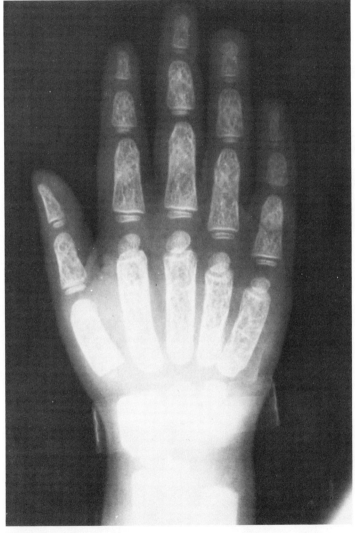

Figure 7

**Fig. 7:** Thalassemia major. Marrow hyperplasia has resulted in under-tubulated rectangular bones, decreased density, thin cortices, and decreased but coarse trabeculae.

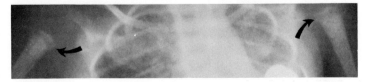

Figure 8

**Fig. 8:** Lucent metaphyseal stress bands (arrows). This finding is nonspecific and can be seen in erythroblastosis, leukemia, tuberculosis, congenital syphilis, or any severe neonatal or infantile illness.

biconcave deformities.[12] Central depression of the vertebral body can also be seen in thalassemia, but it is uncommon.[13] Ribs show marked expansion with cortical thinning and osteoporosis (Fig. 6). Long bone architecture is altered, resulting in a rectangular appearance and sometimes a distal Erlenmeyer flask shape. The bones of the hands have decreased density, thin cortex, few but coarse trabeculae, and a rectangular shape due to marrow hyperplasia (Fig. 7). Short stature commonly results from premature epiphyseal closure. Spontaneous fractures are frequent.

The changes in the heterozygous form are similar but much less severe. Most of the alterations occur in the skull.[14] Patients with heterozygous form combined with hemoglobin S are discussed later.

Hereditary spherocytosis is a disease in which a red cell membrane defect causes sequestration and destruction of red cells in the spleen.[15] Generally the patients are asymptomatic except for an increased incidence of pigmented gallstones. Clinically they are mildly anemic, have indirect hyperbilirubinemia and splenomegaly. The diagnosis is based on the presence of spherocytes of the peripheral smear, and both osmotic fragility and autohemolysis tests.

Moseley describes bone changes secondary to marrow expansion as uncommon.[6] In Young's series of 28 patients, five of whom had radiographic studies, no skeletal abnormalities were found.[16] When changes are present, widened diploic space and thinned cortex in the skull are the most common.

Other hemolytic disorders can result from red cell enzyme deficiencies. The two most well known are glucose-6-phosphate dehydrogenase (G-6PD) and pyruvate kinase deficiency. Skeletal changes have been described in pyruvate kinase deficiency only, and they are uncommon.[17] No exhaustive roentgenographic study has been performed, but when findings occur they usually reflect some degree of marrow hyperplasia (i.e., widened diploic space, thinned skull cortex and osteoporosis).

Isoimmune hemolytic disease of the newborn, erythroblastosis fetalis, occurs when maternal antibodies are transferred via the

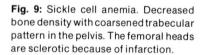

**Fig. 9:** Sickle cell anemia. Decreased bone density with coarsened trabecular pattern in the pelvis. The femoral heads are sclerotic because of infarction.

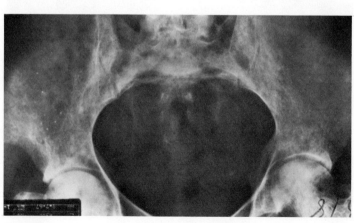

Figure 9

Bone Radiology Case Studies

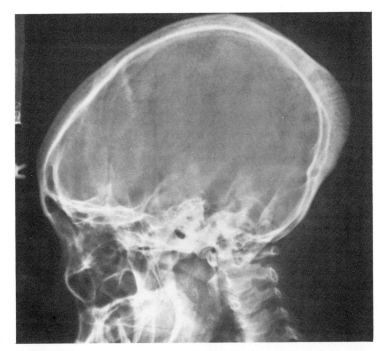

**Fig. 10:** Sickle cell anemia. The calvarial thickening spares the occiput below the torcular herophili. Note the normally aerated sinuses.

**Fig. 11:** Sickle cell anemia. Avascular necrosis of femoral head with typical subcortical lucency plus sclerosis and lucency of the head and neck.

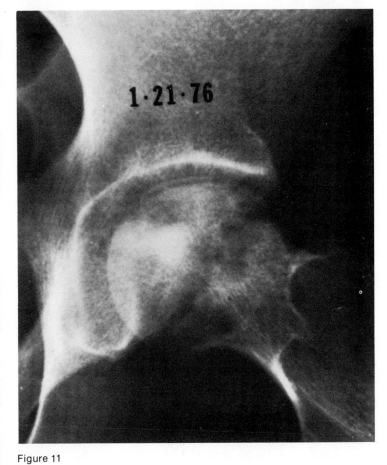

Figure 11

placenta and react with fetal red cells.[18] Most are due to either ABO or Rh incompatibility, with ABO twice as frequent but less severe than Rh. In most cases of Rh incompatibility prior sensitization is necessary, while with ABO incompatibility the disease frequently occurs in the first born. In the severe form babies are jaundiced, pale, have hepatosplenomegaly and anasarca, petechial bleeding and CHF. They are severely anemic. There are no bone changes in nearly one half, while the remainder have transverse lines of decreased density in the metaphysis of the long bones. These changes are nonspecific and can be found after any severe stress including hyaline membrane disease, infantile syphilis, or leukemia (Fig. 8).[19]

*Paroxysmal nocturnal hemoglobinuria* (PNH) is not classified by most as an anemia since it involves all marrow elements. We discuss it here because hemolytic anemia is a component. In PNH, cells are sensitive to the lytic action of complement. It is a noninherited disorder characterized by hemoglobinuria (usually worse at night and presenting initially in less than one quarter of all patients) hemolysis, iron deficiency, venous thrombosis, severe back and abdominal pain, and renal damage.[20] There can be absent or severe anemia, mild granulocytopenia and thrombocytopenia. Diagnosis is made by the Ham's and sucrose hemolysis tests. Central depression of the vertebral body, a finding most commonly seen in sickle cell anemia, has been found in PNH.

**Fig. 12:** Sickle cell anemia. Typical sclerotic cap of the head of humerus indicates infarction.

**Fig. 13:** Sickle cell anemia with hand-foot syndrome. The fingers are swollen, and several bones, especially of the index and little fingers, are widened, lucent and sclerotic, and have periosteal reaction.

Figure 12

Figure 13

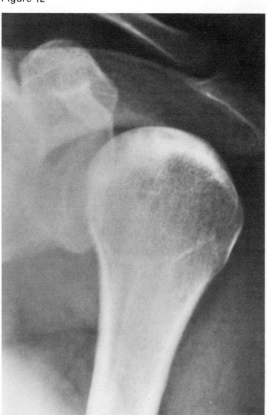

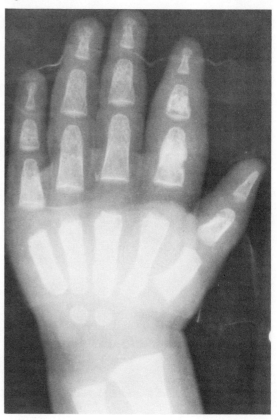

Bone Radiology Case Studies

The *sickling disorders* (of which sickle cell anemia, SS, is the most recognized) result from abnormal globin synthesis (as opposed to alteration of globin synthesis rate seen in thalassemia).[21] These disorders are genetically transmitted and biochemically are characterized by amino acid substitutions in the globin molecule. This causes structural abnormalities in both the molecule and the cell, giving the characteristic sickle shape. The cells have a decreased peripheral life span as a result. The most common abnormal hemoglobins are S, C, D and E. Homozygous S disease (SS or sickle cell anemia), heterozygous S (sickle trait), sickle cell-hemoglobin C disease (S-C) and sickle cell-thalassemia will be discussed. Bone changes in these disorders are more complex than in other anemias and are due to the unique nature of the sickled cell. In addition to the changes secondary to marrow hyperplasia, the manifestations of vascular stasis and occlusion abound in these disorders. Sickled cells cause increased blood viscosity, and bone infarction is common. The severity of the changes correlate with the amount of abnormal hemoglobin.

Of all the hemoglobinopathies, sickle cell anemia (homozygous S) has the most profound clinical presentation. In infants, after the protective fetal hemoglobin level drops, periodic attacks known as crises occur. Between crises patients are relatively asymptomatic. Crises are classified as infarctive (painful), aplastic-megaloblastic, sequestration and hemolytic.

**Fig. 14A & B:** This young child fractured the distal radius (arrow). Extensive destruction and periosteal reaction then developed with no evidence of infection and was attributed to infarction.

Figure 14A

Figure 14B

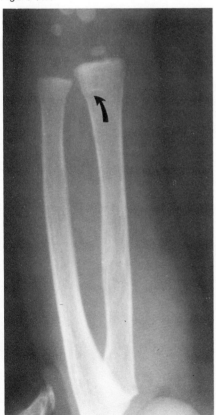

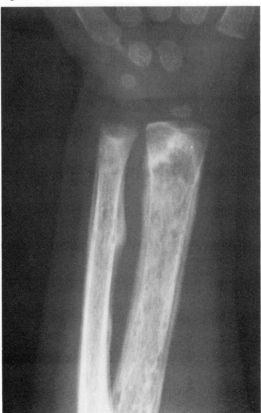

Infarctive crises are characterized by pain resulting from tissue anoxia. Common sites include bone, chest and abdomen. Splenic infarctions are common, and most patients after the age of eight to 10 are asplenic. This is the only crisis in which hemoglobin level does not fall. Aplastic-megaloblastic crises occur during infections when marrow activity is decreased. Sequestration crises occur only in infants and young children with a viable spleen. Hemolytic crises are fortunately rare.

The manifestations of marrow hyperplasia are similar to the other anemias but seldom as profound as beta-thalassemia major. There is medullary cavity widening, osteoporosis, cortical thinning and prominent trabecular patterns (Fig. 9). In a review of skull radiographs in 194 patients, 25% had decreased bone density, 22% had widened diploic space and a decrease in the outer table width (Fig. 10), while only 5% had "hair-on-end" striations.[22] As with all the other anemias the base of the occiput is spared, as well as facial bones. Generalized osteoporosis with a prominent trabecular pattern occurs in the remainder of the skeleton.

Osteonecrosis secondary to vascular occlusion is perhaps the most well known complication.[23,24] Although more common in SC disease, epiphyseal infarcts of the capital femoral (Fig. 11) and proximal humeral epiphysis (Fig. 12) are frequent in SS disease.[25] Often these are bilateral. Dactylitis is characterized by necrosis of the small tubular bones of the hands and feet in children between six

**Fig. 15:** Sickle cell anemia. Growth arrest of thumb and ring metacarpals.

**Fig. 16:** Sickle cell anemia. Central depressions of the vertebral end plates (arrows). This finding is usually, but not always, due to sickle cell anemia.

Figure 15

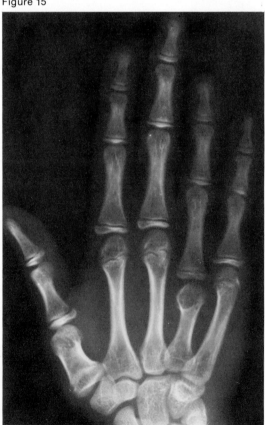

Figure 16

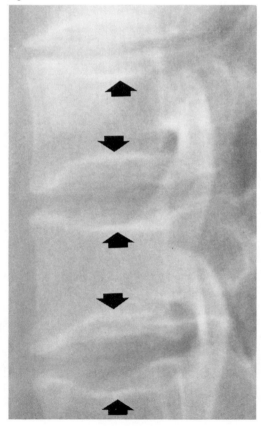

Bone Radiology Case Studies

months and two years. Also known as the hand-foot syndrome, it is clinically evident by hand and foot swelling, pain, fever and decreased range of motion (Fig. 13). Differentiation from osteomyelitis may be impossible. Diaphyseal infarctions, especially in the proximal femur, proximal humerus, distal femur, and proximal tibia occur commonly (Fig. 14). Infarctions may be so extensive that the resulting sclerosis resembles blastic metastases or Paget's disease.[26]

Growth disturbances are frequent and include epiphyseal-metaphyseal changes and spinal deformities as a result of epiphyseal damage (Fig. 15). Long bones may be shortened or misshaped. Tibiotalar slant may occur, but is nonspecific. Changes in the spine have led to a cornucopia of confusing and misleading terms. Reynolds has done much to reduce this confusion and explains the changes.[12] The fish vertebra (or cod fish vertebra) refers to the biconcave deformity found in patients whose bone is softened. It is most common in senile osteoporosis but can be found in numerous disorders of which sickle cell anemia is only one. This biconcave vertebra resembles the vertebra found in fish. Central depression of the vertebra is a distinct finding with a different etiology. Presumably it results from long standing ischemia and secondary growth inhibition. It is distinct from the biconcave changes in that it spares the periphery of the end plates, i.e., it is localized in the centrum (Figs. 1B, 16). The defect is square or rectangular, symmetric across the joint space, involves the spine diffusely, and is unrelated to weight bearing. Interestingly, patients with much milder forms of anemia (e.g., SC disease and sickle trait) often show profound changes. This finding is more specific than the biconcave deformity but has been reported in spherocytosis, osteoporosis, thalassemia, Gaucher's disease, homocystinuria, and PNH.[27,28]

Another unique complication of SS disease is the propensity for infection, including osteomyelitis and septic arthritis. According to Barrett-Connor, infection is the most common cause of death in patients with SS disease.[29] In her series of 250 infections in 166 patients, 29 episodes of osteomyelitis occurred in 21 patients. Salmonella predominated in this series. Diggs states that over 50% of osteomyelitis is secondary to this organism. Unfortunately the infection is multifocal and difficult to eradicate. Septic arthritis is less common. As with other anemias, fractures are common. Hemarthrosis and joint effusions are difficult to distinguish from septic arthritis.

Heterozygous sicklers (trait) are asymptomatic except under stress, and consequently have few bone changes. Marrow expansion does not occur. Spine changes have been described, and aseptic necrosis of the femoral head has been reported.[25]

In SC disease the patient is heterozygous for both hemoglobin S and hemoglobin C. Clinically the patients are intermediate between sickle trait and disease. In Barton's series of 117 patients, 46 were asymptomatic while 64 had symptoms of abdominal, bone and joint pain.[30] Changes due to marrow hyperplasia, osteonecrosis of the femoral and humeral heads, and in the spine occur but with less frequency than in SS disease.

Sickle-thalassemia patients are heterozygous for hemoglobin S and beta thalassemia as well. As with SC disease the clinical and roentgen findings vary. It is important to remember that all of the bone changes are attributable to the sickle aspect of the disease and that they in no way resemble changes in thalassemia.[31]

*—Mark Baker, MD*

# References

1. Erslev AJ: Aplastic anemia, in Williams W (ed): *Hematology,* ed 2. New York, McGraw-Hill, 1977, p 258.
2. Fanconi G: Familial constitutional panmyelocytopathy, Fanconi's Anemia (F.A.)—I. Clinical Aspects. *Semin Hematol* 1967; 4:233.
3. Juhl JH, Wesenberg RL, Gwinn JL: Roentgenographic findings in Fanconi's Anemia. *Radiology* 1967; 89:646.
4. Minagi H, Steinbach H: Roentgen appearance of anomalies associated with hypoplastic anemias of childhood: Fanconi's anemia and congenital hypoplastic anemia (erythrogenesis imperfecta). *Am J Roentgenol* 1966; 97:100.
5. Hall J: Thrombocytopenia with absent radius (TAR). *Medicine* 1969; 48:411.
6. Moseley J: Skeletal changes in anemia. *Semin Roentgenol* 1974; 9:169.
7. Fairbanks VF, Beutler: Erythrocyte disorders—anemias related to disturbances of hemoglobin synthesis. Iron deficiency, in Williams W (ed): *Hematology,* ed 2. New York, McGraw-Hill, 1977, p 363.
8. Britton HA, Canby JP, Kohler CM: Iron deficiency anemia producing evidence of marrow hyperplasia in the calvarium. *Pediatrics* 1960; 25:621.
9. Agarwal KN, Dhar N, Shah MM: Roentgen changes in iron deficiency anemia. *Am J Roentgenol* 1970; 86:635.
10. Weatherall DJ: The thalassemias, in Williams W (ed): *Hematology,* ed 2. New York, McGraw-Hill, 1977, p 391.
11. Caffey J: Cooley's anemia: A review of the roentgenographic findings in the skeleton. *Am J Roentgenol* 1957; 78:381.
12. Reynolds J: A re-evaluation of the fish vertebra sign in sickle cell hemoglobinopathy. *Am J Roentgenol* 1966; 97:693.
13. Cassaday JR, Berdon WE, Baker DH: The "typical" spine changes of sickle cell anemia in a patient with thalassemia major (Cooley's anemia). *Radiology* 1967; 89:1065.
14. Sfikakis P, Stamatoyannopoulos G: Bone changes in thalassemic trait. *Acta Haematol* 1963; 29:193.
15. Cooper RA, Jandl JH: Hereditary spherocytosis, in William W (ed): *Hematology,* ed 2. New York, McGraw-Hill, 1977, p 453.
16. Young LE, Izzo MJ, Platzer RF: Hereditary spherocytosis I. Clinical, hematologic and genetic features in 28 cases with particular reference to osmotic and mechanical fragility of inoculated erythrocytes. *Blood* 1951; 6:1013.
17. Becker MH, Genieser NB, Piomelli S, et al: Roentgenographic manifestations of pyruvate kinase deficiency hemolytic anemia. *Am J Roentgenol* 1971; 113:491.
18. Swisher SW, Travis SF: Isoimmune hemolytic disease of the newborn, in Williams W (ed): *Hematology,* ed 2. New York, McGraw-Hill, 1977.
19. Janus WL, Dietz MW: Osseous changes in erythroblastosis fetalis. *Radiology* 1949; 53:59.
20. Rosse WF. Paroxysmal nocturnal hemoglobinuria, in William W (ed): *Hematology,* ed 2. New York, McGraw-Hill, 1977, p 560.
21. Lehmann H, Huntsman RS, Costy R, et al: Sickle cell disease and related disorders, in William W (ed): *Hematology,* ed 2. New York, McGraw-Hill, 1977, p 495.
22. Sebes JI, Diggs LW: Radiographic changes in the skull in sickle cell anemia. *AJR* 1979; 132:373.

23. O-Hara AE: Roentgenographic osseous manifestations of the anemias and leukemias. *Clin Orthop* 1967; 52:63.

24. Diggs LW: Bone and joint lesions in sickle-cell disease. *Clin Orthop* 1967; 52:119.

25. Hill MC, Oh KS, Bowerman JW, et al: Abnormal epiphyses in the sickling disorders. *Am J Roentgenol* 1975; 124:34.

26. Resnick D: *Hemoglobinopathies and Other Anemias in Diagnosis of Bone and Joint Disorders*. Resnick D, Niwayama G (eds). Philadelphia, W.B. Saunders, 1981, pp 1885-1913.

27. Rohlfing B: Vertebral end plate depression: Report of two patients without hemoglobinopathy. *Am J Roentgenol* 1977; 128:599.

28. Hansen G, Gold R: Central depression of multiple vertebral end-plates: A "pathognomonic" sign of sickle hemoglobinopathy in Gaucher's disease. *Am J Roentgenol* 1977; 129:343.

29. Barrett-Connor E: Bacterial infection and sickle cell anemia. An analysis of 250 infections in 166 patients and a review of the literature. *Medicine* 1971; 50:97.

30. Barton CJ, Cockshott WP: Bone changes in hemoglobin SC disease. *Radiology* 1962; 88:523.

31. Reynolds J, Pritchard JA, Ludders D, et al: Roentgenographic and clinical appraisal of sickle cell B-thalassemia disease. *Am J Roentgenol* 1973; 118-378.

# Study 7

This 27-year-old man is experiencing foot pain following a minor injury. He has had intermittent pain in the same foot following prolonged exercise since age 12. There is marked limitation of inversion of the foot on physical examination. *Your diagnosis? What additional views of the foot would you obtain?*

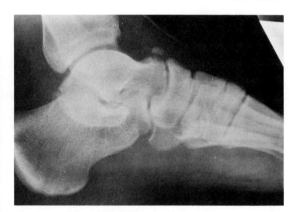

**Fig. 2:** Lateral view of foot.

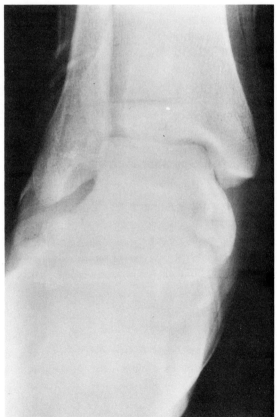

**Fig. 1:** AP view of ankle.

# Diagnosis: Congenital Tarsal Coalition

Congenital coalition of the tarsals is an important and often cryptic cause of foot pain. Tarsal coalition can be congenital or can develop secondary to trauma, infection, or arthritic inflammation. Congenital coalition is almost always an isolated abnormality but has been found in patients with symphalangism, minor anomalies of the little finger such as clinodactyly and gross limb anomalies such as phocomelia and hemimelia.[1] Tarsal coalition has been a feature of a few rare congenital syndromes including Apert's syndrome, Crouzon's syndrome, and Nievergelt-Pearlman syndrome, and is found in Morquio's disease.[2,3]

Union of tarsal anlage has been observed in the fetus leading to the conclusion that congenital coalition is due to failure of segmentation of the primitive mesenchyme that forms the tarsals.[4]

Congenital coalition of tarsal bones is found in the form of a syndesmosis, synchondrosis, or synostosis. The condition may be bilateral. The union is fibrous or cartilagenous early in life, and often becomes ossified later.[5] Bony union is easily seen with proper radiographic views, but cartilagenous and fibrous union cause subtle radiographic findings which can be easily overlooked.

The incidence of tarsal coalition in the general population is unknown. The reported incidence of tarsal coalition at autopsy, of military personnel and from a children's clinic, varied from .03% to 0.9%. The anomaly is transmitted as an autosomal dominant. One report detailed the findings in 98 parents and siblings of 31 patients with tarsal coalition. These 98 relatives were screened with physical examination and radiographs. Thirty-eight (39%) out of 98 persons screened had tarsal coaltion. None of these relatives were symptomatic.[6] Tarsal coalition is an important cause of foot pain, however. It is the most common cause of a rigid, painful flat foot.

The most common types of congenital tarsal coalition unite the calcaneus with the navicular or the talus with the calcaneus. Of 197 coalitions in four reported series, 98 (50%) were calcaneo-navicular and 85 (43%) talo-calcaneal.[4,6-8] Rare types include talo-navicular (Fig. 5), calcaneal-cuboid, cubo-navicular, naviculo-cuneiform (Fig. 6), and massive fusion. In this group of 197 feet, there was one foot which had both talo-calcaneal and calcaneo-navicular fusion.

Instead of joint fusion there may be an intact joint with an anomalous bony mass fusing two tarsals or a bony mass projecting from a single tarsal in such a way that motion is limited (Fig. 3).[5]

Congenital tarsal fusion seldom causes symptoms during infancy and early childhood. At this stage the coalition is fibrous or cartilagenous, and limitation of motion is minor. Rigidity increases with progressive ossification of the anomaly and symptoms usually appear near the time of adolescence.[9-11]

Pain is seldom severe and often occurs following prolonged exercise, unusual stress, or minor injury. Rest brings relief. Flat foot is a very common finding but is not always present (Fig. 2). There

58

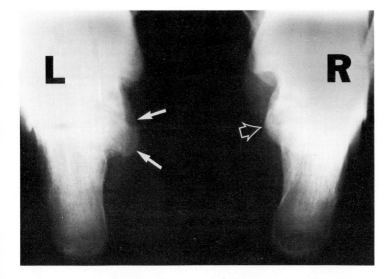

Fig. 3: Feet of patient in Figs. 1, 2—45° angled PA view of sub-talar joints. A bony mass at the left sustentaculum tali (solid arrows) obscures the middle talo-calcaneal joint. The right is normal (open arrow). The bony mass is seen at medial talus in Fig. 1, and there is talar beaking in Fig. 2.

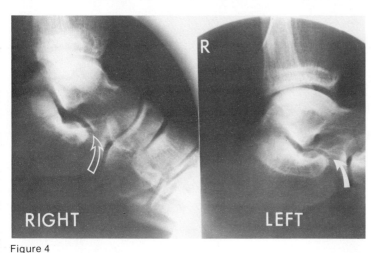

Figure 4

Fig. 4: Lateral view of feet. The bony mass of the sustentaculum tali seen in Fig. 3 is projected posterior to the narrowed middle talo-calcaneal joint (closed arrow). Compare to the normal right foot (open arrow).

may be varying degrees of valgus deformity at the subtalar and mid-tarsal joints. Mid-tarsal and/or subtalar movement is decreased or absent.

Intermittent spasm of the peroneal muscles provoked by overactivity is a frequent finding. Anterior tibial spasm is found less frequently.[4,11] This clinical constellation has been called peroneal spastic flat foot, peroneal flat foot, adolescent rigid foot, spastic flat foot, and rigid valgus foot. While most of these patients have congenital tarsal coalition, other etiologies include traumatic, infectious, and arthritic tarsal fusion; osteochondral fracture of the talar head; and degenerative change of the anterior talo-calcaneal joint.[12,13]

The radiographic diagnosis of tarsal coalition requires well positioned views and, in some cases, tomography. Initial study should include AP, lateral, and 45° oblique views of the foot, plus a 45° angled PA view of the posterior and middle talo-calcaneal joints. The angle of the oblique view of the foot may have to be

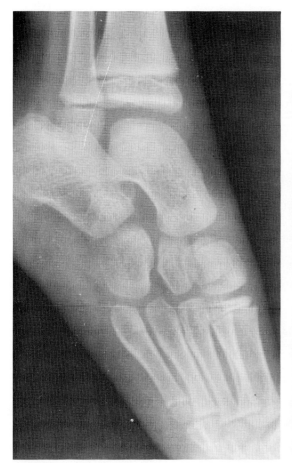

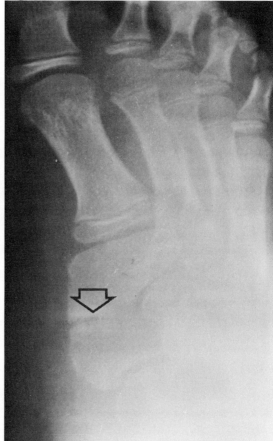

Figure 5                                    Figure 6

**Fig. 5:** Talo-navicular synostosis. This rare type of coalition is seldom symptomatic. The opposite foot had talo-navicular synostosis also.

**Fig. 6:** A rare naviculo-cuneiform coalition in 9-year-old child (arrow). There is non-bony fusion indicated by a narrowed joint space, sclerosis, and irregular cortical margins. (Degenerative changes could result in a similar radiographic appearance). (Courtesy of Dr. Edwin Harris.)

**Fig. 7A:** Oblique view of the foot. Calcaneo-navicular coalition in a 12-year-old child (arrow). There is sclerosis and a narrow, irregular space between the calcaneus and navicular. (Courtesy of Dr. Edwin Harris.)

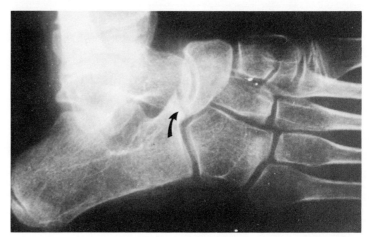

Figure 7A

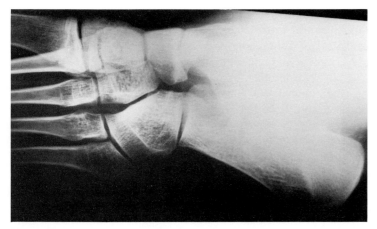

Figure 7B

varied in order to demonstrate optimally the relationship of the calcaneous and navicular, since overlap due to positioning can simulate calcaneo-navicular fusion.

Bony *calcaneo-navicular coalition* (Fig. 7) is usually obvious in the oblique view of the foot, but again, care must be taken to avoid mistaking overlap of the bones for synostosis. Multiple obliquities may be necessary. Fibrous or cartilagenous fusion is more difficult to detect. Decreased space between the two bones, irregular and indistinct cortical margins, sclerosis, and hypoplasia of the talar head all indicate abnormality.[8,10]

*Talo-calcaneal coalition* is almost always suggested by one or more "secondary" findings seen on the lateral radiograph of the foot.[10,14] These are:

1. *Talar Beak* (Fig. 8). A bony spur or beak projects from the distal superior margin of the head of the talus.(This bony spur must be located at the very distal end of the superior surface at the talus since a more proximal spur can be seen normally. This is especially true in athletes, and is caused by traction of the insertion of the joint capsule (Fig. 9).[15] The talar beak is caused by abnormal motion between the talus and navicular secondary to fixation of the subtalar joint. This sign is not specific and has been seen in acromegaly, hypermobile flat foot, following casting of club foot, post Grice procedure, and in rheumatoid arthritis.

   The talar beak has occasionally been in calcaneo-navicular coalition, but if a patient with a calcaneo-navicular coalition has beaking and surgery is contemplated, a careful search for talo-calcaneal fusion should be made since the two fusions can co-exist in rare cases.[10,12]

2. *Widened lateral process of the talus*(Fig. 14A). The calcaneus is forced into a valgus position causing the lateral process of the talus to impact on the sulcus calcaneus with resultant deformity.

3. *Narrowed posterior talo-calcaneal joint.* The posterior joint is narrowed due to decreased subtalar motion. This can be simulated by slight obliquity of the foot in the lateral view.

When lateral radiography shows one or more secondary signs of talo-calcaneal coalition, a careful search for fusion of a talo-calcaneal joint should be made. The complex articulation between the calcaneus and talus consists of two or three joints (Fig. 10, 11). The posterior joint and middle (sustentacular) joint are separated by the diagonal sulcus calcaneus. These two joints are usually parallel, and make about a 45° angle with the long axis of the calcaneus.

The angled PA view of the posterior and middle talo-calcaneal joints must be parallel to the joint surfaces to avoid misdiagnosis (Fig. 12). An X-ray beam angle of 45° is an average figure. If this angle does not demonstrate the joints well, the angle of the posterior joint can be easily measured on the lateral radiograph, and the x-ray tube positioned at the measured angle. In some patients the posterior and middle talo-calcaneal joint surfaces are not parallel and two different angled views will be needed.

The anterior talo-calcaneal joint is almost horizontal with only slight medial and inferior tilt. The anterior joint is most difficult to demonstrate, but fortunately, fusion of the anterior joint is rare. Posterior joint fusion is also unusual. The large majority of talo-calcaneal fusions involve the middle joint (Fig. 13).

Bony middle talo-calcaneal joint fusion can often be suspected on lateral or oblique films of the foot (Fig. 8, 14A) and confirmed by the PA angled view. If fusion is fibrous or cartilagenous, the joint space is visible, but often narrow with irregular cortical margins and indistinct joint margins (Fig. 4, 6, 14C). The normal posterior and middle joints in the angled PA view are horizontal and parallel (Fig. 12). A joint space fused by fibrous or cartilagenous tissue, in this view, may show a posterior and medial tilt (Fig. 15).

In cases in which the diagnosis of tarsal coalition is in doubt, or when the joints cannot be properly demonstrated with routine radiographs at various angles, longitudinal tomograms are invaluable (Fig. 14B, 14C). The width of the foot is measured at the level of the sustentacular joint (anterior and inferior to the medial malleolus). Sections are made at 1 cm, 1.5 cm, and 2 cm less than this distance, and a final section is made at one-half the measured distance.[10] The first section is through the middle (sustentacular) joint, the second and third cut through the anterior joint and the midline section is through the posterior joint.

The anterior facet poses a special problem in imaging since its articular surface is not only horizontal, but tilted medially. There may be a spurious appearance of fusion on lateral tomography. Coronal tomograms have been used to demonstrate the anterior talo-calcaneal joint.

There has been a report of patients with painful rigid feet who had secondary radiographic signs suggesting tarsal coalition, but no radiographic evidence of joint fusion (no tomograms were done). At surgery, there were bony protuberances blocking movement. Most of these extended upward from the posterior sustentaculum tali and obstructed talar movement.[5] These bony masses were either subtle and overlooked, or not visible on preoperative radiographs. Coronal tomograms would demonstrate this type of lesion. A bony

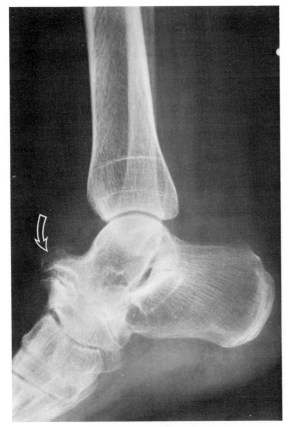

Figure 8

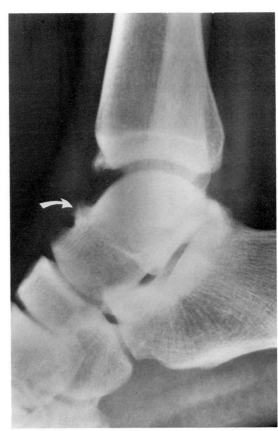

Figure 9

bar bridging the posterior calcaneus and talus across the location of the os trigonum has occurred. Another case was reported with a normal middle talo-calcaneal joint and a thin bony bar bridging the medial aspect of the joint.[13]

A peculiar ball and socket appearance of the ankle has been reported in patients with tarsal coalition, a short limb, and absence of at least one toe. The articular surface of the talus became spheroid and the talar mortis concave resulting in a ball and socket appearance. Most patients were asymptomatic despite the strikingly abnormal appearance of the ankle.[16]

There is considerable variation in therapy recommended for tarsal coalition. Excellent results are reported with early resection of calcaneo-navicular coalition, but conservative management is also advocated.[11,12] Talo-calcaneal coalition is seldom resected because secondary degenerative changes are almost always present at the time of diagnosis. Non-surgical management consists of treatment with heel wedges, arch supports, walking casts, and manipulations under anesthesia. If these measures are not successful in relieving pain, triple arthrodesis is done.[12]

**Fig. 8:** Large talar beak (arrow) in a woman with tarsal coalition. The beak extends from the most distal talus. There are degenerative changes at the talo-navicular joint also.

**Fig. 9:** Small, more proximal talar beak is a normal variant located at the insertion of the joint capsule. Similar beak is located at tibial insertion of capsule.

## Summary

Persistent foot pain in an older child or adolescent should suggest the possibility of congenital tarsal coalition, especially if the child

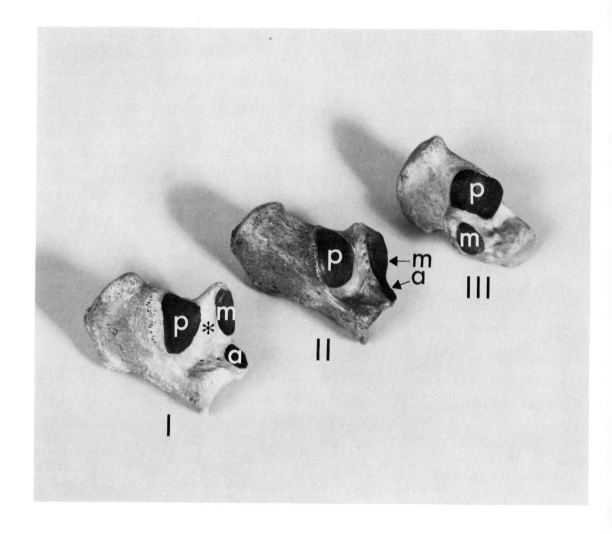

**Fig. 10:** Two right and one left calcaneus. The calcaneal sulcus (asterisk) divides the sub-talar joint into posterior and anterior compartments. The posterior compartment contains the posterior facet (P). The anterior compartment contains the middle facet (M) of the sustentaculum tali and the anterior facet (A). The anterior facet may be an independent articular surface (calcaneus I), may be a continuation of the middle facet (calcaneus II) or may be absent (calcaneus III).

limps or there is rigidity of the foot. In addition to AP and lateral views, screening radiographs should include an oblique view of the foot and an angled PA view of the posterior and middle talo-calcaneal joints. Because the radiographic findings are often subtle, they are easily missed or misinterpreted. If the initial views are taken in assembly line fashion, some abnormalities will not even be demonstrated. The anatomy of the foot varies from patient to patient. In order to display this anatomy optimally, radiographs must be monitored during the examination or repeated with altered foot position or x-ray tube angulation when necessary. If the talo-calcaneal joints cannot be demonstrated well despite multiple views at various angles, if radiographic findings are equivocal, or if there is strong clinical suspicion of coalition despite normal radiographs, longitudinal tomograms should be done. In the rare cases of anterior talo-calcaneal joint coalition and bony protuberances without coalition, coronal tomograms may be useful (Fig. 15).

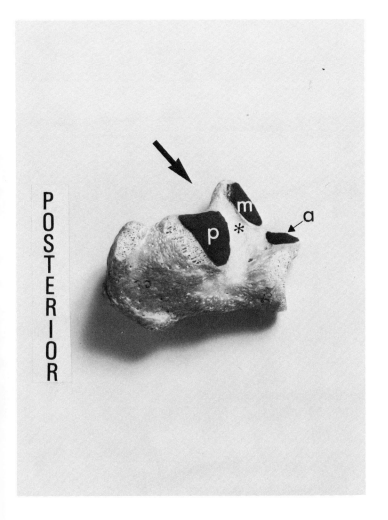

**Fig. 11:** Calcaneus viewed from its lateral aspect. Asterisk = sulcus calcaneus. The posterior facet (P) and middle facet (M) are parallel and make about a 45° angle with the longitudinal axis of the calcaneus. The PA x-ray beam (Large arrow) must be angled at 45° to demonstrate these joint surfaces. Notice that the anterior facet (A) is almost horizontal and therefore will not be seen with the angled PA view.

## References

1. Challis J: Hereditary transmission of talo-navicular coalition in association with anomaly of the little finger. *J Bone Joint Surg* 1974; 56A:1273.
2. Craig CL, Goldberg MJ: Calcaneocuboid coalition in Crouzon's syndrome. *J Bone Joint Surg* 1977; 59A:826.
3. Murakami Y: Nivergelt-Pearlman Syndrome with impairment of hearing. *J Bone Joint Surg* 1975; 57B:367.
4. Harris RI: Retrospect-peroneal spastic flat foot. *J Bone Joint Surg* 1965; 47A:1657.
5. Harris RI: Rigid valgus foot due to talocalcaneal bridge. *J Bone Joint Surg* 1955; 37A:169.
6. Leonard MA: The inheritance of tarsal coalition and its relationship to spastic flat foot. *J Bone Joint Surg* 1974; 56B:520.
7. Gillespie R, Raja D, Cummings W: Tarsal coalition revisited. *J Bone Joint Surg* 1974; 56B:587.
8. Braddock GT: A prolonged follow-up of peroneal spastic flat foot. *J Bone Joint Surg* 1961; 43B:734.
9. Harris RI, Beath T: Etiology of peroneal spastic flat foot. *J Bone Joint Surg* 1948; 30B:624.

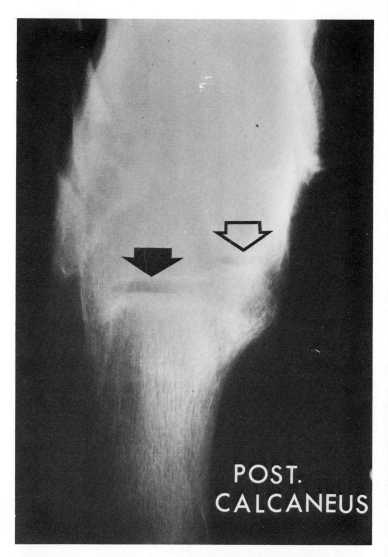

**Fig. 12:** 45° angled *PA* view of posterior (solid arrow) and middle (open arrow) talo-calcaneal joints. The joints are normal.

POST. CALCANEUS

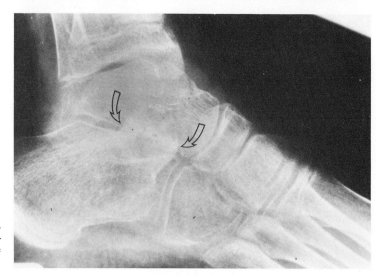

**Fig. 13:** 45° oblique view of the foot. There is synostosis of the middle talo-calcaneal joint (arrows). (Courtesy of Dr. Edwin Harris).

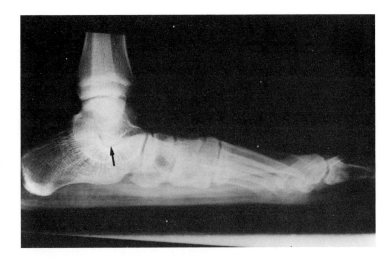

**Fig. 14A:** Coalition of the middle talo-calcaneal joint in an 11-year-old child. Lateral view. The foot is flat and the lateral process of the talus is broadened (arrow).

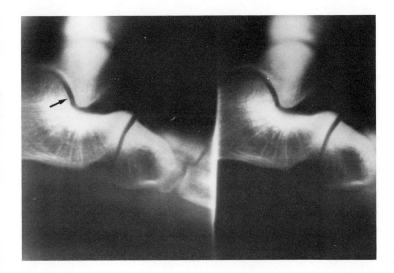

**Fig. 14B:** Longitudinal tomograms of the foot. The posterior talo-calcaneal joint is normal (arrow).

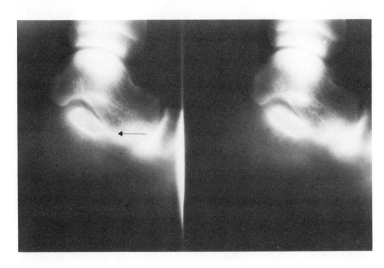

**Fig. 14C:** More medial longitudinal tomograms of the foot. The middle talo-calcaneal joint is narrow and there is local anterior synostosis (arrow).

10. Conway JJ, Cowell HR: Tarsal coalition: Clinical significance and roentgenographic demonstration. *Radiology* 1969; 92:799.
11. Dwyer FC: Causes, significance and treatment of stiffness of the subtaloid joint. *Proc Royl Soc Med* 1976; 69:97.
12. Cowell HR: Talocalcaneal coalition and new causes of peroneal spastic flat foot. *Clin Orthop* 1972; 85:16.
13. Outland T, Murphy ID: The pathomechanics of peroneal spastic flat foot. *Clin Orthop* 1960; 16:64.
14. Beckly DE, Anderson PW, Pedegana IR: The radiology of the subtalar joint with special reference to talo-calcaneal coalition. *Clin Radiol* 1975; 26:333.
15. Keats TE, Harrison RB: Hypertrophy of the talar beak. *Skeletal Rad* 1979; 4:37.
16. Channon GM, Brotherton BJ: The ball and socket ankle joint. *J Bone Joint Surg* 1979; 61B:85.

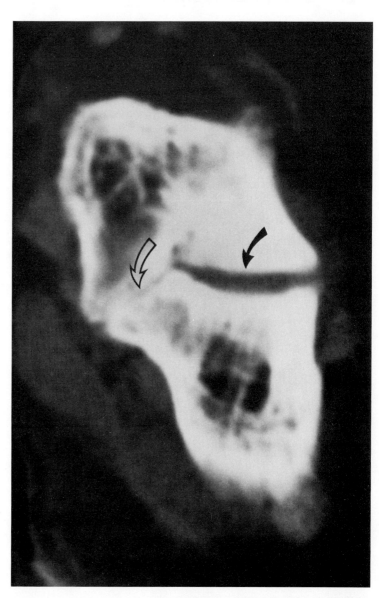

**Fig. 15:** Coronal computed tomography displays normal posterior subtalar joint (solid arrow) and obliterated, tilted middle joint (open arrow). Coronal sections could also (arrow) identify bony protuberances.

# Study 8

This 14-year-old boy has been limping slightly for several weeks and has pain in the anteromedial right knee. *Your Diagnosis?*

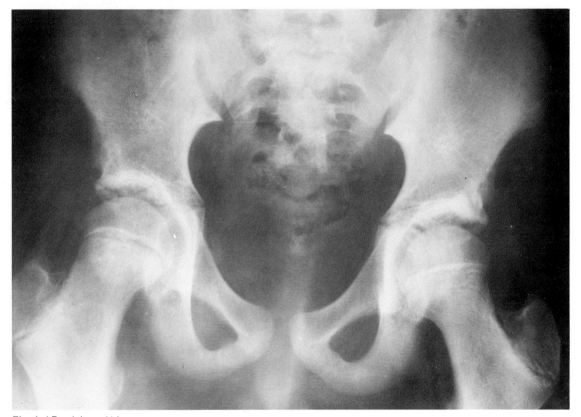

**Fig. 1:** AP pelvis and hips.

# Diagnosis: Slipped Capital Femoral Epiphysis

Slipped capital femoral epiphysis (SCFE) is most common in the period of rapid growth in adolescence. Males are more commonly affected, and the peak incidence (13-16 years) is a year or two older than in females. Patients are often obese, and may have underdeveloped genitals. Occasionally patients are tall and thin. SCFE is bilateral in 15 to 25% of patients.

Cartilage separation occurs between the zones of hypertrophy and provisional calcification.[1] While the location of the problem is documented, etiology remained unproven. There may be multiple factors, including: structural changes of the epiphysis and physis, oblique position of physis, rapid growth, normal adolescent atrophy of periosteum, obesity, and endocrine imbalances, especially increase in growth hormone and decrease in sex hormone. Endocrine imbalance has not been biochemically documented.

While the large majority of patients who have been studied have had normal endocrine systems, there have been increasing numbers of reports of patients with endocrine problems and associated SCFE.[2]

## Diseases Reported in Patients with SCFE

1. Chronic renal failure.
2. Hypothyroidism[3]
3. Craniopharyngioma
4. Primary hyperparathyroidism
5. Acromegaly
6. Rickets
7. Pituitary pathology
8. Turner's syndrome
9. Klinefelter's syndrome
10. Radiation therapy

Patients may limp and have pain in the groin, thigh, and / or knee. Limitation of adduction, flexion, and internal rotation are physical findings along with thigh atrophy and shortening plus slight flexion deformity.

## Radiographic Findings and Grading

### Preslip

The only finding is a widened physis which may have irregular margins.

### Minimal (less than 1 cm)

Widened physis may be the only finding on frontal view (Fig. 1). Lateral view is mandatory in order to avoid missing minimal posterior-inferior displacement (Fig. 2).

### Moderate (less than 2/3 width neck):
### Severe (more than 2/3 width neck)

Other findings include disruption of Shenton's line and osteoporosis of inferior medial metaphysis of femoral neck. In

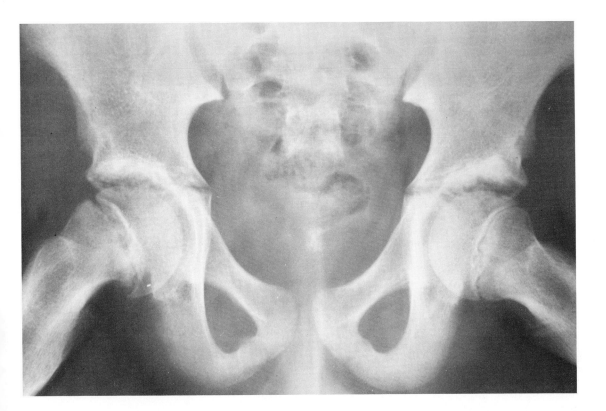

chronic cases, callus and sclerosis are found at the posterior inferior femoral neck and the neck appears short and wide due to anterior bowing.

**Fig. 2:** Lateral view of femurs with minimal posterior slipped right capital femoral epiphysis. Figure 1 showed widened physis, but did not demonstrate the posterior displacement of the epiphysis seen here.

## Complications

Avascular necrosis occurs only after reduction in severe cases with incidences of 25 to 35% reported after open reduction. Degenerative joint disease and deformity are late complications. Chondrolysis has averaged about 8% of 2,000 reported cases.[4] Radiographs first show osteoporosis and irregular subchondral bone, and later joint space narrowing with sclerosis. Symptoms may persist despite rewidening of the joint space with passage of time.[5] Actually, most patients have narrowing of the joint space after treatment which improves with time. Pain, limitation of motion with narrowing to less than one-half the original width, is probably pathologic however.[4]

### References

1. Howorth M, Ferguson A: Pathology etiology and treatment of slipping of the capital femoral epiphysis. *Clin Orthop* 1966; 48:33.
2. Ogden J, Southwick W: Endocrine dysfunction and slipped capital femoral epiphysis. *Yal J Biol Med* 1977; 50:1.
3. Crawford A, MacEwen G: Slipped capital femoral epiphysis with hypothyroidism. *Clin Orthop* 1977; 122:135.
4. Ogden J, Simon T: Cartilage space width in slipped capital femoral epiphysis. *Yale J Biol Med* 1977; 50:17.
5. Tillema D, Golding J: Chondrolysis following slipped capital femoral epiphysis in Jamaica. *J Bone Joint Surg* 1971; 53:1528.

# *DENSITY*

Altered bone density is a common feature of bone and joint disease. The plain radiograph is insensitive to bone loss. In a vertebra, for example, destruction of cancellous bone is not seen until at least one-third of the bone is gone. In general, trabecular loss, thin cortices, and prominent vertebral end plates indicate loss of bone density on plain radiographs. Nuclear medicine I-125 transmission scans of the radius and the ulna and computed tomography of the spine can accurately determine appendicular and axial bone density.

Generalized decreased bone density is not equated with osteoporosis because the decreased bone density found in hyperparathyroidism, osteomalacia, multiple myeloma, and other diseases looks identical to that found in osteoporosis; findings such as subperiosteal resorption or pseudofractures must be present to suggest a specific radiologic diagnosis. Local decreased bone density may be due to disuse. Periarticular density loss indicates hyperemia in joints affected by inflammatory arthritis.

Patterns of focal bone destruction reflect the aggressiveness of the underlying process. A single well defined *geographic* area of destruction indicates an indolent process, even more so if there is a sclerotic margin. The entire perimeter, however, must be evaluated in estimating activity. Multiple coalescent medium-sized holes present a motheaten appearance which indicates an active process, while innumerable tiny holes permeating the bone indicate a very aggressive lesion.

Generalized osteosclerosis can be the result of a variety of disorders including hematologic disease, metastases, hypercalcemia, or fluorosis. Focal sclerosis is commonly the result of metastases, infarcts, and degenerative joint disease.

This 61-year-old man has had pain in the anterior chest of four months duration. A mass fixed to the sternum is tender to palpation. *Your diagnosis?*

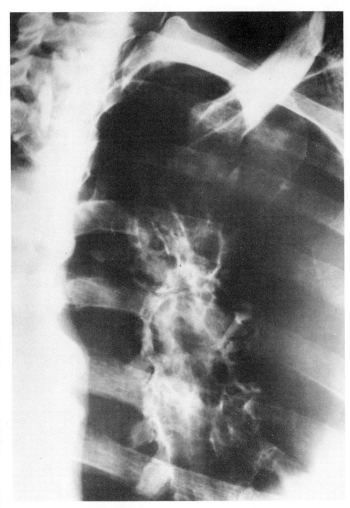

**Fig. 1:** Oblique view of sternum.

# Diagnosis: Solitary Plasmacytoma of Sternum

The sternum is a rare site for a primary malignant neoplasm. The most common sternal lesion is bone metastasis, followed in frequency by primary malignant neoplasm and inflammatory disease. Least common are benign neoplasms.[1]

Sternal lesions often cause pain, a palpable mass or both. These nonspecific findings occur with both neoplastic and inflammatory disease.

Inflammatory diseases affecting the sternum include osteomyelitis, tuberculosis, fungal diseases and Echinococcus disease.

Again, metastases are the most common sternal lesions. The majority of metastases are from kidney, thyroid and breast primaries and in lymphoma.[1] In the case presented here the lesion is

Figure 2

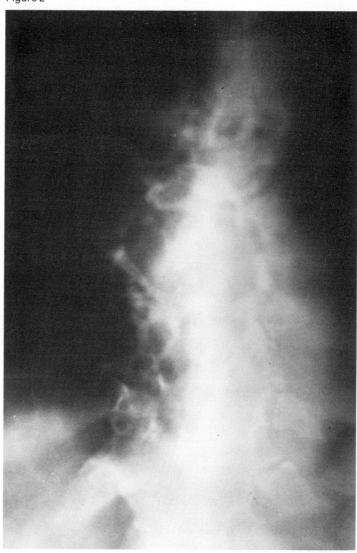

**Figs. 2, 3:** AP and lateral tomograms of the sternum demonstrate widespread bone destruction and expansile nature of the plasmacytoma.

not only osteolytic, but also expansile. Bone metastases may have this appearance, and thyroid or kidney metastases are most commonly the cause of gross expansion of bone. One striking feature of thyroid and kidney metastases is that they may be extremely vascular. These metastases may even be pulsatile on physical examination. Rarely expansile metastases have been reported with breast and lung primaries, pheochromocytoma and melanoma.[2]

The most common primary sternal malignancy is chondrosarcoma. This tumor may expand bone also, but is often identified by multiple discrete calcifications characteristic of cartilage calcification. Plasmacytoma, reticulum cell sarcoma and osteosarcoma have occurred as sternal primaries in descending order of frequency. Most of the very rare benign neoplasms are enchondromas or osteomas.[1]

Figure 3

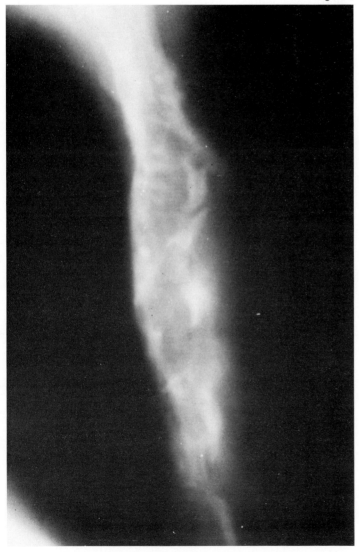

Up to 10% of patients with plasma cell myeloma present with solitary skeletal lesions. Median survival in multiple myeloma is two to three years. There is a question as to whether solitary myeloma is merely early multiple myeloma or a separate entity with a better prognosis. In a series of 248 patients, 78 presented with solitary skeletal lesions. Only 11 survived five years with no spread of disease. Fifty-eight developed multifocal or generalized disease.[3]

More stringent criteria for solitary myeloma are: (1) a solitary skeletal lesion, (2) normal bone marrow elsewhere, (3) normal serum electrophoresis (except for small amounts of monoclonal immunoglobulins which have been caused by solitary plasmacytomas and disappeared after treatment[4]) and (4) absent Bence Jones proteinuria. Even with these criteria, most patients develop generalized disease. In a series of 47 patients with solitary spinal plasmacytomas, five patients survived 4 to 14 years.[5]

If a patient with the above criteria isn't considered to have a solitary lesion unless two years elapse without spread, survival is even better. Of 12 patients, three survived, five, 12, and 19 years, and nine developed spread after 2 to 10 years.[6] Surgery and radiotherapy have each been used as sole treatment with long-term survival reported with each modality.

The most common location of solitary myeloma is the spine. The lesion usually begins in the vertebral body and is purely lytic with frequent bony expansion. Pedicles are involved late, as opposed to metastasis to the spine, which often involves the pedicles early. The long bones and flat bones are other common sites for plasmacytoma. In the flat bones, these tumors are frequently expansile.

## References

1. Vieta JO, Maier MC: Tumors of the sternum. *Surg Gynecol Obstet* 1962; 114:513.
2. Greenfield GB: *Radiology of Bone Disease.* Philadelphia, Lippincott, 1975.
3. Griffiths DL: Orthopaedic aspects of myelomatosis. *J Bone Joint Surg* 1966; 48B:703.
4. Snapper I, Kahn A: *Myelomatosis.* Baltimore, University Park Press, 1971.
5. Valderrama JA, Bullough PG: Solitary myeloma of the spine. *J Bone Joint Surg* 1960; 50B:82.
6. Meyer JE, Schulz MD: Solitary myeloma of bone. *Cancer* 1974; 34:438.

# Study 10

This 13-year-old girl has had pain in the middle finger of her right hand for several months and it is getting worse. She is afebrile. *Your diagnosis?*

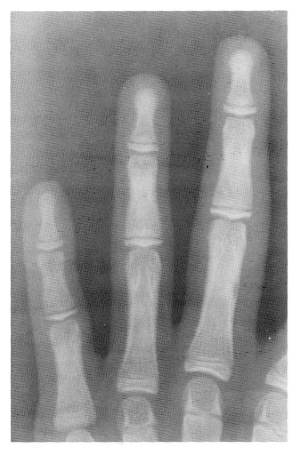

Fig. 1: AP view shows middle, ring, and little fingers of the right hand.

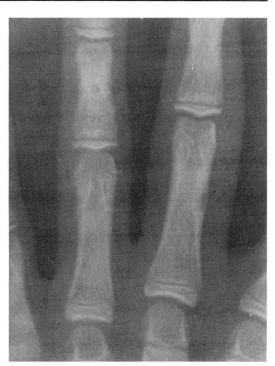

**Fig. 2:** AP view shows closeup of the proximal phalanx of the middle finger.

# Diagnosis: Osteoid Osteoma

This patient has a soft tissue swelling of the middle finger (Fig. 1). There is a small oval lucency in the lateral cortex of the proximal phalanx at its midpoint. There is minimal cortical thickening and minimal convexity of the cortical margin at the level of the lucent nidus (Fig. 2). This paucity of reactive bone is frequent in osteoid osteomas of the hand.

Primary bone neoplasms of the hand are very unusual. Among about 12,000 bone tumors representing a summation of those reported in several large series, there were 468 (4%) tumors of the hand.[1-4] Less than 10% originated in the carpals. Of these 468 neoplasms of the hand, only 39 (8%) were malignant. This collected group of bone neoplasms of the hand included:

## Benign
Enchondroma (305)
Osteochondroma (33)
Osteoid osteoma (23)
Osteoblastoma (19)
Chondroblastoma (16)
Chondromyxoid fibroma (15)
Giant cell tumor (13)
Aneurysmal bone cyst (5)

## Malignant
Chondrosarcoma (21)
Osteosarcoma (6)
Ewing's sarcoma (5)
Malignant giant cell (3)
Parosteal osteosarcoma (2)
Malignant histiocytoma (1)
Histiocytic lymphoma (1)

Osteoid osteoma is predominantly a lesion of the young. About 80% of patients are between the ages of 5 years and 25 years. Cases reported in the extremes of life, however, include an 8-month-old infant and a 70-year-old man. Male patients are affected four times more often than female patients.[1-3]

Most lesions are located in the femur and tibia. Just about every bone in the body has been the site of an osteoid osteoma, but the jaw, calvarium, clavicle, ribs and sternum are very rare sites. There were 363 osteoid osteomas among the 12,000 bone tumors reported, and 23 (6%) of these were located in the hand. The proximal phalanx is involved most commonly. In the wrist the navicular is affected most frequently.[5]

The typical patient complains of persistent aching pain. The pain may be intermittent, but often increases gradually in severity over a period of weeks to years. Worsening of the pain at night and relief with aspirin are characteristic of osteoid osteoma. Although aspirin can relieve symptoms in some patients, there is some dispute over how often this occurs.[2] Pain is not relieved by immobilization.

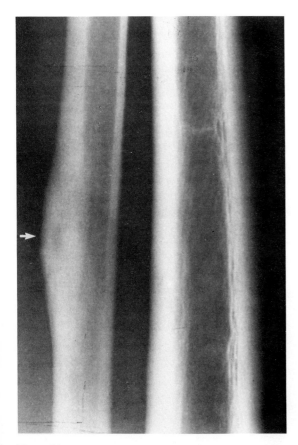

Figure 3A

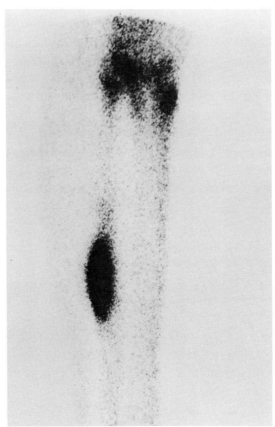

Figure 3B

Occasionally a patient with a typical bone lesion is pain-free. Swelling is common, especially in the fingers, but there is no redness. There is no fever. There may be tenderness to palpation over the area of the tumor nidus.[6,7]

The roentgenographic appearance of osteoid osteoma varies with the location of the neoplasm in the bone. The actual tumor or nidus is seen most often as a lucency less than 1.5 cm in diameter. The lucent nidus sometimes contains a central density. If the central density is large the remaining peripheral lucency of the nidus results in a ringlike ("ring sequestrum") appearance. In some cases the entire nidus is dense rather than lucent. The density of the nidus in these cases can be equal to, less than, or greater than, normal bone.

When the nidus is located in cortical bone there is usually extensive surrounding sclerosis and cortical thickening due to periosteal new bone formation (Figs. 3A, 3B). In these cases tomograms may be needed to identify the small nidus that is obscured by adjacent sclerotic bone. When the nidus is located in cancellous bone there is much less sclerosis, and it may be distant from the nidus (Figs. 4, 5A, 5B). Tumors in a subperiosteal or intra-articular position often have no accompanying sclerosis. A small rounded soft tissue mass and periosteal reaction are found with a subperiosteal lesion. The intra-articular lesion can result in a joint effusion and simulate arthritis.[8]

**Fig. 3A:** Cortical osteoid ostema of fibula. Cortical thickening with lucent nidus below arrow.

**Fig 3B:** [99m]Technicium diphosphonate bone scan with avid uptake in mid-fibula.

When osteoid osteomas are located in the phalanges or metacarpals there may be sclerosis and expansion of the bone. Subperiosteal and cancellous osteoid osteomas are more common in the femoral neck, vertebrae, and small bones of the hand and foot. The cancellous or rare subperiosteal lesion may be subtle on roentgenograms when the nidus is small and there is no surrounding sclerosis. Enlargement of the digits and premature fusion of epiphyses have been reported with osteoid osteomas of the hand.

Nuclear medicine studies regularly image these tumors. In cases presenting diagnostic problems angiography is helpful. The nidus is quite vascular, which differentiates it from a focus of bone destruction due to osteomyelitis.

The histologic diagnosis of osteoid osteoma depends upon identification of the nidus. In a series of 140 patients with pain and clinical diagnosis of osteoid osteoma who had surgery, the pathologist failed to identify a nidus in 54 (two patients had Brodie's

**Fig. 4:** Medullary osteoid osteoma of distal femur with lucent nidus and slight sclerosis.

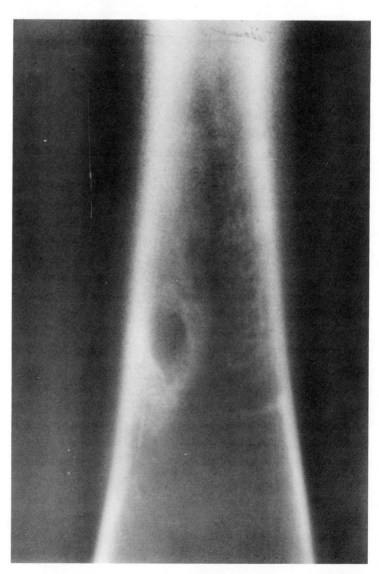

Bone Radiology Case Studies

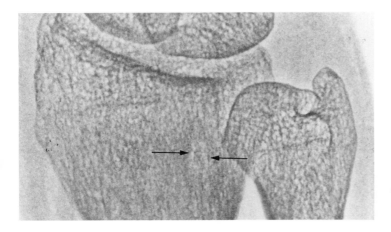

**Fig. 5A:** Medullary osteoid osteoma of distal radius. The dense central nidus results in a subtle ring appearance (arrows) in this xerogram.

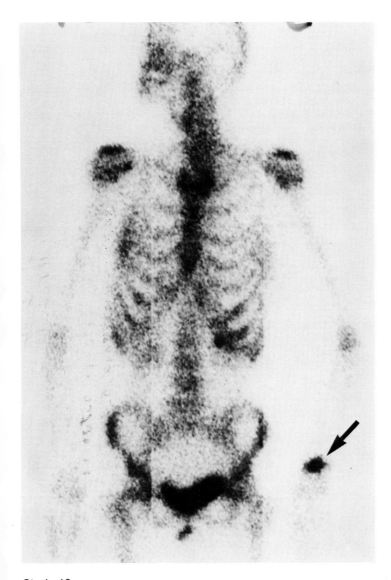

**Fig. 5B:** Avid uptake of radionuclide (arrow). (Courtesy of Richard Marsan, M.D.).

abscesses). A central nidus was visible preoperatively in 51 of these 54 patients. In 29 of these 54 operated patients without histologic confirmation of osteoid osteoma, symptoms were relieved after surgery. Eighteen patients who had persistent symptoms following surgery were re-operated. Thirteen of these re-operated patients were cured and typical nidi were found in seven.[9]

If there is no nidus in the surgical specimen, the nidus may not have been removed. Such patients may have recurrent symptoms. Intra-operative radiographs and specimen roentgenograms are useful in confirming that resected or curetted bone has included the nidus. In other cases it would seem that the pathologist was unable to identify a nidus even though it had been removed.[1]

### References

1. Dahlin D. *Bone Tumors.* Springfield, Charles C. Thomas, 1978.
2. Huvos A. *Bone Tumors.* Philadelphia, WB Saunders, 1979.
3. Netherlands Committee on Bone Tumors. *Radiologic Atlas of Bone Tumors.* Baltimore, Williams and Wilkins, 1966.
4. Mangini U. Tumors of the skeleton of the hand. *Bull Hosp Joint Dis* 1967; 28:61.
5. Carroll R. Osteoid osteoma in the hand. *J Bone Joint Surg* 1953; 35A:888.
6. Kendrick J, Everts C. Osteoid osteoma—A critical analysis of 40 tumors. *Clin Orthop* 1967; 54:51.
7. Spjut H, Dorfman M, et al. *Tumors of Bone and Cartilage.* Washington DC, Armed Forces Inst Path, 1970.
8. Edeiken J, DePalma A, Hodes P. Osteoid osteoma (roentgenographic emphasis). *Clin Orthop* 1966; 49:201.
9. Sim F, Dahlin D, Beabout J. Osteoid osteoma: Diagnostic Problems. *J Bone Joint Surg* 1975; 57A:154.

# Study 11

This 23-year-old man has had an ache of the right knee for three months. It is intermittent and worse at night. The only positive physical finding is tenderness on palpation of the proximal tibia. Admission laboratory values are normal. *Your diagnosis?*

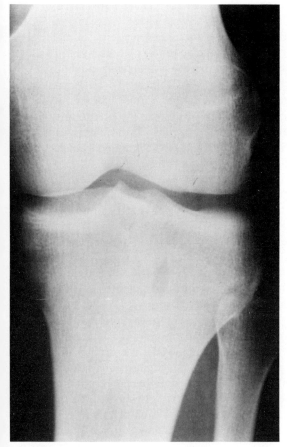

**Fig. 1:** AP right knee.

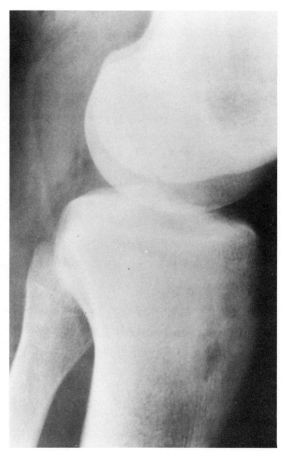

**Fig. 2:** Lateral right knee.

# Diagnosis: Subacute Osteomyelitis

Cases of osteomyelitis can be divided into three groups based on pathogenesis: (1) most common, associated with direct spread from a focus of infection contiguous to the bone, (2) associated with peripheral vascular disease—usually in diabetics, and (3) least common, hematogenous bone infection.[1] Osteomyelitis is also defined as acute or chronic. A minority of patients with hematogenous osteomyelitis have an atypical course which is termed subacute pyogenic osteomyelitis or Brodie's abscess. While the prognosis of this condition is very good, the diagnosis may be difficult.

In subacute osteomyelitis there is no acute attack. There are no systemic effects in most patients. The course of the disease is prolonged and insidious. Symptoms are present for weeks to months or even years, and there may be spontaneous remissions during that time. Most patients have mild to moderate pain at a single site—a localized ache. This may occur at night and be relieved by aspirin, similar to osteoid osteoma. The majority of patients are children and adolescents, with a higher incidence in males. The metaphyseal areas of long bones are most commonly affected.[2,3]

On physical examination there is often localized tenderness to palpation. Soft tissue swelling is less frequent. The patient is usually afebrile and the white blood cell count normal. The sedimentation rate may be slightly elevated. Radiographs are almost always abnormal.[4] Positive cultures of the abscess in these cases usually yield *Staphylococcus aureus* and rarely *S albus* or Gram negatives. However, there may be no bacterial growth.

The indolent course in subacute osteomyelitis is probably due to a combination of host resistance and low virulence of the infecting organisms resulting in the infection being kept focal and then walled off. The central lesion in acute osteomyelitis is necrotic and contains pus cells. The central lesion in subacute osteomyelitis is lined with granulomatous tissue and leukocytes. The process has been contained and is surrounded by a capsule of connective tissue. The adjacent cancellous tissue is compressed and often sclerotic. There is no subperiosteal spread.[5,6]

Radiographic abnormality is almost always present. A single site is involved, but there are rare reported cases of bilateral symmetric lesions.[7] The metaphyses of the tibia and femur are most frequently involved. A diaphyseal location is uncommon and more apt to be seen in the adult (Figs. 5A, 5B).[3] Epiphyseal location has been reported but is least common. Epiphyseal lesions can be solitary or result from metaphyseal infection crossing the physis.[4] Subacute osteomyelitis is also found in the vertebrae and calcaneous.[2]

Since the infection is well contained, there is seldom any periosteal reaction. Sequestra are rarely present. Most patients have one or several lytic areas, often with sclerotic rims or faint sclerosis of the surrounding bone.

Subacute osteomyelitis may mimic a bone neoplasm. In the

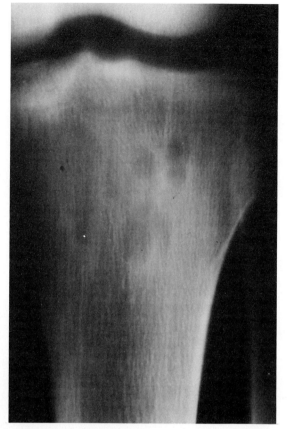

**Fig. 3:** AP tomogram right tibia.

**Fig. 4:** Lateral tomogram right tibia.

metaphyseal area an unusually large, poorly defined lytic area has been mistaken for osteosarcoma.[8] A metaphyseal lucency with a sclerotic rim can resemble a chondroblastoma or chondromyxoid fibroma. Purely lucent defects can be mistaken for eosinophilic granuloma or metastases. The unusual diaphyseal location of subacute osteomyelitis can result in periosteal reaction, and when seen in a child, can mimic Ewing's sarcoma. The most frequent diagnostic problem, however, is differentiating Brodie's abscess from osteoid osteoma. Mistakes have been made in both directions. The solitary cavity with surrounding sclerosis resembles an osteoid osteoma. This appearance plus a history of night pain is even more of a problem.[2,4] In this last situation angiography has proven valuable, demonstrating no vascularity in an abscess cavity but increased vascularity in the nidus of osteoid osteoma.

The presentation and course of acute osteomyelitis can be altered by antibiotic therapy that is not sufficient to be curative. This can happen when there is a misdiagnosis of osteomyelitis, inadequate antibiotic therapy of known osteomyelitis or when osteomyelitis develops in a patient receiving antibiotics for an unrelated condition.[9] This antibiotic modified osteomyelitis may resemble a Brodie's abscess clinically and radiographically.

Preferred treatment of subacute osteomyelitis with cavitation is surgery and antibiotic therapy. Surgery is therapeutic and also

**Figs. 3, 4:** Well defined defects with sclerotic borders present in Figures 1 and 2 are better seen on these tomograms. Surgical biopsy report was: fragments of fibrous tissue heavily infiltrated by chronic inflammatory cells and fragments of granulation tissue infiltrated by mononuclear cells, consistent with Brodie's abscess. Culture of fluid obtained at surgery grew *Salmonella*. Although rare, this organism has been reported in otherwise healthy people with osteomyelitis and in patients with subacute osteomyelitis.[2]

provides tissue for histology and fluid for culture. Antibiotic therapy alone may be followed by recurrence.[2-4]

## References

1. Waldvogel FA, Medoff G, Swartz MN: Osteomyelitis: A review of clinical features, therapeutic considerations and unusual aspects. *New Engl J Med* 1970; 282:198.
2. Harris NH, Kirkaldy-Willis WH: Primary subacute pyogenic osteomyelitis. *J Bone Joint Surg* 1965; 47B:526.
3. King DM, Mayo KM: Subacute hematogenous osteomyelitis. *J Bone Joint Surg* 1969; 51B:458.
4. Kandel SN, Mankin HJ: Pyogenic abscess of the long bones in children. *Clin Orthop* 1973; 96:108.
5. Gledhill RB: Subacute osteomyelitis in children. *Clin Orthop* 1973; 96:57.
6. Jaffe HL: *Metabolic, Degenerative, and Inflammatory Diseases of Bones and Joints.* Philadelphia, Lea & Febiger, 1972.
7. Giedion A, Holthusen W, Masel LF, et al: Subacute and chronic "symmetrical" osteomyelitis. *Ann Radiol* 1972; 15:329.
8. Cabanala ME, Sim FH, Beabout JW, et al: Osteomyelitis appearing as neoplasms. *Arch Surg* 1974; 109:68.
9. Davis LA: Antibiotic modified osteomyelitis. *Am J Roentgenol* 1968; 103:608.

**Fig. 5A:** Subacute osteomyelitis of tibial diaphysis. The tibia is sclerotic and widened.

**Fig. 5B:** Serpigenous lucency, demonstrated here by tomography, is characteristic of subacute osteomyelitis and excludes osteoid osteoma. (Courtesy of Andrew Berkow, M.D.)

Figure 5A

Figure 5B

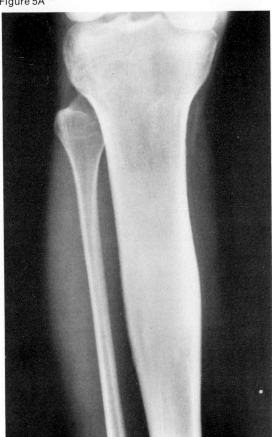

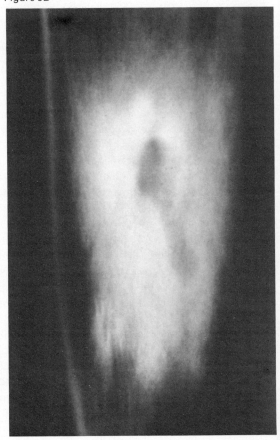

Bone Radiology Case Studies

# Study 12

This 42-year-old man has had back pain for more than one year. He has multiple sharply defined lytic lesions of the pelvis and anterior erosion of L2. *Your diganosis?*

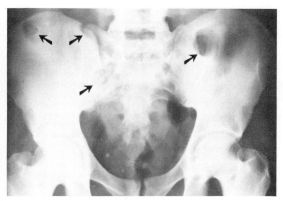

**Fig. 1:** AP view of pelvis. (Arrows indicate lytic lesions.)

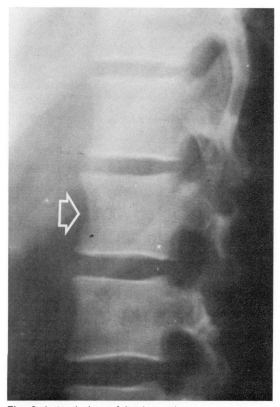

**Fig. 2:** Lateral view of lumbar spine. (Arrow indicates anterior erosion of L2.)

*Note: Figs. 1, 2, 4, 5, 6, 7 courtesy of Arnold Seitam, MD, V.A. Hospital, Hines, Illinois.*

# Diagnosis: Skeletal Tuberculosis

This patient has disseminated skeletal tuberculosis. Figure 1 shows sharply defined lytic lesions of the sacrum and both iliac bones. Figure 2 shows that the anterior surface of L3 is abnormally concave because of erosion by subligamentous tuberculosis. Disseminated tuberculosis is an uncommon form of the disease, and is found most often in noncaucasian children.[1-3] The individual bone lesions frequently appear "cystic," as in this patient.

All cases of tuberculosis are reportable in the U.S.A. There has been a steady decline in reported pulmonary tuberculosis since the early 1960s, while the rate of extrapulmonary tuberculosis has remained constant. Pulmonary tuberculosis declined from 48,000 cases/year in 1964 to 27,000 cases/year in 1974, while extrapulmonary tuberculosis remained at about 4,000 cases/year during the same interval. In 1976, 14% of all reported cases of tuberculosis were extrapulmonary.[4]

An epidemiologic study of 13 states from 1969-1973 reported 676 cases of bone and joint tuberculosis, representing about 10% of all extrapulmonary tuberculosis.[4] Almost half of the patients had involvement of the vertebral column; the hip and knee were next most commonly affected. There was a higher incidence of skeletal tuberculosis in non-caucasians, and most of the patients were more than 35 years old. In other recent studies an increasing percentage of bone and joint tuberculosis was found in older age groups.[5,6]

A summation of two studies published in the early 1950s disclosed a total of 386 patients with 478 tuberculous skeletal lesions.[7,8] The most common sites of involvement were:

| | |
|---|---|
| Spine | 209 |
| Cervical | 10 |
| Thoracic | 113 |
| Lumbar | 86 |
| Sacroiliac joints | 47 |
| Knee | 41 |
| Hip | 27 |
| Rib | 18 |
| Disseminated | 54 |

Only 30% of these 386 patients had roentgenographic evidence of active pulmonary tuberculosis. Genitourinary tract tuberculosis was present in 20%.

Tuberculous infection caused by ingesting *Mycobacterium bovis* is no longer found in the U.S.A. Most bone and joint infections are caused by inhaling droplets containing *Mycobacterium tuberculosis*. It is generally assumed that bone and joint lesions are the result of hematogenous spread from a pulmonary focus of infection, even though most patients with skeletal tuberculosis have normal chest roentgenograms.

Atypical *Mycobacterium* species, including *M. kansasii* (Fig. 3), *M. fortuitum, M. marinum,* and *M. intracellulare,* rarely affect the skeletal system. These organisms most often involve the tendon

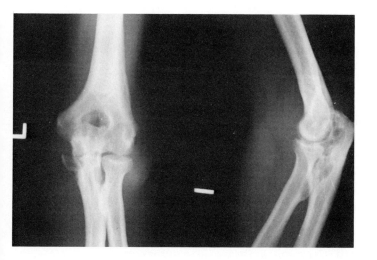

**Fig. 3:** Views of the left elbow show destructive lesions caused by *M. kansasii.* (Reprinted with permission from Zvetina JR, Reyes CV. Mycobacterium kansasii infection of the elbow joint. J Bone Joint Surg 1979; 61A(7):1099-1102.)

sheaths of the hand and wrist, probably due to direct inoculation associated with trauma. Hematogenous spread, with involvement of larger joints and the spine, has been reported, however.[1] Roentgenographic findings are similar to those of disease caused by *M. tuberculosis.*

Skeletal tuberculosis is an indolent process. One series compared a total of 150 cases of spinal tuberculosis, pyogenic osteomyelitis of the spine, and spinal column neoplasia.[6] About 80% of the patients with tuberculosis had symptoms for more than six months, while 40% had symptoms for more than one year. Only 2% of patients with other forms of osteomyelitis had symptoms for more than one year, while almost 80% had symptoms for less than three months.

The onset of symptoms usually is insidious. Pain is a common symptom, and there may be swelling or joint effusion. Systemic signs and symptoms may or may not be present. Patients may be seen initially because of soft tissue "cold" abscesses, sometimes without evidence of bone involvement.[9] Paraplegia caused by spinal tuberculosis has been reversed following decompression and chemotherapy.[10]

Smears or cultures of joint fluid and abscesses or surgical specimens provide the definitive diagnosis. Culture is needed to differentiate *M. tuberculosis* from other species of tuberculosis. Often the diagnosis of bone and joint tuberculosis is not initially considered, however, and delay in proper diagnosis may extend to months or even years.[10,11] Up to 20% of patients do not have positive tuberculin skin tests.[12]

About half of all bone and joint tuberculosis is spinal. Usually infection begins in the anterior part of a vertebra near the superior or inferior cortex, with spread to the intervertebral disc and adjacent vertebra. On roentgenogram there is early loss of the cortical margin of the vertebra, then narrowing of the disc space with symmetric involvement of the adjacent vertebrae (Fig. 4A). With further destruction there is anterior wedging, and a sharply angled gibbus deformity may occur (Fig. 4B). A soft tissue mass is seen commonly in the cervical and thoracic spine (Fig. 5A), but cannot be identified in the lumbar spine because there is no air to outline it. Erosions of the anterior vertebral bodies (Fig. 2) occasionally result from spread of infection under the anterior longitudinal ligament of the spine. (Similar defects can be caused by enlarged lymph nodes or an aortic aneurysm).[1] Involvement of the pedicles and neural arch is rare.[13]

In general there is less sclerosis in tuberculosis than in other types of osteomyelitis, but frequently it is impossible to differentiate tuberculosis of the spine from pyogenic infections or fungal infections. A large abscess (Fig. 5A), especially if calcified (Fig. 5B), is very suggestive of tuberculosis, but these are late findings.[14] Tuberculous involvement of a solitary vertebral body has mimicked the vertebra plana of histiocytosis X, neoplasm, and Schmorl node defects.[14] Some reports indicate more florid and atypical findings in non-caucasians with spinal tuberculosis.[1,15]

Articular lesions are second in frequency to spine lesions (Figs. 6, 7). Most patients have monarticular disease with long standing symptoms. Classic roentgenographic findings include osteoporosis, marginal erosions in non-weight bearing areas, and late joint space narrowing. There may be synovial thickening and effusion. Often patients are thought to have some type of arthritis.[16]

Synovial tuberculosis in children causes hyperemia, resulting in epiphyseal overgrowth in the knee. Hyperemia caused by juvenile rheumatoid arthritis and hemophilia is associated with identical changes.

**Fig. 4A:** Lateral view of the thoracic spine shows destruction of the margins of adjacent vertebrae, more marked anteriorly, and disc space narrowing.

**Fig. 4B:** Lateral view of the lumbar spine shows marked destruction and sclerosis of L2, destruction of L1, disc narrowing, and early gibbus formation.

Figure 4A

Figure 4B

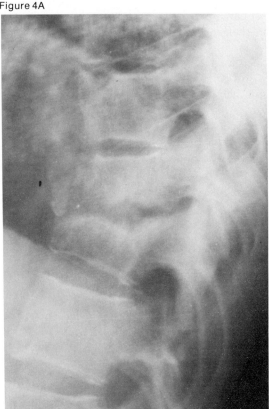

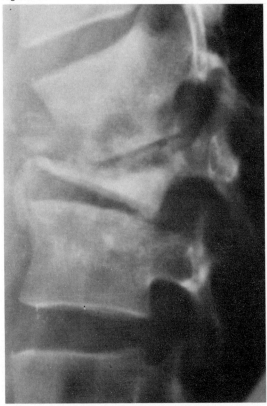

In the hip, roentgenographic findings usually are similar to those found in pyogenic infections, but joint space narrowing is delayed because of absence of proteolytic enzymes.

The sacroiliac joints may be widened because of bone destruction, and accompanying bone sclerosis is more common than in other joints. If both sacroiliac joints happen to be involved, findings usually are asymmetric.

Tuberculous osteomyelitis usually is metaphyseal because of the configuration of the metaphyseal blood vessels (Fig. 8). Striking roentgenographic findings may be evident in the long bones of the hands. Tuberculous dactylitis is more frequent in children, but does occur in adults.[17] Spina ventosa (Figs. 9A, 9B), a form of tuberculous dactylitis, refers to a phalanx, metacarpal, metatarsal, or other long bone with an expanded appearance. This appearance is not specific for tuberculosis, however, and is found in children with sickle cell anemia, granulomatous disease of childhood, and congenital syphilis. Fibrous dysplasia and enchondroma may resemble tuberculous dactylitis, but they do not cause the soft tissue swelling or periostitis found in tuberculosis. Furthermore, discrete cartilage calcifications often are present in enchondromas, while patients with fibrous dysplasia may have cafe-au-lait spots.

### References

1. Chapman M, Murray RO, Stoker DJ: Tuberculosis of the bones and joints. *Semin Roentgenol* 1979; 14:266.

**Fig. 5A:** AP view of the thoracic spine shows narrowing of the T10-11 disc interspace and a large tuberculous paraspinal "cold" abscess (arrows).

**Fig. 5B:** AP view of the lumbar spine shows destruction of L2 and calcifications (arrows) in a soft tissue abscess.

Figure 5A

Figure 5B

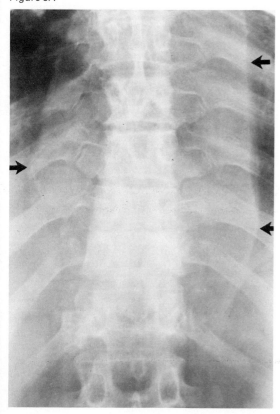

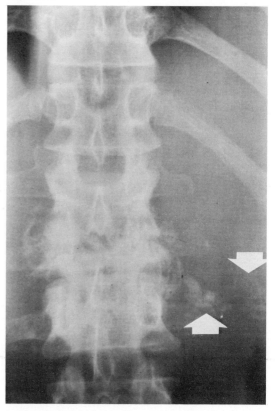

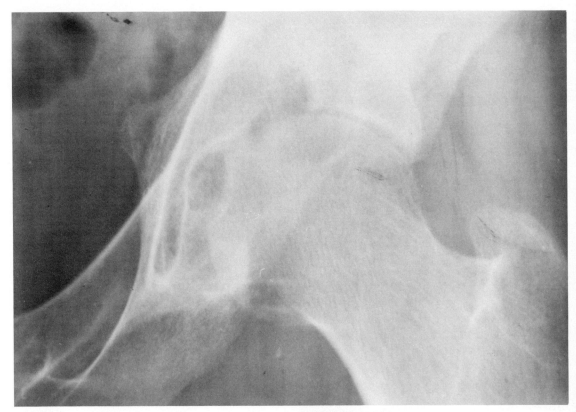

Figure 6

**Fig. 6:** AP view of the hip shows joint space narrowing and well-defined destructive lesions of the femoral head and acetabular rim.

**Fig. 7:** AP view of a hip shows more advanced destruction of the femoral head.

Figure 7

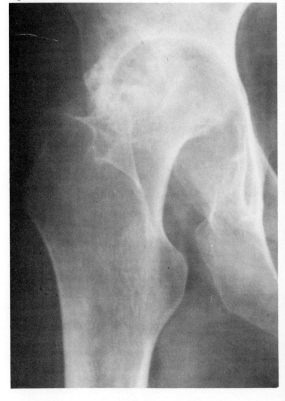

Bone Radiology Case Studies

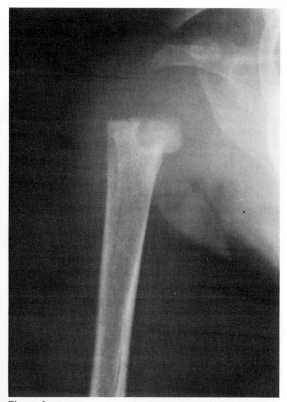

Figure 8

**Fig. 8:** AP view of the shoulder in a child shows metaphyseal destruction with joint space involvement, causing lateral subluxation of the humerus. The metaphyseal site is a common location for early tuberculous bone infection.

**Fig. 9A:** AP view of the hand of a young child with the spina ventosa type of tuberculous dactylitis that is "expanding" a proximal phalanx. Note the soft tissue swelling.

**Fig. 9B:** AP view of the opposite hand shows slight expansion and minimal periosteal reaction of the second metacarpal.

Figure 9A

Figure 9B

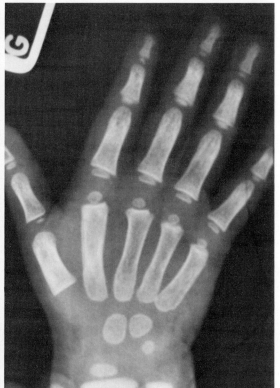

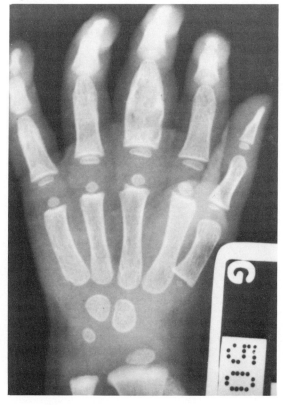

2. McTammany JR, Moser KM, Houk VN: Disseminated bone tuberculosis: Review of the literature and presentation of an unusual case. *Am Rev Resp Dis* 1963; 87:889.

3. O'Conner BT, Oswestry WM, Sanders R: Disseminated bone tuberculosis. *J Bone Joint Surg* 1970; 52:537.

4. Farer LS, Lowell AM, Meador MP: Extrapulmonary tuberculosis in the United States. *Am J Epidemiology* 1979; 109:205.

5. Paus B: The changed pattern of bone and joint tuberculosis in Norway. *Acta Orthop Scand* 1977; 48:277.

6. Paus B: Tumour, tuberculosis and osteomyelitis of the spine. *Acta Orthop Scand* 1973; 44:372.

7. Poppel MH, Lawrence LR, Jacobson HG, et al: Skeletal tuberculosis. *Am J Roentgenol* 1953; 70:936.

8. LaFond EM: An analysis of adult skeletal tuberculosis. *J Bone Joint Surg* 1958; 40A:346.

9. Shaw NM, Basu AK: Unusual cold abscesses. *Brit J Surg* 1970; 57:418.

10. Wolfgang GL: Tuberculous joint infection. *Clin Orthop* 1978; 136:257.

11. Davidson PT, Horowitz I: Skeletal tuberculosis. *Am J Medicine* 1970; 48:77.

12. Bayour A: The spectrum of extrapulmonary tuberculosis. *Western J Med* 1977; 126:253.

13. Bell D, Cockshott WP: Tuberculosis of the vertebral pedicles. *Radiology* 1971; 99:63.

14. Goldman AB, Freiberger RH: Localized infectious and neuropathic diseases. *Sem in Roentgenol* 1979; 14:19.

15. Allen EH, Cosgrove D, Millard F: The radiological changes in infections of the spine and their diagnostic value. 1978; *Clin Radiol* 1978; 29:31.

16. Pritchard DJ: Granulomatous infections of bones and joints. *Orthop Clin N Am* 1975; 6:1029.

17. Feldman F, Auerbach R, Johnston A: Tuberculous dactylitis in the adult. *Am J Roentgenol* 1971; 112:460.

# Study 13

This 41-year-old woman has low back pain. She has no significant medical history and has no other symptoms. *Your diagnosis?*

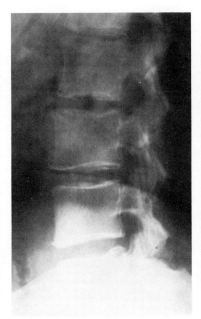

**Fig. 1:** Lateral view of the lumbar spine.

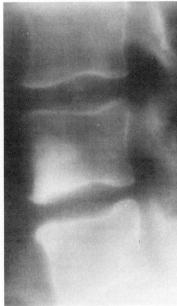

**Fig. 2:** Lateral tomogram of the lumbar spine.

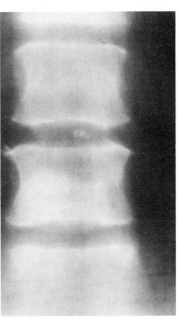

**Fig. 3:** Frontal tomogram of the lumbar spine.

# Diagnosis: Benign Vertebral Sclerosis

The patient whose case is presented (Figs. 1-3) has circumscribed sclerosis of the anterior inferior portion of L4, which is eccentric and extends to the intact anterior and inferior margins of the vertebra. (This type of sclerosis in this location, L4, is characteristic of benign vertebral sclerosis.) The disc space is intact. There is a small osteophyte of L4 and calcification of the L3-4 nucleus pulposus. The patient, a healthy young woman, was considered to have benign vertebral sclerosis. She has remained well and her symptoms have diminished; the sclerotic vertebra has not changed in one year.

Benign vertebral sclerosis is a non-neoplastic, noninfectious segmental sclerosis involving one vertebra or opposing segments of two vertebrae. Almost all cases have involved the lumbosacral spine. The disc space is often abnormal, but the disc may be normal roentgenographically. Only adults are affected, and there is a predilection for women over age 40.[1] Patients with intact disc spaces may be asymptomatic,[2] while those with disc space abnormalities often have mild back pain.[1] In 1957 there was a report of non-neoplastic segmental sclerosis in five patients.[3] Four of the patients had carcinomas and all five were suspected of having osteoblastic metastasis to the spine. Biopsies showed broad trabeculae, mature bone, and no neoplastic cells. One patient came to autopsy and the discs adjacent to the sclerotic vertebra were normal. The sclerosis in these five patients was considered to be of unknown etiology. Another report in 1968[4] discussed nine patients with varying degrees of vertebral sclerosis plus lucency who had resolution of symptoms without antibiotic therapy. Those who underwent biopsy had no tumors and no growth on culture. It was hypothesized, however, that they had a very low grade infection. A third report, in 1976,[1] detailed 22 patients with sclerosis, lucent lesions, or a combination of sclerosis and lucent lesions, none of whom had infection or neoplasm. Vertebral sclerosis alone was present in 11 patients. The L4 vertebral body was involved in 9 of 11 of these patients, and 10 of 11 had disc space narrowing. Thickening of the anterior cortex by periosteal bone formation was present in 8 of 11. Most had no history of a traumatic event, but it was hypothesized that repetitive discovertebral trauma caused their roentgenographic abnormalities.

A common feature in all of these reports was that many patients were suspected of having either metastatic disease or infection, based on the roentgenographic appearance of the spine. Patients with sclerosis, with or without lucent lesions, plus disc space narrowing were felt to have infection, while patients with intact disc spaces were felt to have metastasis.

Benign vertebral sclerosis had been divided into a discogenic type and a nondiscogenic type.[2,3] In the nondiscogenic type the disc space is intact and the patient is usually asymptomatic. The discogenic type of benign sclerosis is associated with disc space narrowing, has a predilection for women over age 40, is associated with symptoms, and is probably the result of repetitive disco-vertebral trauma.[1,5]

The findings in both types are confined to one or two vertebrae and the disc space between them. The sclerotic area is well defined. homogenous, and usually extends to the anterior and inferior margins of the body. The disc space, in addition to being narrowed, may contain gas, and disc material may herniate into the vertebral body, causing lucent defects. Osteophytes may develop. Sclerosis may be present in the superior portion of the adjacent vertebra.[1-4] There is no associated paravertebral mass, and the height of the vertebra is maintained (Fig. 5).

The vertebral body most often affected by discogenic sclerosis is L4, probably because L4-5 is subject to high degrees of rotational stress. All of the findings in the discogenic type of benign vertebral sclerosis can be explained by repeated trauma that affects the junction between the intervertebral disc, anterior longitudinal

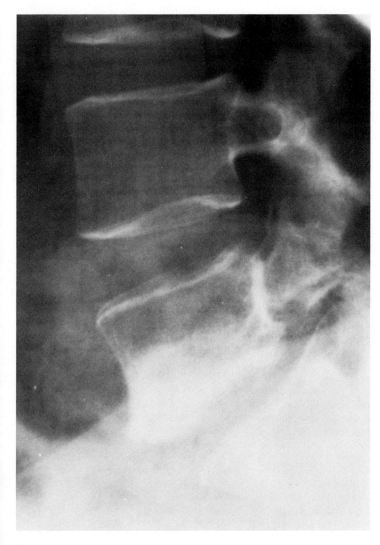

**Fig. 4:** Another patient with vertebral sclerosis of the anterior inferior portion of L5 plus minimal spondylolisthesis.

**Fig. 5A:** The L3-4 disc interspace is narrowed, and there is sclerosis of the adjacent vertebral bodies with lucent areas representing herniated disc material (arrows).

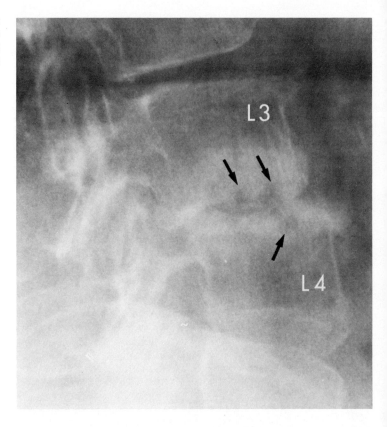

ligament, and vertebral body.

The outer fibers of the annulus fibrosis extend into the vertebral rim in the form of Sharpey's fibers. Repeated trauma causes separation of these fibers from the rim, and the tight connection between the vertebral body and disc is loosened. This permits abnormal motion and allows the intact nucleus pulposus to bulge the annulus fibrosis anteriorly and laterally. The anterior longitudinal ligament, which is attached to the vertebral body just above the vertebral rim, is then stretched by the bulging disc. Repeated trauma and stress to these altered anterior structures result in reactive sclerosis of the vertebral body. Later, small fractures of the end plate allow herniation of disc material into the vertebral body. Disc alterations result in disc space narrowing.

Sclerosis involving one vertebra or two adjacent vertebrae can be due to a number of etiologies, including:

metastasis
lymphoma
primary neoplasm
infection
Paget's disease
Charcot spine[6]
sarcoid[7]
ankylosing spondylitis[8]
rheumatoid arthritis[8]
compact bone island[5,9]

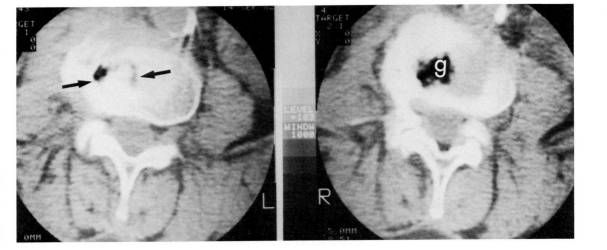

post disc surgery[10]
benign vertebral sclerosis
-with disc abnormality
-without disc abnormality.

**Fig. 5B:** CT. Gas (g) in the disc. Disc material protrudes into the vertebral body (arrows). There is also a right anterolateral osteophyte.

In a patient with segmental anterior sclerosis of a lumbar vertebra, especially when accompanied by adjacent disc space abnormality, benign vertebral sclerosis is a prime consideration. Radionuclide bone scans may be positive due to osteoblastic activity, but a case has been reported in which a bone scan was normal, thus, virtually eliminating the possibility of neoplasm or infection.[11]

### References

1. Martel W, Seeger JF, Wicks JD, et al: Traumatic lesions of the discovertebral junction in the lumbar spine. *Am J Radiol* 1976; 127:457.
2. Feldman FR: Miscellaneous localized conditions of the spine. *Semin Roentgenol* 1979; 14:58.
3. Ackermann W, Schwarz GS: Non-neoplastic sclerosis in vertebral bodies. *Cancer* 1958; 11:703.
4. Williams JL, Moller GA, O'Rourke TL: Pseudoinfections of the intervertebral disc and adjacent vertebrae? *Am J Radiol* 1968; 103:611.
5. Schmorl G, Junghanns H: *The Human Spine in Health and Disease.* New York, Grune and Stratton, 1971.
6. Feldman F, Johnson AM, Walter SF: Acute Axial Neuroarthropathy. *Radiology* 1974; 111:1.
7. Baldwin DM, Roberts SG, Croft HE: Vertebral sarcoidosis. *J Bone Joint Surg* 1974; 56:629.
8. Seaman WB, Wells SJ: Destructive lesions of the vertebral bodies in rheumatoid disease. *Am J Radiol* 1961; 86:241.
9. Epstein BD: *The Spine. A Radiologic Text-Book and Atlas.* Philadelphia, Lea & Febiger, 1976.
10. Lowman RM, Robinson F: Progressive vertebral interspace changes following lumbar disc surgery. *Am J Radiol* 1966; 97:664.
11. Sauser DD, Goldman AE, Kaye JJ: Discogenic vertebral sclerosis. *J Can Assoc Radiol* 1978; 29:44.

# Study 14

The first patient (Fig. 1) has bilateral polyarthralgia. The second patient (Fig. 2) also has bilateral polyarthralgia. They both have the same disease. *Your diagnosis?*

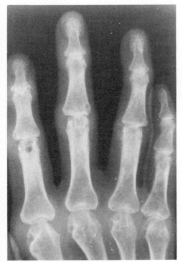 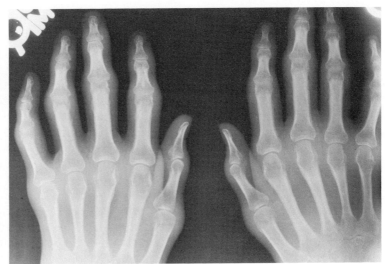

**Fig. 1:** AP view of right hand (Patient One).

**Fig. 2:** AP view of hands (Patient Two).

# Diagnosis: Rheumatoid Arthritis

The hands of the second patient (Fig. 2) demonstrate bilateral symmetric swelling and juxta-articular osteoporosis characteristic of the early radiographic findings in rheumatoid arthritis. The first patient (Fig. 1) has more advanced changes with minimal soft tissue swelling and juxta-articular osteoporosis. There is uniform narrowing of all metacarpophalangeal and proximal interphalangeal joints shown. There are numerous erosions. The distal interphalangeal joints are spared.

Rheumatoid arthritis (RA) is a chronic systemic disease of uncertain etiology characterized by a symmetric inflammatory polyarthritis. There is particular involvement of the small joints of the extremities. The large joints of the extremities and the spine are affected less frequently and generally less severely. Systemic involvement includes blood vessels, lung, muscle, heart, skin and the eyes.

## Etiology

There is much evidence to suggest that the pathogenesis of RA is an immunologic abnormality involving both humoral and cell-mediated responses. Evidence to support this includes:

1. It has been known for some time that the serum and synovial fluid in the majority of patients with RA contain anti-IgG antibodies (rheumatoid factor) and that some patients have anti-nuclear antibodies. (Rheumatoid factor consists of IgM, IgG and IgA antibodies but only IgM is measured in routine laboratory testing.)[1] It should be noted that serum rheumatoid factor is not specific for RA but can be present in many other chronic diseases including tuberculosis, subacute bacterial endocarditis, and systemic lupus erythematosis; also, patients with these diseases and positive serology for rheumatoid factor do not manifest a chronic arthritis as seen with RA.[1,2]

2. Decreased levels of complement components have been found in the synovial fluid in a large number of patients with RA.[3]

3. Deposits of immune complexes have been demonstrated within phagocytic synovial cells and the synovial membrane of patients with RA.[4]

4. B cell and T lymphocytes are both present in the synovium of patients with RA and cells capable of antibody dependent cell-mediated cytotoxic reactions are also present.[5]

5. T cell products such as migration-inhibiting factor have been demonstrated in the synovium of patients with RA. There is also evidence to support the contention that susceptibility to the immunologic abnormality resulting in RA is genetically related and determined by gene products of the patient's major histocompatibility system.[6]

It is thus suggested that RA is an abnormality of immune response to an unidentified antigen in a genetically susceptible patient. The immunopathogenesis of RA may be as follows: an unidentified antigen, possibly a virus, combines with the patient's IgG and initiates anti-IgG antibodies. These antibodies combine with the patient's IgG to form immune complexes which activate the complement system and stimulate chemotactic migration of leukocytes. The leukocytes phagocytize the immune complexes and release lysosomal enzymes which cause articular injury. Superimposed on this process is damage due to cell-mediated immune reactions. Systemically there is a malfunction of the inflammatory and surveillance function of cellular immune responses which is responsible for the patient's vasculitis.[6]

## Pathology

The pathologic changes in RA are characterized by a diffuse proliferative synovitis. Hypertrophy of the synovium which becomes highly vascular and contains many lymphocytes is

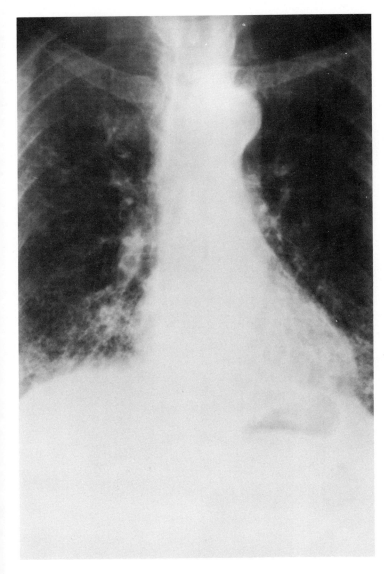

**Fig. 3:** There is diffuse interstitial lung disease indicating rheumatoid lung. The patient had rheumatoid nodules of the skin which are common in patients with lung involvement.

referred to as pannus formation. This pannus extends over the articular cartilage and destroys it along with the subchondral bone. The earliest involvement of bone is at the joint margins where bone is still within the synovial capsule but not protected by overlying articular cartilage. Mechanical trauma of joint use erodes the pannus, causing bleeding and subsequent formation of granulation tissue. In long standing severe cases the entire joint space is destroyed and replaced by bony ankylosis. Before bony ankylosis occurs joint instability and subluxation are common. They are due to structural weakness of the joint capsule and surrounding ligaments caused by chronic inflammation and imbalance of opposing muscle groups.

Another characteristic finding in RA is the rheumatoid nodule located in subcutaneous tissue commonly at pressure points along bones. These nodules may also be found in lung parenchyma, pleura and myocardium. They consist of an area of central necrosis surrounded by a pallisade of monocytic cells. The nodules are probably the result of small vessel vasculitis.

Necrotizing vasculitis involving the large or small arteries may result in pathologic changes ranging from asymptomatic perivascular accumulations of lymphocytes to thrombus which result in vascular insufficiency or infarction.[7]

The lungs may contain rheumatoid nodules, as already

**Figs. 4A, 4B:** Bilateral symmetric changes characteristic of rheumatoid arthritis. Osteoporosis and distribution of lesions in wrist, metacarpophalangeal joints, and proximal interphalangeal joints with sparing of the distal joints is typical. Also note ulnar deviation of right fingers.

Figure 4A

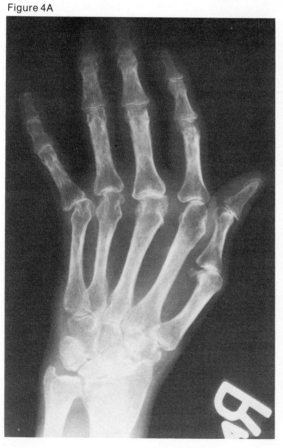

Figure 4B

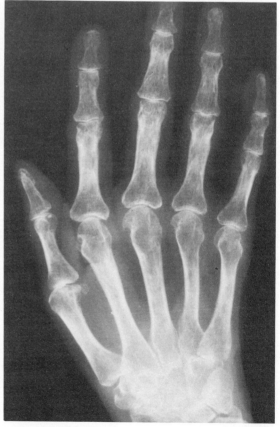

Bone Radiology Case Studies

mentioned, but more commonly there is diffuse interstitial fibrosis (Fig. 3). Nonspecific pleuritis and myocarditis may develop. The pleural fluid is characterized by low glucose, elevated lactic dehydrogenase, and decreased complement. Valvular heart disease indistinguishable from that of rheumatic fever may occur. Occular manifestations include uveitis and keratoconjunctivitis sica (Sjogren's syndrome).

## Clinical

The American Rheumatism Association has compiled diagnostic criteria for RA.[8] When three or four findings are present the diagnosis is probable, with five or more findings present the diagnosis is more definite.

**American Rheumatism Association**
**Diagnostic Criteria for**
**Rheumatoid Arthritis**
- Morning stiffness
- Joint tenderness or pain on motion
- Soft tissue swelling of at least one joint
- Soft tissue swelling of a second joint within three months
- Soft tissue swelling of symmetric joints
- Subcutaneous nodules

**Fig. 5:** Radiocarpal and widespread intercarpal joint space narrowing with multiple erosions including a tiny erosion of the tip of the ulnar styloid which is often an early finding in rheumatoid arthritis.

**Fig. 6:** Focal cortical loss (arrow) indicating early erosion on radial side of a distal metacarpal.

Figure 5

Figure 6

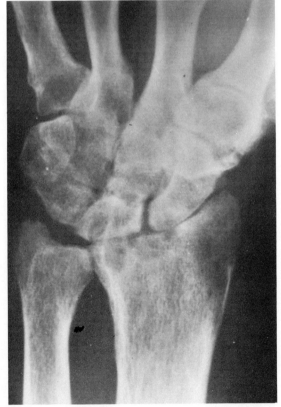

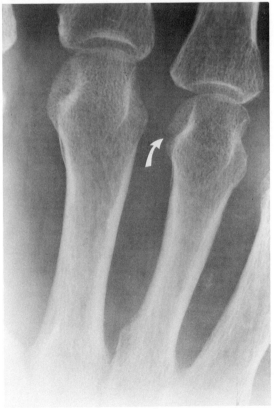

- Radiographic changes
- Rheumatoid factor detected
- Poor mucin precipitate from synovial fluid
- Histologic changes of rheumatoid arthritis in synovial membrane
- Histologic changes of rheumatoid arthritis in subcutaneous nodules

RA usually presents with joint stiffness which is characteristically worse upon awakening. Joint stiffness may be preceded by a period of fatigue, weakness and vague arthralgias. The hands and feet are usually affected first. The polyarthralgia is most often bilateral and symmetric. Early in the disease, however, arthralgia may be monarticular or assymetric.[9]

The involved joints are enlarged and tender with slight erythema. Adjacent muscle atrophy accentuates the fusiform appearance. Later when the inflammatory process involves the synovial lining of tendon sheaths, volar subluxation with ulnar deviation may occur. Bony ankylosis and irreversible subluxations and flexion contractures occur in severe disease. The clinical course is unpredictable with remissions and exacerbations. Relentless progression is present in only a small percent of patients.

Although most common in the hands, wrists, and feet, RA may affect any synovial joint. The ankles, knees, hips, elbows, and shoulders are involved in a smaller number of patients. When the

**Fig. 7:** Advanced rheumatoid arthritis with severe carpal involvement, subluxations, and "pencil in cup" appearance of the interphalangeal joint of the thumb (arrow).

**Fig. 8:** Rheumatoid arthritis with "swan-neck" deformities. Such deformity which is not fixed is seen in systemic lupus erythematosis. Erosions and joint space narrowing seen here are seldom seen in SLE.

Figure 7

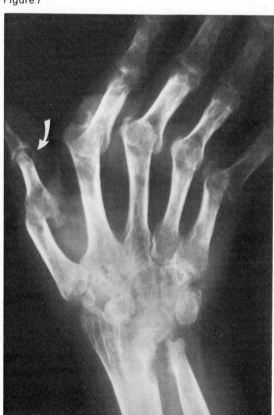

Figure 8

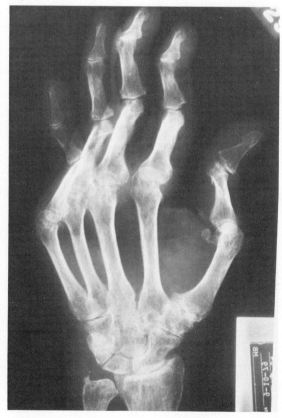

spine is involved the cervical region is most commonly affected with the possibility of serious subluxations compressing the spinal cord. Sacroilitis may occasionally occur but is of little clinical significance. Also unusually affected but of more serious importance is arthritis of the cricoarytenoid joints which may lead to upper airway obstruction.[10]

Giant cysts may develop in the popliteal region of the knee and less often in the shoulder when synovial fluid is forced into bursae. When these cysts extend into the calf they may mimic thrombophlebitis clinically. Ultrasound will demonstrate the cystic nature of the lesion causing enlargement of the calf and arthrography will confirm the diagnosis.

Rheumatoid nodules are commonly found on the extensor surface of the elbow. They are firm, nontender, and may be freely moveable.

Systemic findings are often related to arthritis. Chronic ulcers of the lower extremeties due to vascular insufficiency and digital infarcts have been described. Thrombosis of large vessels has resulted in myocardial, cerebral, and mesenteric infarcts.

## Radiology

Radiographs provide important diagnostic information in patients when the diagnosis of RA is in doubt. When the diagnosis of RA is already established, some rheumatologists would not

**Fig. 9:** Multiple distal metatarsal erosions most severe in metatarsals 4 and 5.

**Fig. 10:** Osteoporosis and severe uniform narrowing of the tibiotalar joint typical of rheumatoid arthritis.

Figure 9

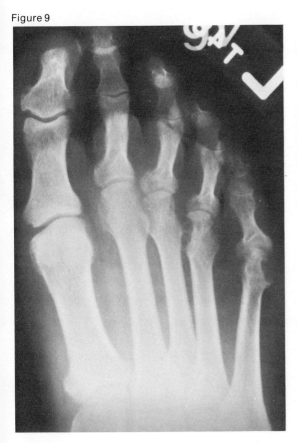

Figure 10

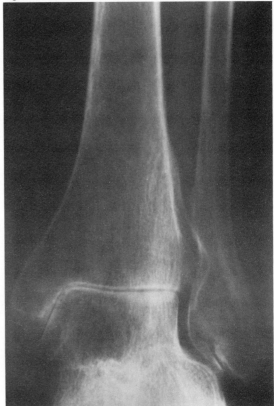

obtain radiographs; others would use them as an objective baseline study.[67] Gallium citrate provides a sensitive means of documenting synovitis but is seldom used.

A semi-quantitative assessment of the severity of RA by the method of Larsen demonstrates a correlation between years of disease and grade of roentgenographic findings.[11] A significant correlation has also been shown between clinical activity, assessed at four month intervals, and progressive radiographic findings.[12] There are some reports that the dominant hand is more severely affected in RA in accordance with the concept that the mechanical forces of stress are a contributing factor to joint injury.[13] This concept is further substantiated in patients with hemiplegia. They may have unilateral changes of RA on the side with normal movement and sparing of the paralyzed side.

The earliest roentgenographic finding in RA is fusiform soft tissue swelling around joints corresponding to the initial synovitis and effusion. These soft tissue changes in turn call attention to joints which require close inspection for early manifestations of RA. Hyperemia due to the pannus results in juxta-articular osteoporosis (Fig. 2). Later the pannus erodes the articulating cartilage and intracapsular bone producing uniform joint space narrowing, and marginal "bare area" osseous erosions. Erosions are usually not seen until symptoms have been present for several months. Intraosseous cysts may develop, rarely before the cartilage is

**Fig. 11:** Typical uniform narrowing of the knee joint in rheumatoid arthritis. Lack of sclerosis and osteophytes also distinguish this joint involvement from osteoarthritis.

**Fig. 12:** Large intraosseous cyst (arrows) in a patient with rheumatoid arthritis with no joint space narrowing.

Figure 11

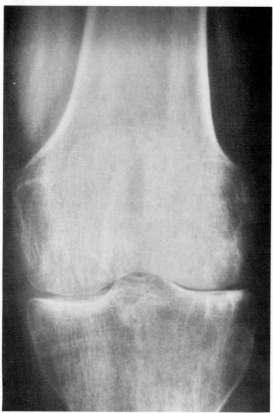

Figure 12

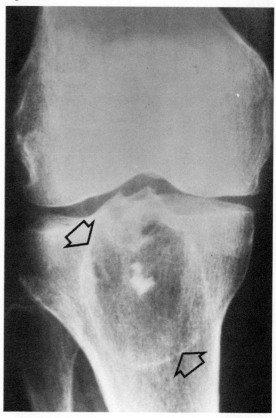

Bone Radiology Case Studies

destroyed. As the inflammatory process affects the joint capsule and ligaments, subluxations occur which are manifested roentgenographically. In long standing disease severe destructive changes may occur producing a "cup and pencil" appearance although in many cases the appearance is one of non-specific end stage joint disease. Although it is not unusual for a pathologic specimen to demonstrate intra-articular cartilagenous and bony fragments, loose bodies are rarely demonstrated roentgenographically.[14] Periosteal new bone is uncommonly present in RA and when it does occur, it is slight and usually subtle (Fig. 2).

## Hand and Wrist

The hand and wrist are commonly affected early in RA. Soft tissue swelling, osteoporosis, erosions, and joint space narrowing are usually bilateral and symmetric in contrast to sero-negative polyarthridities which are often asymmetric and involve only a few joints (Fig. 4). The joints of the wrist are most frequently involved followed by the metacarpophalangeal joints and proximal interphalangeal joints. The metacarpophalangeal joints of the ring and middle finger are typically affected earliest and most frequently.[15] The distal interphalangeal joints are minimally involved in contradistinction to osteoarthritis and psoriatic arthritis. In the wrist the ulnar styloid often is the earliest site of involvement. The distal portions of the radius and ulna, the

**Fig. 13:** Typical axial (along axis of femoral neck) migration of femoral head in rheumatoid arthritis. Note absence of osteophytes or sclerosis.

**Fig. 14:** Slight acetabular protrusion. Note axial migration of the femoral head with superior and medial aspect of the joint space still present.

Figure 13

Figure 14

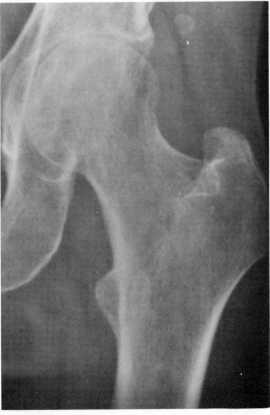

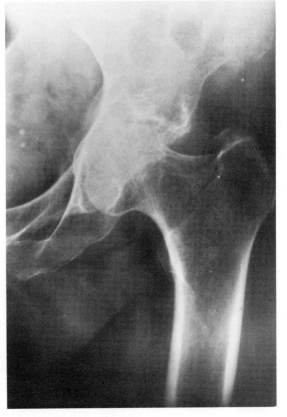

**Fig. 15:** Rheumatoid arthritis in the elbow joint commonly causes effusion which displaces the intracapsular fat pads (arrows). Note cystic lesion of the ulna.

**Fig. 16:** Erosion of the lateral aspect of the head of the humerus which is displaced slightly superiorly.

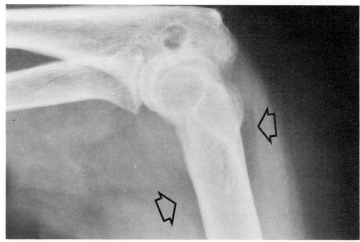

Figure 15

Figure 16

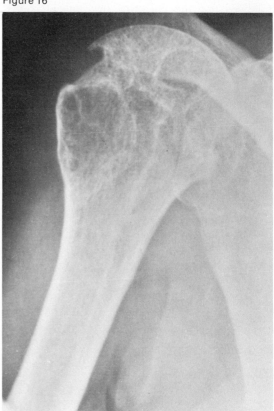

triquetrum, pisiform, and midsection of the radial aspect of the scaphoid are also commonly involved early (Fig. 5).[16] Initially there is only soft tissue swelling at affected joints. In the case of the ulnar styloid, swelling is due to synovitis of the extensor carpi ulnaris tendon. The marginal osseous erosions which occur at sites covered by synovium but not protected by cartilage typically are first seen at the radial aspect of the metacarpal heads. The earliest change is

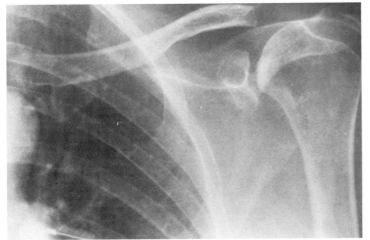

**Fig. 17:** Severe erosion of the distal and proximal clavicle and the head of the humerus plus osteoporosis. The head of the humerus has migrated superiorly due to involvement of the rotator cuff.

**Fig. 18:** Abnormal distance between anterior cortex of the odontoid and posterior cortex of the arch of the atlas (arrows) indicating subluxation.

Figure 17

Figure 18

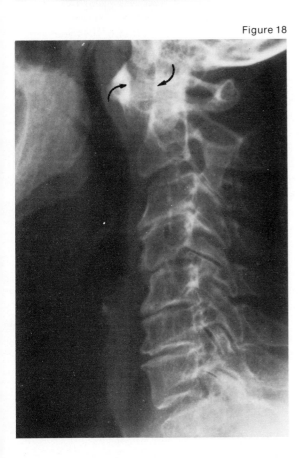

conversion of the dense cortical rim of the subarticular cortex to a dot-dash appearance. Later there is focal absence of cortex (Fig. 6) and then an actual bony defect. As the pannus proliferates destruction becomes more severe with narrowing (penciling) of the distal metacarpal or proximal phalanx. The proximal articulation of the corresponding phalanx widens and deepens (cupping) (Fig. 7). The end stage is non-specific mutilating arthritis. The carpal bones sharing a common synovium (except for the triquetrum) may be universally and severely involved with a "bag of bones" appearance (Fig. 7).

Subluxations commonly occur as the inflammatory process involves the joint capsule and adjacent ligaments and tendons. Synovitis at the proximal interphalangeal joint allows lateral slippage of the extensor tendons resulting in flexion deformities of the proximal interphalangeal joints producing a "boutonniere deformity."

Synovitis at the metacarpophalangeal joint prevents the normal slide of flexor tendons. Attempts at flexion pull the phalanx off the metacarpal and change the direction of pull distally resulting in flexion of the distal interphalangeal joint and hyperextension of the proximal interphalangeal joint producing a "swan-neck" deformity (Fig. 8).[17] Synovitis involving the radio-carpal ligaments allows instability of the scaphoid which becomes volar-flexed. The subsequent shortening of the radial carpal height leads to supination of the carpus with radial deviation of the metacarpals and ulnar deviation of the fingers (Figs. 4A, 7).[18]

## Foot

The earliest sign of RA in the foot is soft tissue swelling of the first and fifth toes due to bursal swelling. Erosions of the lateral aspects of the heads of the fifth metatarsals and uniform joint space narrowing of all the metatarsophalangeal joints are other early findings (Fig. 9). Erosions of the metatarsal heads, with the exception of the fifth, typically first appear medially. Proximal interphalangeal joint space narrowing and later erosive changes are especially prominent in the great toe. As in the hand the distal interphalangeal joints are relatively spared. All of the articulations of the mid foot may be involved.

With progression of the disease, joint destruction and resorption of bone may produce the pencil-in-cup appearance as seen in the hands. Bony ankylosis is uncommon and more frequently affects the tarsal bones than the phalanges. Subluxations may occur including hallux valgus deformity and fibular deviation of the second, third, and fourth toes. Flexion contractures at the proximal interphalangeal joints produce "hammer toe" deformities.

## Ankle

Marked involvement of the ankle in RA is infrequently demonstrated roentgenographically. Symmetric narrowing of the talotarsal joint (Fig. 10) may be accompanied by bony erosions. Plantar calcaneal spurs and posterior calcaneal erosions due to retrocalcaneal bursal involvement are not uncommon. Similar erosions occur in seronegative polyarthritidies and lipoid-dermatoarthritis.

## Knee

In the knee a large effusion caused by synovitis may greatly distend the intercommunicating bursa (Baker's cyst). The disten-

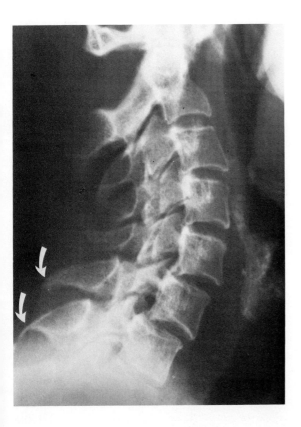

**Fig. 19:** Pointed spinous processes of C6 and 7 are very suggestive of rheumatoid arthritis (arrows). Note minimal subluxation at C6-7 and abnormal C7-T1 apophyseal joint.

sibility of the bursa delays articular erosion. Knee joint narrowing is symmetric with absence of marginal osteophytes which typify osteoarthritis (Fig. 11). Patellofemoral joint space narrowing may be present also. Marginal osseous erosions are found in the tibia and fibula. Large intraosseous cysts may occur (Fig. 12).

## Hip

Hip disease occurs relatively late in rheumatoid arthritis in less than one-third of patients and mostly in those over 50 years of age.[19] Bilaterally symmetric involvement is common. Osteoporosis is frequent. Radiographically the joint effusion may be difficult to detect. There is symmetric articular cartilage destruction producing axial migration of the femoral head (Fig. 13). This is in contrast to superior or medial migration commonly found in osteoarthritis. Relatively early involvement of the acetabulum with collapse and protrusio acetabuli has raised the possibility that synovial invasion causes this deformity (Fig. 14). Marginal osseous erosions commonly involve the femoral head, and subchrondral cysts, sometimes large, may be present. As many as 40 percent of patients with roentgenographic evidence of RA have signs of avascular necrosis; however, these patients have often received steroid treatment and the exact association is unclear.[19]

## Elbow

Joint effusions of the elbow are demonstrated by displacement of

**Fig. 20:** Sacroiliac joint involvement in rheumatoid arthritis. Bilateral poorly defined and irregular cortical margins and unilateral sclerosis.

**Fig. 21:** View of the temporomandibular joint. The joint fossa (open arrows) is enlarged and the condyloid process articular surface (closed arrows) truncated and deformed.

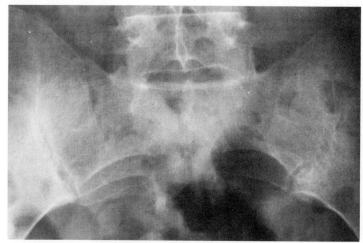

Figure 20

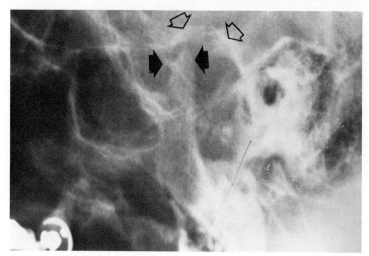

Figure 21

the fat pads, posteriorly from the olecrenon fossa or anteriorly from the radial and coronoid fossae (Fig. 15). This finding is found with any process which causes distention of the elbow joint. Juxta-articular osteoporosis and uniform joint space narrowing also occur early in the disease. Marginal osseous erosions including characteristic erosion of the supinator groove of the ulna are found.[20] Subchondral cysts which are large and disproportionate to the degree of joint space narrowing may simulate gout. Subcutaneous nodules may be fixed and can rarely cause pressure erosions of adjacent bone.

## Shoulder

The soft tissue mass of a distended subdeltoid bursa is an early sign of RA. As is typical of other joints subarticular osteoporosis, uniform joint space narrowing, subchondral cysts and marginal erosions are characteristic findings Erosions of the humeral head and glenoid fossa predominate (Fig. 16). Resorption of the distal clavicles is common (Fig. 17). Erosion of the sternal end of the clavicle is difficult to see because of overlapping anatomy. Weakening of the joint capsule and rotator cuff due to chronic synovitis may result in superior subluxation of the humeral head indicated roentgenographically by increased separation of the inferior lip of the glenoid fossa and the inferior portion of the humeral head (Fig. 17).

## Spine

The cervical spine is most often involved. The atlantoaxial, discovertebral, and the apophyseal joints may all be involved.[21] There is a synovial-lined bursa separating the odontoid from the atlas and transverse ligament. When chronically inflamed, the bursa may erode the odontoid and increase the likelihood of fracture. Subluxation of the odontoid due to ligamentous laxity may be superior into the foramen magnum or more commonly posterior in relation to the atlas. These subluxations may result in compression of the spinal cord. In the adult a separation between the odontoid and the anterior arch of the atlas greater than three mm is generally accepted as abnormal (Fig. 18). A flexion view should be obtained to demonstrate atlantoaxial subluxation which is not always demonstrated in a neutral position. Subluxations below the antlantoaxial articulation may be isolated to one level (Fig. 19) or occur in combination at several levels. It is not uncommon for subluxations to occur at one site, typically the mid cervical region, while levels above and below it are ankylosed. Again flexion and extension views give helpful information. The vertebral end plates may be eroded along with intervertebral disc space narrowing.[21] There may be reactive end plate sclerosis. Erosion of the apophyseal joints results in irregularity of articular surfaces. Erosions of the lower cervical spinous processes result in a "sharpened pencil" appearance (Fig. 19). The upper cervical spinous processes may become compressed together due to disc space narrowing and chronic pressure effect.

Although abnormalities of the sacroiliac joints have been described,[22] sacroiliitis is rarely of clinical significance. Asymmetric erosions, joint space narrowing and juxta-articular sclerosis are seen in these patients (Fig. 20).

The erosive osteitis pubis of akylosing spondylitis is uncommonly seen in RA. Juxta-articular sclerosis, erosions, and subluxations have been described.[23]

RA may involve the temporo-mandibular joint with erosions of the mandibular head and widening of the temporo-mandibular fossa resulting in difficulty with mastication (Fig. 21).

—*John McCaffrey, MD*

## References

1. Christian CL, Paget SA: Rheumatoid Arthritis, in Samter M (ed): *Immunological Diseases*. ed 3. Boston, Little Brown & Co, 1978, p 1061.
2. Horwitz LA. Laboratory diagnosis of rheumatoid diseases. *Postgraduate Medicine* 1980; 67(5):193-200.

3. Winchester RJ, et al: Gamma globulin complexes in synovial fluids of patients with rheumatoid arthritis. *Clin Exp Immunol* 1970; 6:689-705.

4. McDuffie FC: Immune complexes in the rheumatic diseases. *J Allergy Clin Immunol* 1978; 62:37.

5. Abrahamson TG, et al: Antibody-dependent cytotoxicity mediated by cells eluted from synovial tissues of patients with rheumatoid arthritis and juvenile rheumatoid arthritis. *Scan J Immunol* 1977; 6:1251-1261.

6. Paget SA, Gibofsky A: Immunopathogenesis of rheumatoid arthritis. *Am J Med* 1979; 67:961-970.

7. Robbins SL: *Pathologic Basis of Disease*. Philadelphia, WB Saunders, 1974, p 1469.

8. Ropes MW: Revision of diagnostic criteria for rheumatoid arthritis. *Bulletin on rheumatic diseases*. Vol 9, No. 4. Arthritis and Rheumatism Foundation, 1958, pp 175-176.

9. Resnick D, Niwayama G: *Diagnosis of Bone and Joint Disorders*. Philadelphia, WB Saunders, 1981, p 909.

10. *Harrison's Principles of Internal Medicine*. ed 8. Thron GW, Adams RD, Braunwald E, Isselbacher KJ, Petersdorf RG, (eds). New York, McGraw Hill, 1977, p 2052.

11. Yano M, Kimura C, Iu K: Re-evaluation of the radiograpical classification of rheumatoid arthritis. *The Ryumachi* 1979; 19(3):188-194.

12. Young A, Corbett M, Brook A: The clinical assessment of joint inflammatory activity in rheumatoid arthritis related to radiological progression. *Rheumatology & Rehabilitation* 1980; 19(1):14-19.

13. Mattingly PC, Matherson JA, Dickson RA: The distribution of radiological joint damage in the rheumatoid hand. *Rheumatology & Rehabilitation* 1979; 18(3):142-147.

14. Moldofsky PJ, Dalinka MA: Multiple loose bodies in RA. *Skeletal Radiol* 1979; 4:219-222.

15. Poznanski AK. *The Hand in Radiographic Diagnosis*. Philadelphia, WB Saunders, 1974, p 519.

16. Resnick D: Radiology for rheumatoid disorders. *Comp Ther* 1979; 5(8):48-54.

17. Forrester DM, Brown JC, Nesson JW: *The Radiology of Joint Disease*, ed 2. Philadelphia, WB Saunders, 1978, pp 42-44.

18. Talesnik J: Rheumatoid synovitis of the volar compartment of the wrist: Its radiological signs and its contribution to wrist and hand deformity. *The J of Hand Surgery* 1979; 4(6):526-535.

19. Bossingham DH, Schorn D, Morgan GW, Mowat AG: Progression of hip disease in rheumatoid arthritis. *Rheumatology & Rehab* 1978; 17(3):170-178.

20. Foster DR, Park WM, McCall IW, et al: The supinator notch sign in RA. *Clinical Radiology* 1980; 31:195-199.

21. Park WM, et al: The radiology of rheumatoid involvement of the cervical spine. *Skeletal Radiol* 1979; 4:1-7.

22. DeCarvallo A, Graudal H: Sacroiliac joint involvement in classical or definite rheumatoid arthritis. *Acta Radiologica Diagnosis* 1980; 21(3):417-422.

23. Scott DL, et al: A comparative radiolgical study of the public symphysis in rheumatic disorders. *Annals of Rheumatic Disease* 1979; 38:529-534.

# Study 15

This three-year-old child has a fever of unknown origin. There is pain and swelling over multiple joints (Fig. 1). *Your diagnosis?*

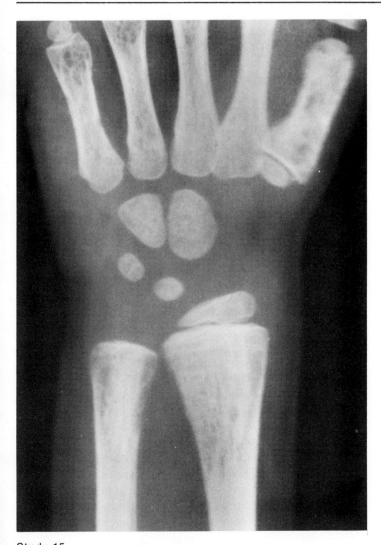

**Fig. 1:** AP view of wrist and metacarpals.

# Diagnosis: Acute Lymphocytic Leukemia

In Figure 1 there are multiple coalescent lytic lesions of the thumb, ring, and little metacarpals. There is subtle destruction of the distal shaft of the radius, and lytic areas of the distal ulna.

## Lymphoreticular Disorders

The lymphoreticular disorders include all neoplastic diseases that involve cells of the lymphocyte line. In this category, acute lymphocytic leukemia, Hodgkin's and non-Hodgkin's lymphoma, and the plasma cell dyscrasias can affect bone.

*Acute lymphocytic leukemia* is primarily a neoplastic disease of childhood involving the abnormal proliferation of lymphocyte precursors (nongranulocytic white blood cells).[1] The clinical presentation is similar to acute myelogenous leukemia (AML) with the exception of more lymphadenopathy and hepatosplenomegaly. Lymphocytic blast cell counts are markedly elevated, while the red cells, granulocytes and platelets are decreased. In recent years dramatic long term remissions have been obtained.

In the literature it is said that bone changes are common (50-70%) in childhood leukemia.[2,3] The studies do not indicate whether the leukemia is lymphocytic or myelogenous. If we assume that most of the childhood cases cited are of the lymphocytic type, then bone changes are common in this disease. Changes include diffuse decreased bone density (Fig. 1), metaphyseal dense or lucent bands (Figs. 2,3), multiple or solitary lytic lesions (Fig. 4) and, less commonly, periostitis and osteosclerosis (Fig. 5). In addition, sutural diastasis secondary to meningeal leukemic cell infiltration can occur. Arthralgias and arthritis can result from leukemic infiltration of the synovium. With thrombocytopenia, hemarthrosis can occur.

Lymphomas, as opposed to leukemias, are solid neoplastic tumors involving lymphoreticular cell lines. These are generally divided into the Hodgkin's and non-Hodgkin's types. A more detailed classification of these is controversial and currently in flux.

*Hodgkin's disease* is a neoplasm distinguished from all other lymphomas by the presence of the Reed-Sternberg cell, without which a diagnosis cannot be made.[4] There is a bimodal age incidence, the first in early adulthood, the second after 50 years of age. Most patients present with painless adenopathy and may have symptoms of fever, chills, night sweats, weight loss and pruritis. Diagnosis is made by node biopsy. Radiographic bone changes are seen in 10 to 25%.[5,6] Sclerotic (Fig. 6), lytic or mixed lesions (Figs. 7, 8) are seen in the vertebra, pelvis, skull, ribs and long bones. An "ivory" vertebra can be seen.

*Non-Hodgkin's lymphoma* includes the lymphocytic, histocytic and undifferentiated types. With the exception of Burkitt's lymphoma, these are diseases of older adults, generally over the ages of 40 to 50 years old. Again they are characterized by painless adenopathy. Bone changes are seen in approximately 20% of

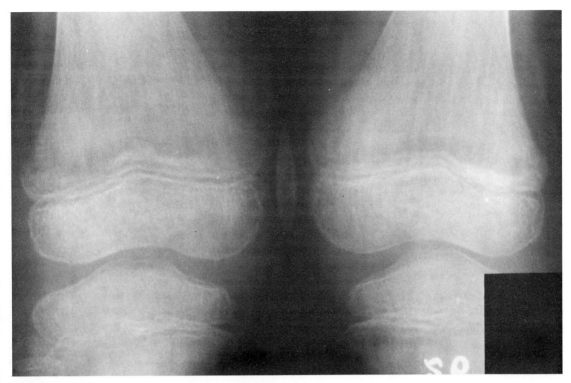

Figure 2

Figure 3

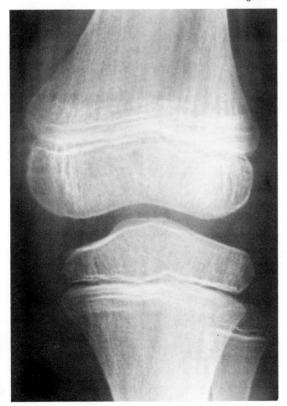

**Figs. 2, 3:** Acute leukemia: The lucent metaphyseal bands in Figure 2 became sclerotic after treatment (Fig. 3). During infancy and early childhood, lucent metaphyseal bands are nonspecific and may be the result of any severe stress. After age two the bands are more apt to be the result of leukemic infiltrate. Sclerosis after therapy is common. Alternating lucent and sclerotic stripes may also occur.

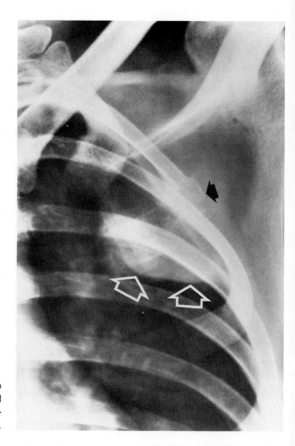

**Fig. 4:** Acute leukemia: Solitary lytic rib lesion (black arrow) of the anterior third rib with sharply marginated extra-pleural soft tissue mass (white arrows).

patients.[5,7] Braunstein noted that bone changes were more frequent in patients with poorly differentiated cell types.[7] The lesions are predominately lytic and involve the vertebra, skull, pelvis (Fig. 9), ribs and extremities (Fig. 10). Sclerotic changes do occur but with less frequency than in Hodgkin's disease (Fig. 10).

The plasma cell dyscrasias are neoplasms arising from the malignant transformation and proliferation of a B-cell lymphocyte.[8] Clones of cells are produced and are characterized by their ability to produce monoclonal proteins (ie, immunoglobulins). Included in these disorders are multiple myeloma, solitary plasmacytoma, Waldenström's macroglobulinemia and heavy chain disease. The classification of these entities depends upon the specific abnormal protein as delineated on serum and urine protein electrophoresis.

*Multiple myeloma* is most common.[8] It is characterized by abnormal proliferation of mature and immature plasma cells that synthesize abnormal amounts of monoclonal immunoglobulins (IgG, IgA, and IgE) or kappa or lambda light chains. Mean age of diagnosis is 62 years old, with an equal sex incidence. Patients commonly present with skeletal pain, but may have nonspecific constitutional complaints. The disease is progressive with numerous complications including hypercalcemia, infection, progressive renal failure and neurologic dysfunction. Diagnosis is made by bone marrow examination and protein electrophoresis of

120

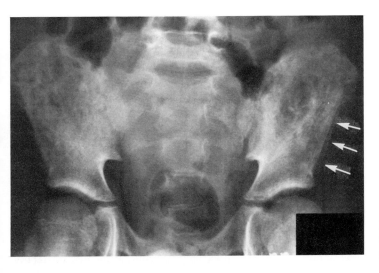

**Fig. 5:** Acute leukemia: Mixed sclerotic and lytic lesions of both iliac bones and periosteal reaction on the left (arrows).

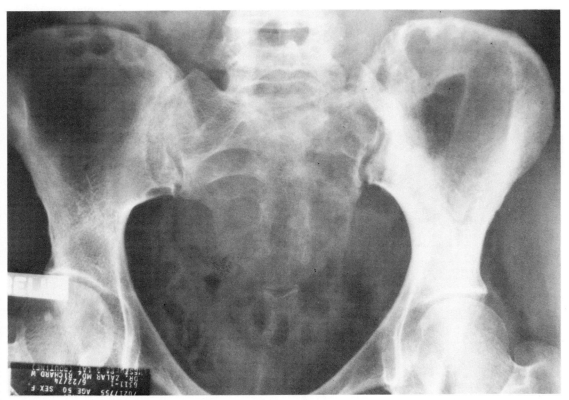

**Fig. 6:** Hodgkin's disease: Sclerotic lesion left iliac bone. Lytic lesion left side of sacrum (note absence of margins of sacral foramina on left).

the urine and serum.

Skeletal changes are striking and account for a large percentage of morbidity. These changes are due to direct invasion of bone by plasma cells, as well as the osteoclast stimulating factor produced by these cells.[9] The most common radiographic changes are diffuse, symmetric osteoporosis and osteolysis.[10,11] Rarely, sclerotic lesions occur.[12,13] The predominant sites involve the axial skeleton: vertebral bodies, ribs, skull, pelvis and femur (Figs. 11, 12). In long tubular bones, subcortical circular or elliptical lucencies cause a scalloped appearance (Fig. 13). Whereas the individual lytic lesions are often indistinguishable from metastases (Fig. 14), the scalloped appearance is very characteristic of myeloma. Skull lesions are common. Numerous small, uniform size "punched out" lucencies are said to be characteristic, but metastases, especially from breast carcinoma may be indistinguishable. Multiple myeloma may also cause a few lytic lesions of varying size simulating metastasis (Fig. 15). Multiple myeloma may be complicated by bone lesions due to amyloidosis, which is more common in the light-chain variety of the disease.

*Solitary plasmacytoma* is a focal lesion composed of an abnormal clone of plasma cells. There is controversy as to whether this entity is distinct from multiple myeloma or is part of a spectrum. Most patients if followed will develop multiple myeloma. Some have no abnormal bone marrow exams and have no serum or urine

**Figs. 7, 8:** Hodgkin's disease: Mixed sclerosis and lysis of distal femur.

Figure 7

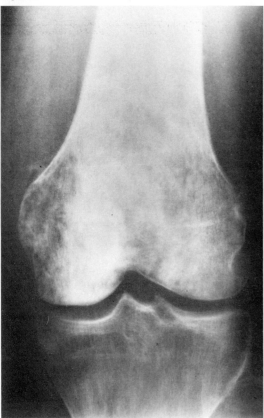

Figure 8

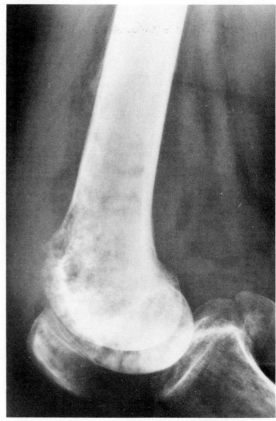

Bone Radiology Case Studies

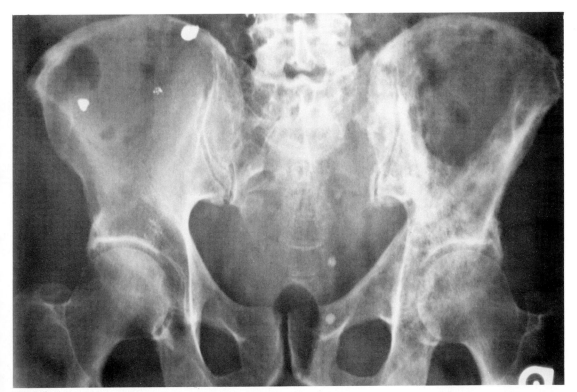

Figure 9

electrophorectic changes. The spine and pelvis are the most common sites.[14] Lesions are generally lytic and expansile. Lesions of the spine cause initial lytic changes followed by collapse. They may extend across the disc space and involve the adjacent vertebral body. The axial skeleton may be involved (Fig. 16). Rarely, multiple myeloma occurs as a soft tissue lesion.

*Waldonström's macroglobulinemia* is characterized by the production of excessive amounts of IgM. The mean age of diagnosis is 60 years of age, and patients present with fatigue, bleeding, weight loss, hepatosplenomegaly, ocular changes and adenopathy. Because the IgM molecule is large and aggregates easily, the serum viscosity is markedly increased (hence the name macroglobulinemia). The neurologic and visual symptoms are referable to this hyperviscosity. Bleeding is caused by impaired platelet function and coagulation impairment.

Bone changes are similar to those in multiple myeloma.[15] Decreased bone density with trabecular coarsening is common. Lytic lesions occur in 10 to 15% of patients.

— *Mark Baker, MD*

**Fig. 9:** Histiocytic lymphoma: Involvement of left iliac bone with mixed sclerosis and lysis. There is destruction of the left sarcum (note loss of definition of left sacral foramina while the corresponding right foramina are preserved).

### References

1. Henderson ES: Acute lymphocytic leukemia, in Williams W (ed): *Hematology*, ed 2. New York, McGraw-Hill 1977, p 992.
2. Simmons CR, Harle TS, Singleton EB: The osseous manifestations of leukemia in children. *Radiol Clin N Am* 1968; 6:115.
3. Thomas LB, Forkner CE Jr, Frei E, et al: The skeletal lesions of acute leukemia. *Cancer* 1961; 14:608.

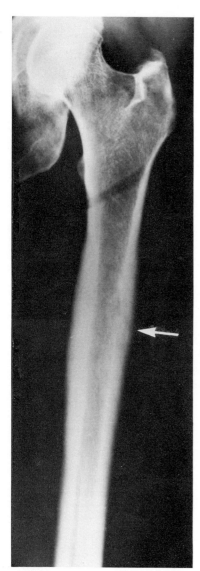

Figure 10

4. Desforges JF, Rutherford OJ, Pico A: Hodgkin's disease. *N Engl J Med* 1979; 302:1212.
5. Vieta JO, Friedell HL, Craver LF: A survey of Hodgkin's disease and lymphosarcoma in bone. *Radiology* 1942; 39:1.
6. Grossman H, Winchester PH, Bragg DG, et al: Roentgenographic changes in childhood Hodgkin's disease. *Am J Roentgenol* 1973; 117:354.

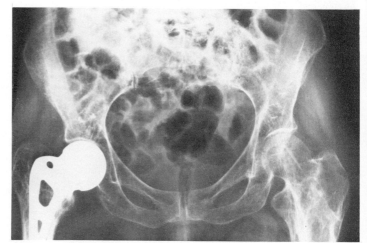

Figure 11

Figure 12

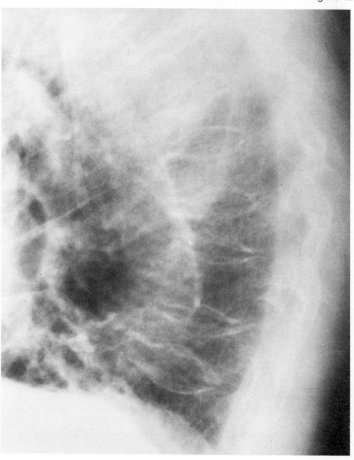

**Fig. 10:** Lymphocytic lymphoma: Sclerosis and a small amount of lysis (arrow) of the upper shaft of the femur.

**Fig. 11:** Multiple myeloma: Profound decreased bone density. This is the most common radiographic finding in this disease.

**Fig. 12:** Multiple myeloma: Severe decreased bone density of the thoracic spine with multiple compression fractures.

7. Braunstein EM, White SJ: Non-Hodgkin's lymphoma of bone. *Radiology* 1980; 135:59.
8. Bergsagel DE: Plasma cell neoplasms—general considerations, in Williams W (ed): *Hematology*, ed 2. New York, McGraw-Hill 1977, p 1087.
9. Mundy GR, Raisz LG, Cooper RA, et al: Evidence for the secretion of an osteoclast factor in myeloma. *N Engl J Med* 1974; 291:1941.
10. Mezaros WT: The many facets of multiple myeloma. *Semin Roentgenol* 1974; 9:219.
11. Heiser S, Schartzman JJ: Variation in the roentgen appearance of the skeletal system in myeloma. *Radiology* 1952; 58:178.
12. Himmelfarb E, Sebes J, Rabinowitz J: Unusual roentgenographic presentations of multiple myeloma. Report of three cases. *J Bone Joint Surg* 1974; 56A:1723.
13. Clavisse PDT, Staple TW: Diffuse bone sclerosis in multiple myeloma. *Radiology* 1971; 99:327.
14. Gootnick LT: Solitary myeloma. Review of sixty-one cases. *Radiology* 1945; 25:849.
15. Vermess M, Pearson KD, Einstein AB, et al: Osseous manifestations of Waldenström's macroglobulinemia. *Radiology* 1972; 102:497.

**Fig. 13:** Multiple myeloma: Lytic lesions of the entire humerus. Endosteal scalloping is quite characteristic of the disease.

**Fig. 14:** Multiple myeloma: The lytic lesion of the proximal radius is slightly expansile. Metastasis from primary neoplasms in the kidney, thyroid, lung or breast, plus malignant melanoma or pheochromocytoma metastases could give a similar appearance.

Figure 13

Figure 14

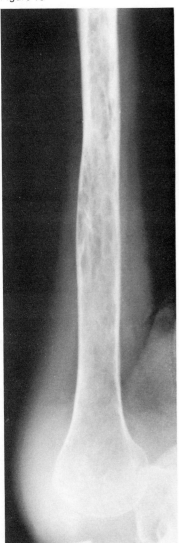

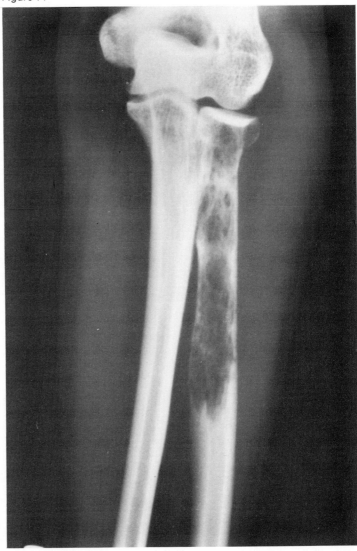

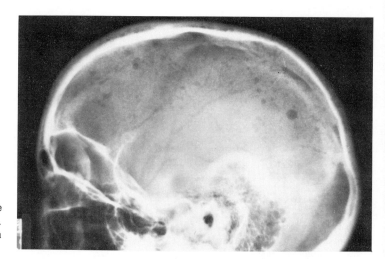

**Fig. 15:** Multiple myeloma: There are multiple sharply defined lytic lesions. Metastases to the skull could have a similar appearance.

**Fig. 16:** Solitary plasmacytoma of the humerus: This 60-year-old woman was pouring water from a large pitcher when she suddenly developed arm pain. The lesion expands the bone and has broken through the cortex in several areas.

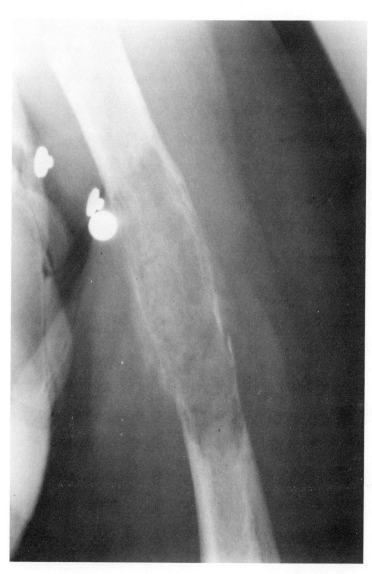

# *CORTEX AND TRABECULAE*

The cortex can be thinned, thickened, discontinuous, or destroyed.

The most common cause of generalized thinned cortex is osteoporosis, but thinning may be the result of other metabolic diseases. Many focal processes within the bone or in the adjacent soft tissue cause focal thinning. A scalloped endosteal surface is most frequently the result of myeloproliferative diseases, especially multiple myeloma. Thick cortex can be the result of generalized processes such as Paget's disease, fibrous dysplasia, or congenital diaphyseal dysplasias. The presence of focal processes within the bone or in adjacent soft tissue may be indicated by focal cortical thickening. A discontinuous cortex is usually due to a fracture. Cortical destruction most often indicates infection or malignancy.

The cortex may have a longitudinal striated appearance when rapid bone resorption via osteoclastic activity in osteones exceeds the ability of osteoblasts to replace bone. A single longitudinal lucency in the cortex producing a split appearance may be the result of bone production on the endosteal side of the cortex in osteomyelitis or sickle cell anemia.

Diseases which result in loss of small trabeculae, such as thalassemia or osteomalacia, are often associated with thickening of the remaining trabeculae, especially along lines of stress. Thickened trabeculae are also characteristic of Paget's disease, while trabecular destruction is commonly due to infection or neoplasm. Incomplete and impacted fractures are often marked by subtle, disordered trabeculae.

# Study 16

This 54-year-old man had a grand mal seizure while watching a movie in a theater. He has had no past medical problems. He was brought to the emergency department because of pain in both shoulders. Attempted movement of his arms caused severe pain. *Your diagnosis?*

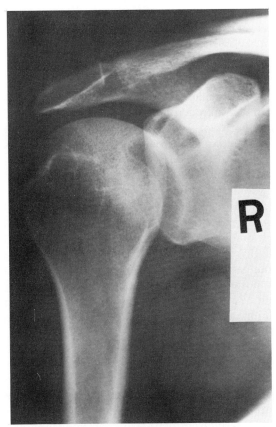 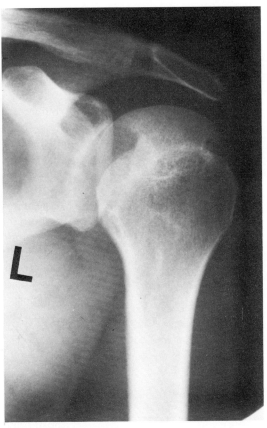

**Fig. 1:** Anteroposterior roentgenogram of the right shoulder.

**Fig. 2:** Anteroposterior roentgenogram of the left shoulder.

# Diagnosis: Posterior Shoulder Dislocations

Shoulder dislocations have been classified by Rockwood and Green in the following manner:[1]

### Glenohumeral Joint

Anterior dislocation (subcoracoid, subglenoid, subclavicular, intrathoracic)
  Traumatic
  Atraumatic (congenital, voluntary)
Posterior dislocation (subacromial, subglenoid, subspinous)
  Traumatic
  Atraumatic (congenital, voluntary)
Superior dislocation
Inferior dislocation—"luxatio erecta"

### Clavicular Joints

Acromioclavicular dislocation (anterior, posterior, superior)
Sternoclavicular dislocation (anterior, posterior)
  Traumatic
  Atraumatic (congenital, voluntary)
Total Dislocation of clavicle.

### Dislocation of Scapula

About 80% of all shoulder dislocations are anterior glenohumeral dislocations, 15% are acromioclavicular dislocations, and less than 5% are posterior glenohumeral or sternoclavicular dislocations.[1] The glenohumeral joint is the most commonly dislocated major joint of the body. In a series of 466 shoulder dislocations, 96% were traumatic and 4% atraumatic.[2]

About 2% of glenohumeral dislocations are posterior.[1,2] This type of posterior dislocation is seen infrequently and often is missed on initial examination. Factors contributing to missed diagnosis are: subtle findings on physical examination, subtle findings on anteroposterior (AP) roentgenograms, fracture-dislocation with the fracture dominating the clinical picture, and lack of consideration of a posterior dislocation due to its rarity. The proper diagnosis may not be made for days, weeks, or months. Missed posterior dislocations undiagnosed for long periods have been considered to be "frozen shoulders."

The subglenoid and subspinous types of posterior dislocation are diagnosed easily, but both are rare. In the vast majority of patients with posterior dislocation the humeral head is located below the acromion. A direct anterior blow to the humeral head may cause posterior dislocation but this is a very unusual event. Most posterior dislocations result from internal rotation, adduction, and flexion forces, such as falling on an outstretched arm. Convulsive seizures are a common etiology of posterior dislocation and occasionally may cause bilateral simultaneous dislocations (Figs. 1, 2, 3). Electrical accidents are another etiology. In either case the dislocation is the result of sudden contraction of the shoulder

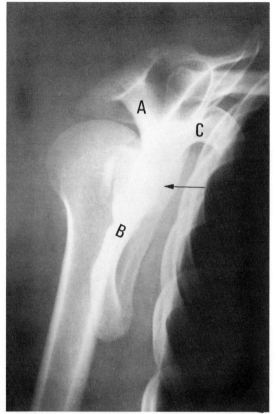

Figure 3

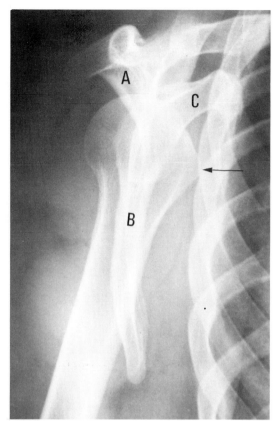

Figure 4

muscles, causing the stronger internal rotators to overpower the weaker external rotators.[1] Atraumatic posterior dislocation may be spontaneous or voluntary in patients with lax joint capsules or congenital bony deficiencies of the humeral head or glenoid.[1] Most patients with recurrent posterior dislocations have the atraumatic type.[3]

A patient with a posterior dislocation holds the upper arm tightly against the side of the chest, and the forearm against the anterior chest or abdomen. Attempts at external rotation or abduction cause severe pain. Fixed internal rotation is always present. Close inspection and comparison of the shoulders may reveal anterior flattening and posterior fullness of the affected shoulder. Occasionally the coracoid process is prominent. These findings may be obscured by a hematoma or be difficult to detect in a patient whose muscles are well-developed.

A posterior dislocation is difficult to identify on AP roentgenograms because the glenoid fossa cannot be seen in tangent and because the humeral head is not completely displaced medial and posterior to the glenoid. Despite this, roentgenographic diagnosis of posterior dislocation can be suggested on the basis of frontal roentgenograms in most cases, and confirmed with additional views in all cases. Routine shoulder roentgenograms usually include AP views with internal and external rotation. There will be fixed internal rotation on AP views of any patient with a posterior

**Fig. 3:** Scapular Y (transscapular) roentgenogram of the right shoulder. (A = acromion, C = coracoid process, B = body of scapula in tangent, arrow = medial margin of humeral head.) The head of the humerus is displaced posteriorly and lies under the acromion. Figures 1 and 2 show impaction fractures of the right and left superior-medial humeral heads produced by impingement on the glenoid rims. The posterior dislocations were treated with closed reduction under general anesthesia.

**Fig. 4:** Scapular Y roentgenogram of a normal shoulder. The head of the humerus is centered over both the glenoid and the junction of the three limbs forming the Y: the acromion (A), coracoid (C), and scapular body in tangent (B). The arrow indicates the medial margin of the humeral head.

**Fig. 5:** AP roentgenogram of a 25-year-old man who fractured his humeral neck in a motorcycle accident. His shoulder is adducted and internally rotated. The cortical line (arrows) medial to the outline of the humeral head is an impaction fracture indicating a posterior dislocation. This is confirmed by the axillary view in Figure 6.

**Fig. 6:** Axillary view (C = coracoid, G = glenoid, A = acromion) of the patient in Figure 5, showing fracture of the humeral neck, posterior dislocation, and impaction fracture of the humeral head produced by the posterior glenoid rim.

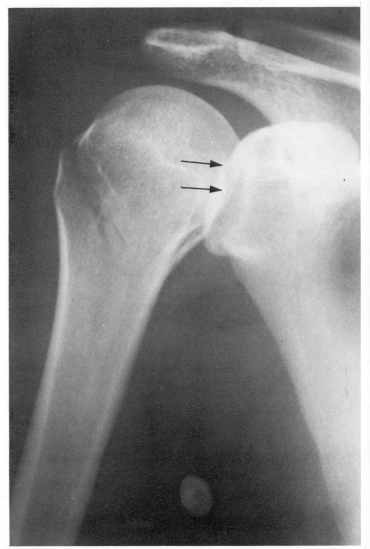

Figure 5

Figure 6

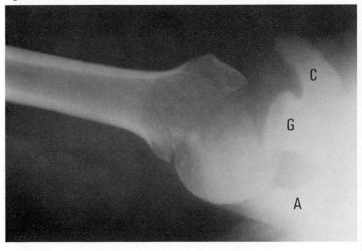

Bone Radiology Case Studies

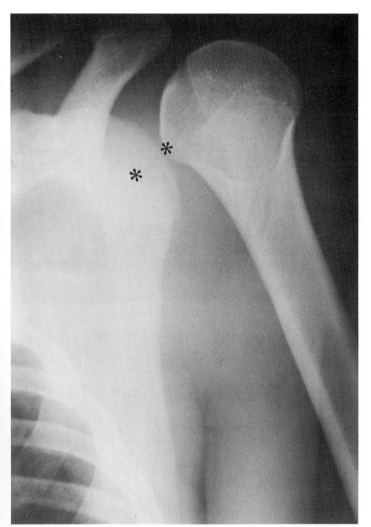

Figure 7

**Fig. 7:** AP roentgenogram of a 24-year-old man who dislocated his shoulder posteriorly in a motocycle accident. The humeral head is displaced laterally, indicating posterior dislocation. A distance > 6mm between the anterior rim of the glenoid and the medial aspect of the humeral head (asterisks) usually is the result of posterior dislocation.

**Fig. 8:** Same patient as in Figure 7, following reduction of dislocation.

Figure 8

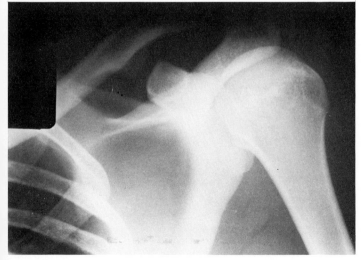

**Fig. 9A:** Lateral transthoracic view. *Normal*: A normal smooth, continuous arch is formed by the posterior cortex of the humerus (open arrows) and the lateral margin of the scapula (closed arrows). The patient was thin, which accounts for this exceptionally clear image.

**Fig. 9B:** *Anterior dislocation:* The arch is widened, and the margins of the scapula (closed arrows) and the humerus (open arrows) are discontinuous.

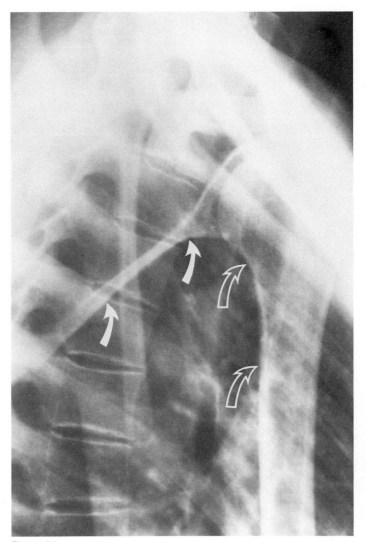

Figure 9A

Figure 9B

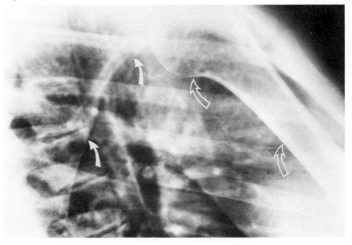

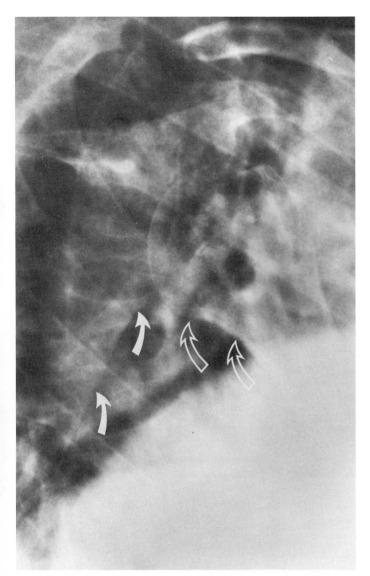

**Fig. 9C:** *Posterior dislocation:* The arch is narrowed, and the margins of the scapula (closed arrows) and the humerus (open arrows) are discontinuous.

Figure 9C

dislocation.[2] The ability to rotate the shoulder externally eliminates the possibility of a posterior dislocation.[1]

On the normal AP roentgenogram the medial humeral head and posterior glenoid fossa overlap, resulting in an ellipse of increased density. This ellipse is smooth and centered in the glenoid fossa from top to bottom. It has been written[1] that an absent or irregular ellipse, an off center ellipse (humeral head displaced superiorly), and loss of a parallel relationship between the medial margin of the head of the humerus and the anterior margin of the glenoid fossa all are indicators of posterior dislocation. However, these findings are not as reliable as the *rim sign* and *trough line*.

Frequently there is an impaction fracture of the anterior humeral head caused by contact with the posterior rim of the glenoid, a "reverse Hill-Sachs fracture." In one series[4] this impaction was visible on AP roentgenograms as a cortical line within the humeral head, parallel to the superomedial articular cortex of the head, in 15 of 20 patients. This line represents the depth of the troughlike impaction fracture caused by the posterior glenoid rim and has been called the *"trough line"* (Figs. 1, 2, 5).[4]

If the dislocated humeral head is behind and lateral to the glenoid, the glenoid may appear vacant because it is not overlapped by the head. It has been stated that a distance greater than 6 mm between the anterior rim of the glenoid and the medial cortex of the head is very suggestive of a posterior dislocation, and this finding has been called a positive *rim sign* (Fig. 7).[5] When dislocation is present, rotation of the patient or impaction of the head of the humerus on the glenoid, however, can cause this measurement to be normal. A false positive *rim sign* may be seen when fluid in the joint space displaces the head laterally.

If a posterior dislocation is suspected on the basis of clinical or radiologic findings, the diagnosis can be confirmed by a lateral roentgenogram of the shoulder. There are several views designed to depict the glenohumeral relationship in the sagittal plane. These include the axillary, scapular Y (transscapular), transthoracic, and true AP views.

The *axillary view* (sitting patient, shoulder abducted, with a vertical x-ray beam) clearly demonstrates the glenoid-humeral head relationship and is also excellent for identifying fractures of the humeral head and glenoid (Fig. 6). Since some abduction is required to obtain the view, however, it may be unobtainable in an acutely injured patient who has limited motion due to pain.

The *scapular Y View* (patient turned 45°, with the anterior affected shoulder touching the cassette and back toward the x-ray tube) displays the scapula as a Y. The acromion and coracoid process form the top of the Y and the body of the scapula, viewed tangentially, forms the stem of the Y. The glenoid rim is a circle centered over the junction of the limbs of the Y. The normal humeral head is centered over the glenoid (Fig. 4). If the glenoid cannot be seen, the humeral head should be centered at the junction of the limbs of the Y. In a posterior dislocation, the head of the humerus is off center and displaced backward to a position under the acromion (Fig. 3). This view is the preferred means for confirming posterior dislocation of the shoulder.

The *transthoracic lateral view* (patient lateral to horizontal x-ray beam, affected arm against the cassette, opposite arm raised) does not require movement of the affected arm. In this view the normal arch formed by the scapula and humerus (Maloney's line) is a rounded dome. A narrow scapulohumeral arch indicates a posterior dislocation. This view may be difficult to interpret, and often the anatomy is obscured by ribs and soft tissue of the upper chest, especially in overweight people (Figs. 9A-C).

The *true AP view* (patient is turned 30° with the posterior aspect of the affected shoulder against the cassette, facing the x-ray tube) demonstrates the glenoid fossa in tangent as a straight line. The angle of the patient may have to be varied to achieve this. With a posterior dislocation, the head of the humerus overlaps the glenoid.

Forces causing posterior dislocation of the shoulder may result in a number of associated fractures in addition to impaction of the head of the humerus. The head, neck or diaphysis of the humerus may fracture. The posterior rim of the glenoid may be fractured (Bankart's fracture). The lesser trochanter may be avulsed. It has been stated that an isolated lesser trochanter fracture is almost pathognomonic of posterior dislocation.[1]

## References

1. Rockwood CA, Green DP: *Fractures.* Philadelphia, JB Lippincott, 1975.
2. Rowe CR: Prognosis in dislocation of the shoulder. *J Bone Joint Surg* 1956; 38A:957.
3. English E, MacNab I: Recurrent posterior dislocation of the shoulder. *Can J Surg* 1974; 17:147.
4. Cisternino SJ, Rogers LF, Stufflebam BC, et al: The trough line: A radiographic sign of posterior shoulder dislocation. *Am J Roentgenol* 1978; 130:951.
5. Arnot JH, Sears AD: Posterior dislocation of the shoulder. *Am J Roentgenol* 1965; 94:639.
6. DeSemet AA: Anterior oblique projection in radiography of the traumatized shoulder. *Am J Roentgenol* 1980; 134:515.

# Study 17

This 8-year-old white boy has had pain in the left hip and knee for six weeks. The pain is worse with walking and he walks with a limp. On physical examination, there is limitation of internal rotation of the left hip. *Your diagnosis?*

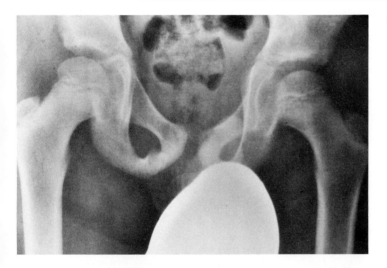

**Fig. 1:** AP view of pelvis and hips.

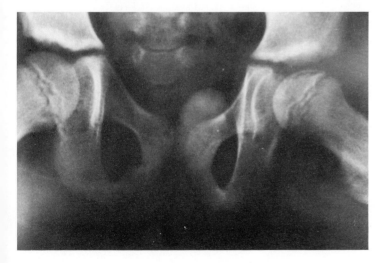

**Fig. 2:** Lateral view of hips.

# Diagnosis: Legg-Calvé-Perthes Disease

Trauma and steroid therapy are the most common causes of avascular osteonecrosis of the femoral head. Other etiologies and associations include:[1]

**Trauma**
    Femoral neck fracture
    Dislocated hip
    Caisson disease
    Radiation

**Iatrogenic**
    Steroid therapy
    Postreduction—slipped capital femoral epiphysis
    Postreduction—congenital dislocated hip

**Systemic Causes**
    Alcoholism
    Pancreatitis
    Diabetes mellitus
    Sickle hemoglobinopathies
    Collagen diseases
    Cushing's syndrome
    Gaucher's disease
    Fabry's disease
    Arteriosclerosis
    Hyperuricemia
    Hyperlipidemia

**Idiopathic**
    Idiopathic adult osteonecrosis of the hip
    Legg-Calvé-Perthes disease
    The etiology of Legg-Calvé-Perthes disease is uncertain, but despite this, it is usually considered a form of a vascular necrosis. It occurs from age 2 to 12, with peak incidence at ages 4 to 8. It is four times more common in boys than in girls. Blacks are rarely affected. There is a familial predisposition. Both hips are involved in 10 to 15% of patients.

There is often a limp, with or without pain. Pain is usually mild, and may be in the hip, thigh and/or knee. The duration of symptoms is usually less than three months, and may be weeks or even days.[2] On physical examination, there is frequent decreased range of motion of the hip, especially internal rotation.

Early radiologic changes occur in the anterolateral part of the epiphysis, and frequently are not seen on AP views, but only on a "frog" view with the leg abducted and externally rotated (Fig. 2).

*Early* radiologic signs include:
    1. Decreased bone age

2. Lateral subluxation of femur (Fig. 1) with medial joint space at least 2 mm wider than opposite hip
3. Lucency of lateral epiphysis (Fig. 1)
4. Subcortical fracture (Fig. 2), soft tissue signs caused by distended joint are difficult to identify prospectively

*Later* findings are:
1. Flattening of epiphysis
2. Loss of volume of epiphysis
3. Fragmentation of epiphysis
4. Sclerosis of epiphysis
5. Metaphysical lucencies

Only about 10% of affected hips return to normal anatomic appearance whatever the treatment.

*Residual* findings are:[4]
1. Flat, widened epiphysis
2. Wide femoral neck
3. Acetabular deformity
4. Late secondary degenerative changes
5. Osteochondrosis dissecans

Several schemes have been used to stage patients according to age, symptoms and x-ray findings.[2,3,6] In general, younger children with few symptoms and few radiologic signs have the best prognosis.

Early diagnosis of Legg-Calve-Perthes disease can be a problem. Acute synovitis is a common cause of hip pain in children and can be indistinguishable from early Legg-Perthes. Both of these diseases

**Fig. 3:** Two months after Figures 1 and 2, and following osteotomy, there is a decreased volume of left femoral epiphysis which is now sclerotic and slightly flattened. Figure 1 shows slight lateral displacement of the upper femur with possible lateral lucency of the epiphysis, while Figure 2 clearly shows a subcortical fracture of the antero-lateral aspect of the epiphysis.)

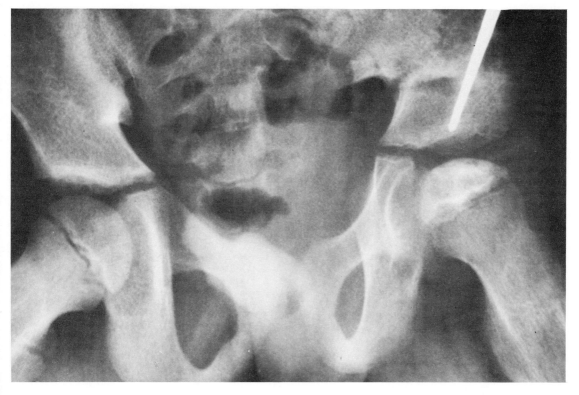

may show only hip subluxation on first radiograph.[7] Radiologic bone changes which identify Legg-Perthes may not appear for several weeks or months after the initial symptoms.

Nuclear medicine has the advantage of early demonstration (within days of onset of symptoms) of bone changes. Several Tc 99m compounds are quite promising for early diagnosis of Legg-Perthes disease. Early in the disease there is decreased activity of the affected hip (ischemia) and later increased activity (repair).[8] Localized decreased activity is uncommon in other types of pathology.

### References

1. Jacobs B: Epidemiology of traumatic and non-traumatic osteonecrosis. *Clin Orthop* 1978; 130:51.
2. Lauritzen J: Legg-Calvé-Perthes disease. *Acta Orthop Scand* 1975; 159 (suppl).
3. Edgren W: Coxa plana. *Acta Orthop Scand* 1965; 84 (suppl).
4. Caffey J: The early roentgenographic changes in essential coxa plana: Their significance in pathogenesis. *Am J Roentgenol* 1968; 103:620.
5. Goldman AB, Hallel T, Salvati EM, et al: Osteochondritis dissecans complicating Legg-Perthes disease. *Radiology* 1976; 121:561.
6. Catterall A: The natural history of Perthes disease. *J Bone Joint Surg* 1971; 530B:37.
7. Jacobs BW: Synovitis of the hip in children and its significance. *Pediatrics* 1971; 47:558.
8. Danigelis JA, Fisher RL, Ozonoff MB, et al:[99]m Tc-polyphosphate bone imaging in Legg-Perthes disease. *Radiology* 1975; 115:407.

# Study 18

This 22-year-old man presented to the emergency room with abdominal pain. Appendicitis was suspected and a supine abdominal film taken. *Your diagnosis?*

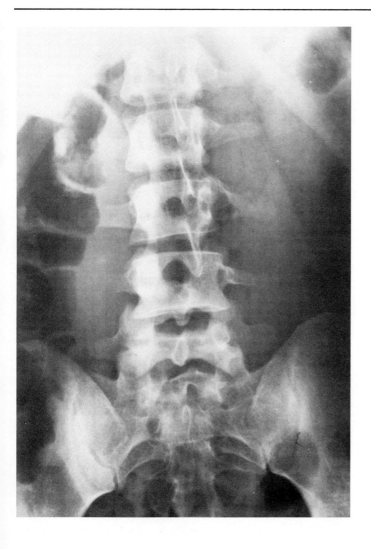

# Diagnosis: Congenital Absence of Vertebral Pedicle

Hypoplastic or absent vertebral pedicles are rare. In a study of 4,200 skeletons, none were identified.[1] This congenital defect is most common in the low cervical spine[2]; next most common in a lumbar location[3]; and least common in the thoracic spine.[4]

The vertebral column is first developed in membrane from mesenchyme surrounding the notochord and dorsally located neural tube. The second stage, chondrification, occurs in the fourth week with formation of paired lateral centers forming the vertebral

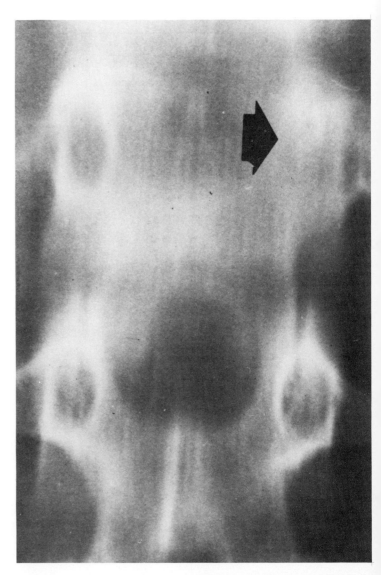

**Fig. 2:** AP laminogram of lumbar spine demonstrating absent left pedicle (arrow). Right pedicle is hyperplastic with thickened cortex demonstrated.

body. Another dorsolateral pair of centers, one on either side of the neural tube, form the neural arch of the vertebra. Fusion of these centers in gestational month 4 results in the cartilagenous vertebra. The third stage, ossification, begins in the third month commencing in the cervical spine and progressing distally. There is an ossification center for the body and separate centers for the right and left neural arch. Unossified cartilage (neurocentral synchondrosis) separates the body from the arch until age 3 to 6 years.[5] Ring epiphyses of the bodies appear about age 7 and fuse at age 12 to 15 years. Secondary ossification centers of the vertebral processes appear about age 16 and fuse about age 25. Abnormal formation and fusion of developmental centers and persistent notochord result in anomalies.

The neural arch consists of pedicles, laminae, superior and inferior articular facets, spinous process, transverse processes and lumbar mammillary processes. Neural arch developmental anomalies include:[5]

1. Spinal bifida: Most common at transitional areas, especially L-5, S-1. Incidence at S-1 is 25%, L-5 is 1 to 2%. Not significant unless wide with meninges and/or cord involved.
2. Spondylolysis: Occurs in about 5% of adults, less in blacks. Common in Mongols and Eskimos. Symptoms with subluxation, unilateral defect.[1]

**Fig. 3A:** AP view lumbar spine shows sclerotic right pedicle of L5.

**Fig. 3B:** Oblique view shows sclerotic right pedicle (open arrow) and left spondylolysis (closed arrow).

Figure 3A

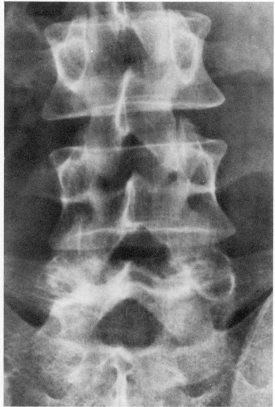

Figure 3B

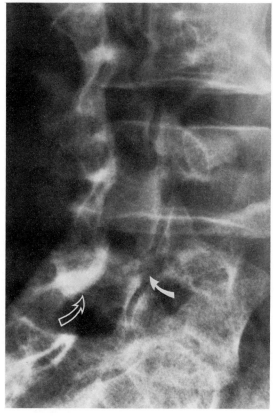

3. Cleft pedicle: Rare, cortical margin excludes acute fracture.
4. Persistent neurocentral synchondrosis.
5. Agenesis, partial or complete.
6. Synostosis, with or without block vertebra.
7. Malformed arch and processes including asymmetry of articular processes, absent processes, unfused secondary ossification centers and accessory processes at base of transverse processes (styloid process).

Hypoplastic and absent pedicles have been considered to be forms of cleft pedicles.[6]

The hypoplastic or absent pedicle probably results from a problem during formation in membrane or cartilage. The patients are usually asymptomatic, although symptoms have been reported with a cervical location.[2]

Absent pedicles may be mistaken for metastasis to bone, since a destroyed pedicle can be the first radiographic sign of vertebral metastasis. Other entities which may affect a pedicle are trauma, osteomyelitis, neurofibromatosis, vertebral artery erosion, spinal canal tumor or cyst, spinal cord tumor and primary bone tumors such as osteoblastoma or aneurysmal bone cyst.

Identification of a hypoplastic or absent pedicle is aided by associated vertebral changes:[7]

1. The contralateral pedicle and lamina may be hypertrophied

**Fig. 4:** Lateral film of a lumbar spine with widened intervertebral foramen (arrow) at level of absent pedicle.

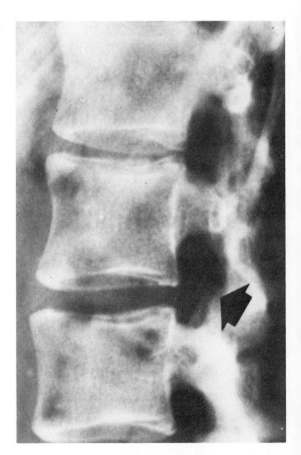

Bone Radiology Case Studies

(Fig. 2). This usually occurs in older patients. This finding can also be seen when there is spondylolysis of the opposite arch[8] or with osteoid ostemoa. (Figs. 3A, 3B).[9]

2. The neural foramen may be enlarged (Fig. 4).
3. The superior articular facet may be oblique instead of vertical.
4. Deformed transverse process.

When a pedicle is absent or abnormal, especially in a young patient, or when the finding is serendipitous, as in this case, think of a congenital etiology and you can avoid an unneeded workup.

The patient presented here did have an appendicitis, although there were no plain film findings. The congenital absence of the lumbar vertebral pedicle was an incidental finding and did not cause any symptoms.

## References

1. Roche MR, Rowe GG: The incidence of separate neural arch and coincident bone variations. *J Bone Joint Surg* 1952; 34:491-494.
2. Danziger J, Jackson H, Bloch S: Congenital absence of a pedicle in a cervical vertebra. *Clin Radiol* 1975; 26:53-56.
3. Morin M, Palacios E: The aplastic hypoplastic lumbar pedicle. *Am J Roentgenol* 1974; 122:639-642.
4. Tomsick TA, LeBowitz ME, Campbell C: The congenital absence of pedicles in the thoracic spine. *Radiology* 1974; 111:587-589.
5. Schmorl G, Junghanns H: *The Human Spine in Health and Disease.* New York and London, Grune and Stratton, 1971.
6. Bardsley JL, Hanelin LG: The unilateral hypoplastic lumbar pedicle. *Radiology* 1971; 101:315-317.
7. Norman WJ, Johnson C: Congenital absence of a pedicle of a lumbar vertebra. *Br J Radiol* 1973; 46:631-633.
8. Sherman FC, Wilkinson RM, Hall JE: Reactive sclerosis of a pedicle and spondylolysis in the lumbar spine. *J Bone Joint Surg* 1977; 59:49-54.
9. Keim HA, Reina EG: Osteoid osteoma as a cause of scoliosis. *J Bone Joint Surg* 1975; 57:159-163.

# Study 19

This 56-year-old man had carcinoma of the prostate gland 11 years ago. He has several draining perineal sinuses. *Your diagnosis?*

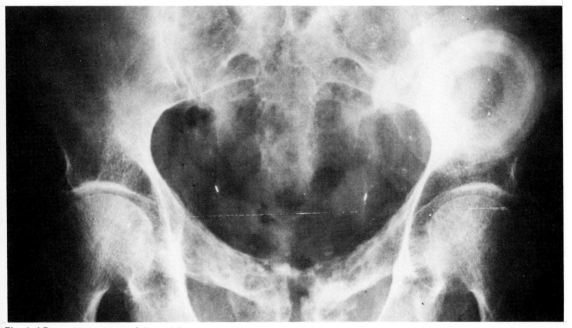

**Fig. 1:** AP roentgenogram of the pelvis.

# Diagnosis: Radiation Bone Damage

Radon seeds were implanted in this patient, followed later by cobalt radiation therapy for prostatic carcinoma more than ten years before Figure 1 was taken. An ileal conduit was necessary because of severe radiation cystitis. The patient developed draining perineal sinuses that have been present for two years. Figure 1 shows symmetric mixed sclerotic and lytic areas of the right and left pubis and ischium. These changes represent radiation bone damage with superimposed osteomyelitis. The small metallic objects are radon seeds, and there is an ileostomy appliance in the RLQ.

Radiation damage to bone has been called radiation osteitis and radiation necrosis. Some feel that, since there is usually no inflammation or necrosis, a more accurate term would be "radiation atrophy of bone."[1] Pathologic information has been obtained from advanced cases so that there is little documentation of the early and progressive microscopic changes of radiation damage in humans. It is believed that there is early necrosis of marrow blood-forming elements, periosteal damage, and death of osteocytes, osteoblasts, and osteoclasts. The death of bone cells leaves an acellular bony structure that initially appears normal on radiographs. Regeneration of the marrow can occur later. Vascular damage consists of endarteritis and progressive obliteration of the vessel lumen, with resultant ischemia.[2]

Damage increases with increasing total dose of radiation, increasing dose per treatment, and size of the radiation port. Low energy kilovoltage radiation results in a greater dose to bone than to soft tissue, due to secondary radiation produced by the calcium in bone. Megavoltage radiation, including cobalt, delivers higher energy radiation. At these higher energies, absorbed doses in bone and soft tissue are equal. High energy megavoltage radiation has superseded low energy kilovoltage therapy; as a result the incidence of radiation bone damage has decreased.[3]

Following completion of radiation therapy there is a latent period during which roentgenograms are normal. Roentgenographic changes generally can be seen two years after completion of radiation therapy. Minimal changes may be seen after one year. Fractures do not usually occur until 2-3 years after completion of therapy. Roentgenographic changes are not seen with a dose less than 3000 rad, while damage is usually seen with a dose over 5000 rad.[4]

The first roentgenographic change is osteoporosis, which is usually patchy rather than uniform. This may gradually become more severe. Osteoporosis appears commonly in long bones, and may be the end result of radiation damage. In other patients repair of dead bone takes place, with resultant thickening of trabeculae and cortex. The appearance is similar to Paget's disease but the expansion of bone seen in Paget's disease does not occur. More severe changes manifest as lytic and sclerotic areas. The cystlike lytic areas are usually small and may have sclerotic rims. This appearance is common in the pelvis. This later, more severe, type of

Bone Radiology Case Studies

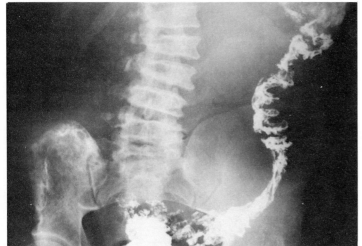

Figure 2

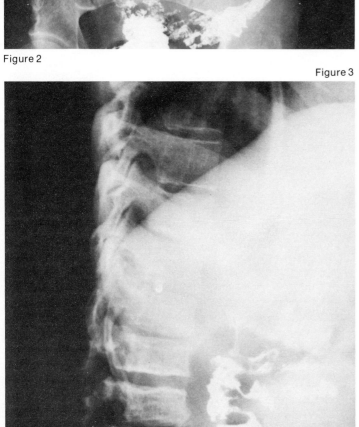

Figure 3

**Fig. 2 and 3:** AP and lateral roentgenograms of the lumbar spine and pelvis. This 24-year-old man had radiation for a right-sided Wilm's tumor in early childhood. The right iliac bone, right sacrum, and right lower ribs are underdeveloped, and there is lumbar scoliosis. The lumbar vertebral bodies are asymmetrically flattened. There is thickening of the trabaculae and cortex of the affected bones. Mixed areas of sclerosis and lucency are found in the iliac bone. These findings are characteristic of radiation damage to growing bone.

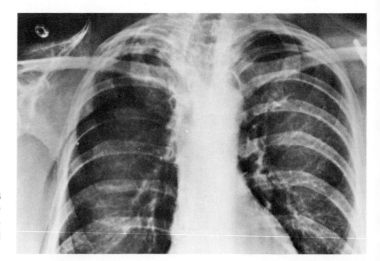

**Fig. 4:** AP roentgenogram of chest 6 years after right radical mastectomy and radiation therapy. There is sclerosis, cortical thickening of ribs 1-4, and an ununited fracture of the first rib.

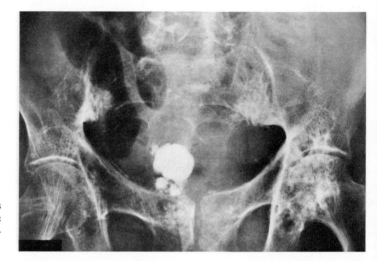

**Fig. 5:** AP roentgenogram of the pelvis in a woman who had radiation for pelvic malignancy. There is avascular necrosis of the left femur.

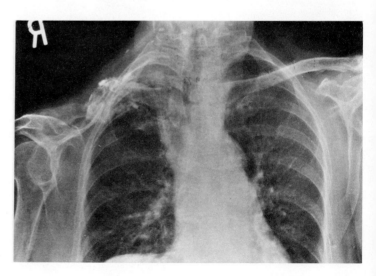

**Fig. 6:** Nonunion of fractured clavicle and loss of volume of right upper lobe following radiation therapy for bronchogenic carcinoma.

damage may be impossible to differentiate from metastasis, especially if the lytic areas are large.[2] Calcification can occur in the soft tissue following radiation when there is necrosis or ulceration (Figs. 4, 5.)

Complications of radiation bone damage are fracture, infection, and radiation-induced sarcoma. Fractures may occur without significant trauma. Delayed union and nonunion are common; however, about 50% of femoral neck fractures heal spontaneously (Fig. 6.).[2,5] Superimposed infection may result in bone destruction and a roentgenographic picture identical to sarcoma. About 200 cases of radiation-induced sarcoma have been reported. Osteosarcoma and fibrosarcoma are by far the most common. The average time span between radiation and subsequent development of a sarcoma is about 10 years, with a range of 3 to 27 years. The relationship of absorbed dose of megavoltage radiation to development of sarcoma is unknown.

Radiation bone damage is stable after five years and, if a roentgenographic change takes place after that time, development of a sarcoma should be considered (if there is no complicating infection or fracture). Radiation bone damage is usually asymptomatic; development of symptoms may also indicate malignancy. Characteristically, bone destruction, tumor osteoid formation, and soft tissue mass are present on roentgenograms. Osteochondroma is the only benign bone tumor induced by radiation.

Radiation of growing bone produces the added problems of growth arrest, scoliosis, and kyphosis. Slipped capital femoral epiphyses, avascular necrosis, and degenerative changes also have been reported after radiation of the extremities in children. Roentgenographic bone changes usually are delayed for at least one year, and scoliosis is not demonstrated until after age 10 (Figs. 2,3).

In general, the deforming effect of radiation is greater in younger children. Little change results from a dose of less than 2000 R to the spine or 1000 rad to the extremities.

### References

1. Howland WJ, Loeffler RK, Strachman DE, et al: Post-irradiation atrophic changes of bone and related complications. *Radiology* 1975; 117:677.
2. Libschitz HI: *Diagnostic Roentgenology of Radiotherapy Change.* Baltimore, Williams and Wilkins, 1978.
3. Kim JM, Chu F, Pope RA, et al: Time dose factors in radiation induced osteitis. *Am J Roentgenol* 1974; 120:684.
4. Bragg DG, Shidnia H, Chu F, et al: Clinical and radiographic aspects of radiation osteitis. *Radiology* 1970; 97:103.
5. Bonfiglio M: The pathology of fracture of the femoral neck following irradiation. *Am J Roentgenol* 1953; 70:449.

# Study 20

This 27-year-old woman complains of pain in the right wrist after minor trauma. *Your diagnosis?*

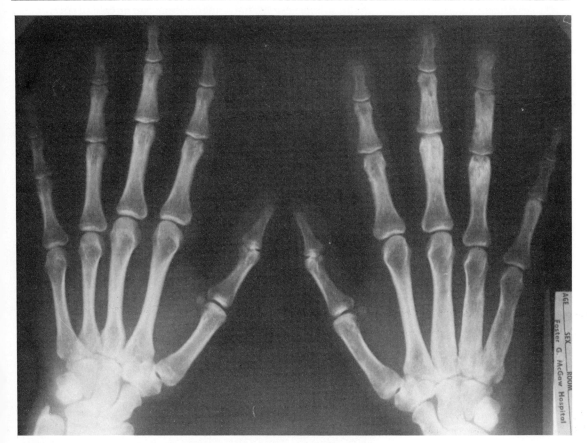

**Fig. 1:** Roentgenogram of a 27-year-old woman.

# Diagnosis: Fibrous Dysplasia

The patient in Figure 1 demonstrates several roentgenographic findings of fibrous dysplasia. There is *bony expansion* of multiple phalanges and metacarpals of the right hand. There is *abnormal lucency* of the ring and little metacarpals. There is *sclerosis* of the phalanges of the index and ring fingers, and there is cortical thinning best seen in metacarpals.

In 1937 Albright described a syndrome with three characteristics:[1]

a. Bone lesions histologically identified as "osteitis fibrosa" which tended to involve one side of the body.

b. Brown non-elevated pigmented areas (café au lait spots) which also had a tendency to be unilateral and on the same side as the bone lesions.

c. Endocrine problems, especially precocious puberty in females.

In 1942 Lichtenstein and Jaffe reported several patients who had multiple bone lesions, but some of whom had no café au lait spots or precocious puberty.[2] They felt that these patients should be considered to have a difficult expression of the same disease which they called fibrous dysplasia of bone. In 1946 Schlumberger described 67 patients who had fibrous dysplasia involving only a single bone.[3] Most writers now refer to three types of fibrous dysplasia (FD):

1. *Monostotic:* Involving a single bone at the time of presentation,

2. *Polyostotic:* Involving several bones, and

3. *Albright syndrome:* The triad of polyostotic fibrous dysplasia, café au lait spots, and precocious puberty.

## Monostotic disease

The usual age of discovery of a single lesion is in the second or third decade of life, although initial diagnosis may be made from childhood to old age.[5] There is a male to female ratio of from 1:1 to 1:3.[6]

**Fig. 2:** Radiodense lesions of fibrous dysplasia involving the sphenoid bone. The patient had diplopia and extra ocular muscle palsy.

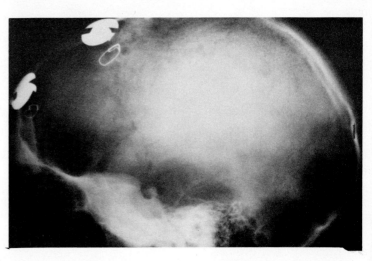

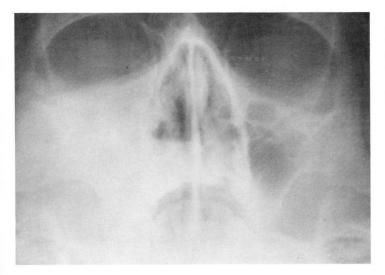

**Fig. 3:** This 23-year-old woman had chronic sinusitis and insidious right facial prominence. There is homogeneous increased density and expansion of the zygoma and maxilla. The maxillary sinus is obliterated by dysplastic bone.

A solitary lesion is not associated with precocious puberty or café au lait spots. The lesion usually becomes arrested at puberty. Harris, however, states that puberty has no affect on the number, size, recurrence, or complications of fibrous dysplasia.[8] Reactivation has also been reported during pregnancy.

The majority of the 67 patients with monostotic FD described by Schlumberger were asymptomatic, and the lesions were discovered as incidental findings on roentgenograms. A minority of patients presented with pathologic fractures, arthritic pain, deformity of facial bones or long bones, or because of a mass associated with an expanded superficial bone such as the clavicle or tibia.

Fourteen of the 67 patients described by Schlumberger had involvement of the skull. The maxilla, mandible, sphenoid, mastoid, and temporal bones were most frequently involved in that order.[4] Fibrous dysplasia involving the skull led to several signs and symptoms. The most common signs related to the local mass effect of the lesion (Fig. 2). Patients had asymmetry of the face, diplopia, partial loss of vision, and proptosis. Cranial nerves II-VIII were involved when there was encroachment on neural foramina.[4] Involvement of the paranasal sinuses may be accompanied by sinusitis (Fig.3).

## Polyostotic Fibrous Dysplasia

In this form of the disease, the onset of symptoms is much earlier than the monostotic form; two-thirds of the patients have symptoms before the age of 10.[7]

The bones most commonly involved are the femur, ilium, tibia, pubis, humerus, fibula, radius, scapula, and clavicle. The lesions tend to involve only one side of the body, often one extremity, although bilateral involvement is not unusual. When the proximal femur is involved, the corresponding ilium is usually involved as well (Figs. 4A, 4B, 8).

Whereas in monostotic disease there is no association with café au lait spots, in polyostotic disease spots are present in one-third of

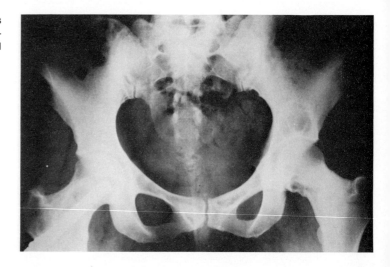

**Fig. 4A:** This 38-year-old woman has multiple FD lesions of the pelvis involving both pubic bones, both femoral necks and the iliac bone.

**Fig. 4B:** A coned down view of the left hip in the same patient demonstrates a pseudofracture (arrow) of the femoral neck.

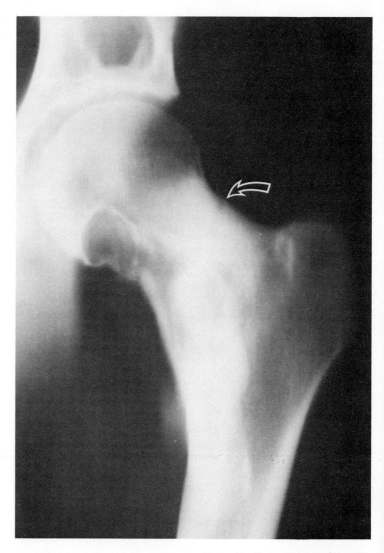

Bone Radiology Case Studies

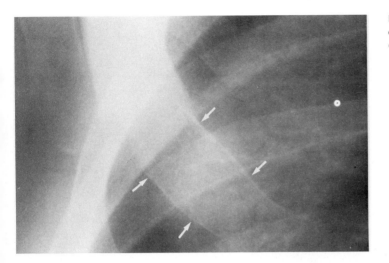

**Fig. 5:** Expansile rib lesion in a 20-year-old male seen on routine chest film. The cortex is thinned (arrows).

patients. Café au lait spots can be seen in other entities (ie, neurofibromatosis), but the contour of the abnormal pigmentation in fibrous dysplasia is distinctive. In fibrous dysplasia the contour is irregularly indented and has been likened to the coast of Maine, while in neurofibromatosis the margin of the spot has a smooth contour that has been likened to the coast of California. The color or histology of these skin lesions is not distinctive. The skin lesions tend to lie over bony lesions, often stop at midline, and are common over the spine and buttocks.

These patients have the same complications as patients with monostotic disease but the frequency and severity of these complications is much higher. In a review by Harris,[8] 85% of 37 patients had a pathologic fracture at some point in their life and 40% had three or more.

## Albright Syndrome

Only six boys with the syndrome have been reported. Premature menstruation begins during the first decade in one-half of girls having the syndrome. Short stature occurs due to early epiphyseal closure. Several other endocrine problems have been reported in Albright syndrome including: Cushing's disease, hyperthyroidism, hyperparathyroidism, acromegaly, and hypogonadism.[9-11] The significance of these later endocrinopathies is uncertain.

## Pathology

The unifying factors in the three categories of fibrous dysplasia are the radiographic and microscopic appearances of the bone lesions. The dysplastic tissue contains mature collagen that is solid, except for degenerative cystic areas containing fluid. The collagenous tissue contains varying amounts of trabecular bone and osteoid. Small amounts of cartilage may also be present.

The appearance of the bone within the lesion is characteristic and differentiates fibrous dysplasia from other fibrous lesions of bone. There are thin bony trabeculae that vary in shape and size. The trabeculae are randomly arranged forming "woven bone." Osteoblasts that form this bone are derived from surrounding fibrous tissue.

**Fig. 6:** FD involving the femoral neck with a homogeneous lucent lesion which has a sclerotic margin. In addition there is a pseudofracture (arrow).

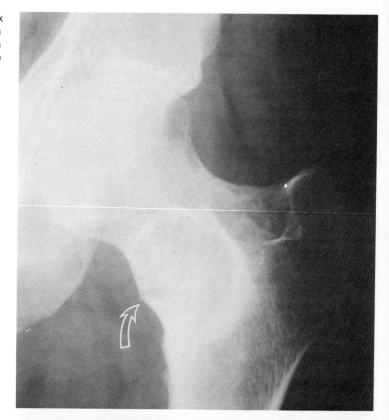

**Fig. 7:** This 13-year-old boy fractured his ulna (arrow). There is extensive fibrous dysplasia of the shaft proximal to the fracture.

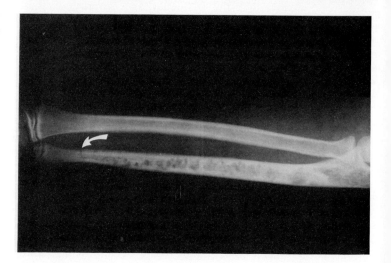

## Radiology

As with the microscopic appearance, there is no way to distinguish the different categories of fibrous dysplasia on the basis of a roentgenogram of a single lesion. In general, monostotic lesions are smaller than the individual lesions found in the polyostotic form. The roentgenographic appearance reflects replacement of medullary bone by dysplastic tissue. If the dysplastic tissue is

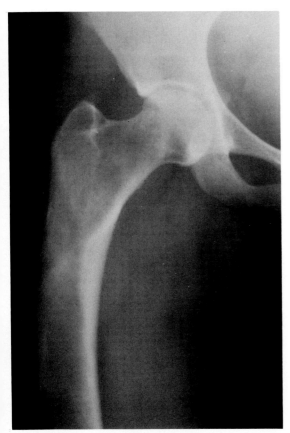

**Fig. 8:** There is bowing of the femur and thinning of the lateral cortex of the proximal shaft. The normal medullary trabeculae are replaced by homogeneous dysplastic bone. The patient had Albright's syndrome and had menarche at age 5.

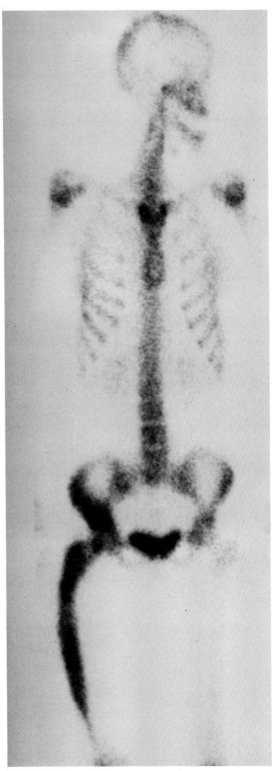

**Fig. 9:** Bone scan of the patient in Figure 7 demonstrating increased activity in the deformed femur and an associated lesion in the right iliac bone.

fibrous, the lesion is very lucent or even cyst like (Figs. 4, 5). If the dysplastic tissue is bony, the lesion is very dense (Figs. 2, 3). Differing amounts of bone, cartilage, and fibrous tissue result in varying radiographic density, but in all cases lesions are homogeneous.

There is a sharp zone of transition between normal bone and dysplastic bone. A sclerotic rim of density fading away from the lesion can often be seen around lucent lesions (Fig. 6). There is commonly expansion of the involved bone with thinning of the endosteal cortex (Fig. 5). When the lesion is dense, endosteal scalloping is obscured and the cortex appears to merge with the dysplastic bone (Fig. 1). The primary site of involvement usually is the metaphyseal-diaphyseal area, but the shaft of the bone may be involved by extensive lesions (Figs. 7, 8). In his initial description Albright said that the epiphysis is now involved by fibrous dysplasia, but Campbell states that the epiphyseal plate may be crossed.[3] There is no periosteal reaction unless the bone is fractured. In these cases, the bone heals in a normal amount of time with bony callus[3] and late cortical thickening.

Pseudofractures are found in fibrous dysplasia (Figs. 4B, 6) but are not distinctive since pseudofractures are also found in osteomalacia, Paget's disease, hyperphosphatasia, hypophosphatasia, osteogenesis imperfecta, and renal osteodystrophy.[9]

The lesions of fibrous dysplasia have shown increased activity on $Tc^{99}m$ MDP bone scans (Fig. 9), presumably due to vascularity of the lesions.

## Treatment

Multiple medical treatments have been used in an attempt to halt progressive lesions. No treatment, including hormonal therapy for Albright syndrome, has been effective.[12] Radiation therapy has also been attempted without benefit. There have been isolated reports of sarcomatous degeneration, both in radiated and non-radiated lesions.[13]

The surgeon may be called upon to treat deformity or fractures due to known FD or to biopsy an undiagnosed lesion. A biopsy site may later be the site of a pathologic fracture unless accompanied by curettage and bone grafts.

The treatment of fractures depends on the bone involved and the extent of the lesion. Most fractures heal with standard treatment, but the proximal femur is a difficult area. Acetabular and femoral deformities are common and can complicate treatment.

Plating of a fracture may be followed by a fracture of the more distal shaft. One or more osteotomies may be necessary to treat the associated deformities. Some deformities in the femoral neck require local resection for the relief of pain.

—*David Gibson, MD*

### References

1. Albright F, Butler A, Hampton A, et al: Syndrome charactersized by osteitis fibrosa disseminata, areas of pigmentation and endocrine dysfunction, with precocious puberty in females. *N Engl J Med* 1937; 216:727-747.

2. Lichtenstein L, Jaffe H: Fibrous dysplasia of bone. *Arch of Pathology* 1942; 33:77-816.
3. Schlumberger HG: Fibrosa dysplasia of single bones (monostotic fibrous dysplasia). *Military Largeon,* 1946; 99:504.
4. Finney HL: Fibrous dysplasia of the skull with progressive cranial nerve involvement. *Surgical neurology* December 1976; 6:341.
5. Spjut H, Dorfman H, Fechser R, et al: *Tumors of bone and cartilage.* Washington DC, Institute of Pathology, 1970.
6. Jaffe H: *Tumors and tumerous conditions of the bone and joints.* Philadephia, Lea & Febiger, 1958.
7. Grabiar S, Campbell C: Fibrous dysplasia. October 1977 18:771.
8. Harris W, Dudley R, Barry R: The national history of fibrous dysplasia. *J Bone Joint Surg* 1962; 44A:207.
9. Shires R, Whyte MP, Avioli LV: Idiopathic hyperthalamic hypogonatrophic hypogonadism with polystotic fibrous dysplasia. *Arch Int Med* October 1979; 193:1187.
10. Richter SM, Maclarin NK, McLaughlin JV, et al: Albright syndrome presenting as thyrotoxicosis: followups of a case. *Pediatrics* January 1979; 63:159.
11. Howard CP, Haylen AB: Hyperthyroidism in childhood. *Clinical Endocrinology and Metabolism* March 1978; 7:127.
12. Case Records of the Massachusetts General Hospital: Case 4-1975. *N Engl J Med* 1975; 292:199.
13. Riddell DM: Malignant changes in fibrous dysplasia. *J Bone Joint Surg* 1969; 46-B:251.
14. Funk JF, Wells RE: Hip problems in fibrous dysplasia. *Clin Orthop* Jan-Feb 1973; 90:77.
15. Greenfield GB: *Radiology of Bone Disease.* Philadelphia, JB Lippincott 1975. 1975.

# Study 21

This 58-year-old man has been in good health. He has had intermittent pain in the distal thigh for more than one year. The pain is not related to activity and has become worse lately. *Your diagnosis?*

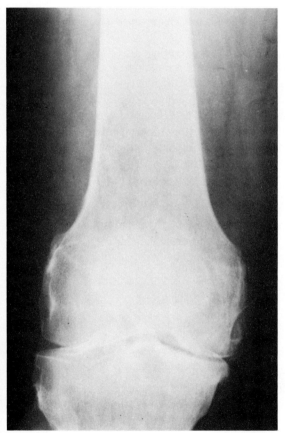

Fig. 1: AP, right femur.

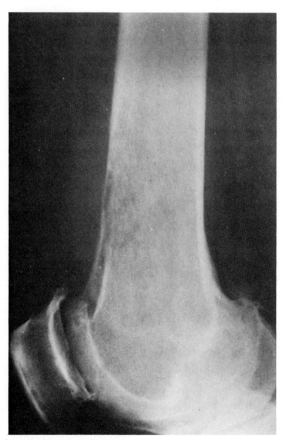

Fig. 2: Lateral, right femur.

# Diagnosis: Primary Lymphoma of Bone

Roentgenograms of patients with disseminated Hodgkin's and non-Hodgkin's lymphoma demonstrate bony involvement in 10-25% of cases. Much less commonly, lymphoma manifests as a primary bone lesion. Primary lymphoma of bone comprises about 5% of all primary bone neoplasms,[1] and has been called reticulum cell sarcoma, histiocytic lymphoma, lymphoma, and non-Hodgkin's lymphoma of bone. Criteria used to assure that a bone lesion is primary rather than secondary are:
1. Histologic study of the bone specimen must indicate lymphoma.
2. A solitary bone is involved.
3. If metastases are present only regional lymph nodes are involved at the time of diagnosis.[2]

Reticulum cell sarcoma of bone is primarily a disease of young and middle-aged adults. About one half of cases occur in the third and fourth decades. Older patients are also affected, but this neoplasm is rare under age ten.[3] Occurrence is slightly greater in men than in women.

The general health of the patient usually is not affected. This neoplasm grows slowly. Even when the local lesion is extensive, systemic signs and symptoms are absent or minimal. In a series of 98 patients the most common complaint was local pain (90%); 30% of the patients had noted a mass. Physical examination disclosed masses in 50%. Duration of symptoms is longer than most primary bone neoplasms; in one report mean duration was 14 months.[3] In another study one-third of the patients had symptoms lasting longer than two years.[4] The mass is usually tender. When the distal bone is involved, a joint effusion can occur. Pathologic fractures are relatively common.

Primary lymphoma of bone is one of the group of round cell tumors of bone. Others in this group include:

Ewing's sarcoma
Primary lymphoma
Disseminated lymphoma
Neuroblastoma
Leukemia
Metastasis
Myeloma
Eosinophilic granuloma

The histology of primary bone lymphoma may be difficult to differentiate from other round cell tumors or even infection. In one series of 21 patients there were initial errors in diagnosis in about one-third. Three were mistaken for eosinophilic granuloma, two for Ewing's sarcoma, and single cases for synovioma, metastatic carcinoma, and fibrous dysplasia.[4]

The proper diagnosis of primary bone lymphoma is especially important because the prognosis for a patient with Ewing's sarcoma is much less favorable than the prognosis for primary lymphoma. Cells in primary lymphoma of bone are larger and contain more cytoplasm, and staining reveals abundant intercellular reticular fibers. There may be admixed lymphocytes, lymphoblasts and Reed-Sternberg-like cells. Ewing's sarcoma cells contain glyogen. Electron microscopy is helpful, but no histologic or histo-chemical findings are absolute.[5] Unlike patients with primary lymphoma of bone, those with Ewing's sarcoma are likely to be younger and have more prominent systemic symptoms.

Bones most frequently affected by primary lymphoma of bone are the pelvis, femur, and humerus. Most cases occur at one of these sites. The ribs, jaw and tibia are less common sites. The hands, feet, and forearm are rarely involved.

The roentgenographic appearance is usually that of a malignant process, but primary lymphoma of bone cannot be diagnosed by roentgenogram. In long bones the diaphysis or metaphysis may be involved. The characteristic finding is bone destruction, which ranges from multiple coalescent patches of destruction ("moth-

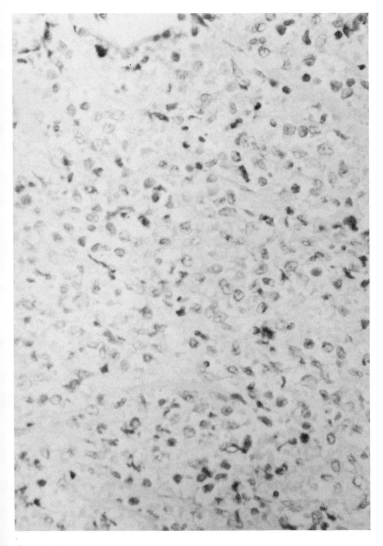

**Fig. 3:** Multiple sections of the surgical specimen showed a very cellular neoplasm. The pleomorphic cells have clear cytoplasm and compact or vesicular nuclei, many indented. There are scattered lymphocytes and groups of lymphocytes. Reticulum stain showed abundant reticular fibers. Diagnosis: Reticulum cell sarcoma of bone. In Figure 1, bone destruction is barely visible. Figure 2 shows permeating bone destruction of the distal femur with almost complete loss of the anterior cortex and an adjacent soft-tissue mass, all consistent with a malignant lesion.

eaten") to almost innumerable small holes riddling the bone (permeative). Often the cortex is involved; the cortex may be broken through completely. Pathologic fracture is relatively common. Periosteal reaction, when present, is not prominent. A soft-tissue mass is common. Calcification does not occur in the soft-tissue tumor mass, but there may be sclerosis of bone in addition to lysis of bone. This increased density represents reactive sclerosis rather than calcification or ossification of the tumor matrix.[3,6,7] Metastases involve regional nodes, other bones, and the lungs, in descending order of frequency.

These neoplasms have an indolent course, with five-year survival in up to 50% of patients.[3,4,6,8] Successful treatment has included surgery, radiation, and a combination of the two. Radiation is regarded as the treatment of choice in most cases.[3,4,6] Chemotherapy has provided prolonged remissions in advanced cases.[8]

### References

1. Spjut HJ, Dorfman HD, Fechner RE, et al: *Tumors of Bone and Cartilage.* Washington DC, Armed Forces Inst Path, 1971.
2. Potdar GG: Primary reticulum-cell sarcoma of bone in western India. *Brit J Cancer* 1970; 24:49.
3. Boston HC, Dahlin DC, Ivins JF, et al: Malignant lymphoma (so-called reticulum cell sarcoma) of bone. *Cancer* 1974; 34:1131.
4. Wang CC, Fleischli DJ: Reticulum cell sarcoma of bone. *Cancer* 1968; 22:994.
5. Rice RW, Cabot A, Johnston AD: The application of electron microscopy to the diagnostic differentiation of Ewing's sarcoma and reticulum cell sarcoma of bone. *Clin Orthop* 1973; 91:174.
6. Shoji H, Miller TR: Primary reticulum cell sarcoma of bone. *Cancer* 1971; 28:1234.
7. Ngan H, Preston BJ: Non-Hodgkin's lymphoma presenting with osseous lesions. *Clin Radiol* 1975; 26:351.
8. Reimer RR, Chabner BA, Young RC, et al: Lymphoma presenting in bone. *Ann Int Med* 1977; 87:50.

# Section V

# *PERIOSTEUM*

When the periosteum is elevated by pus, blood, edema, or neoplastic tissue, its osteogenic inner layer may produce bone which is visible on radiographs. Periosteal new bone formation is sometimes the primary or sole indicator of abnormality, and the radiographic pattern of new bone formation is a good indicator of the aggressiveness of a process. An "expanded" cortex overlies a process indolent enough to allow the periosteum to maintain an intact confining shell despite endosteal osteoclastic bone removal. When the periosteum is lifted by a chronic or self-limited process, the new bone which is formed may eventually result in cortical thickening. Before this new bone blends with the cortex, it may form a thick continuous band of solid periosteal new bone. A thin, single lamina or a laminated appearance are the result of single or multiple episodes of periosteal elevation.

An aggressive process may break through and destroy the central portion of a lifted periosteum, leaving the near and far edges of the lifted periosteum intact and thus producing an interrupted pattern. In some cases the new bone formed by the intact periosteal remnant forms an angle with the cortex; this angle is called a *Codman's triangle*. This sign indicates an aggressive process but is not pathognomonic of malignancy. Spiculated periosteal new bone formation indicates a very aggressive lesion and is often the result of malignancy. Spicules of new bone may be thin and perpendicular to the cortex, radiate from a point, or be thick and slanted. Spiculated new bone may be laid down on Sharpey fibers or radially-oriented periosteal vessels. Amorphous new bone is found with benign and malignant conditions and has an irregular, coarse appearance.

# Study 22

This 13-year-old boy had trivial trauma to his leg six months previously. *Your diagnosis?*

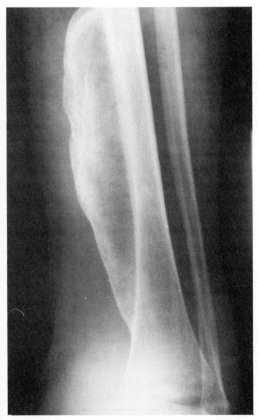

**Fig. 1:** AP roentgenogram of the right tibia and fibula.

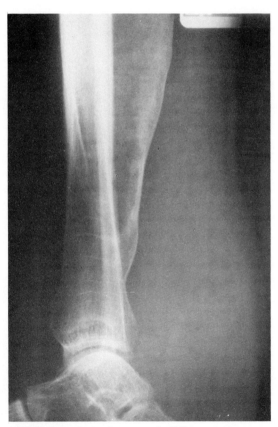

**Fig. 2:** Lateral roentgenogram of the right tibia and fibula.

# Diagnosis: Neurofibromatosis

## Incidence

The neurocutaneous syndromes include tuberous sclerosis, Sturge-Weber syndrome, von Hippel-Lindau disease, ataxia-telangiectasia, and neurofibromatosis (von Recklinghausen's disease). Neurofibromatosis (NF), a hereditary hamartomatous dysplasia, is the most common of these.

Neurofibromatosis can involve all three germ cell layers, and may affect any organ system of the body.[1,2] There is remarkable variation in the extent of the disease. Some patients have only a few inconspicuous skin lesions, no symptoms and live a normal life, while other patients have extensive crippling deformities, develop malignancies, and die young. The incidence of neurofibromatosis is about 1:3000 births. It is transmitted as an autosomal dominant trait with incomplete (80%) penetrance. Up to 50% of cases are mutations.

## Manifestations

The most frequent manifestations of NF result from dysplasias involving neuroectoderm and mesoderm; tan, smooth, sharply defined cafe' au lait skin spots; cutaneous and subcutaneous neurofibromas; central nervous system abnormalities; and skeletal lesions. Definitive diagnosis is based on the presence of two or more biopsy-proven neurofibromas.[1]

Skin lesions include:

    Cafe' au lait spots
    Cutaneous and subcutaneous neurofibromas
    Plexiform neurofibromas
    Giant nevi
    Axillary freckling
    Hemi-hypertrophy.

Cafe' au lait spots are quite common and are an important

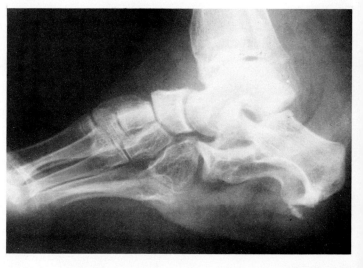

**Fig. 3:** Lateral roentgenogram of the right foot. In Figures 1 and 2 there is elephantoid soft tissue hypertrophy and a large calcified residual of a subperiosteal hematoma. There is dysplastic deformity of the bones of the foot of the same extremity, along with hypertrophied soft tissue. Massive subperiosteal hemorrhage secondary to trivial trauma is a very uncommon feature of neurofibromatosis. It may be due to a loosely attached periosteum. This massive subperiosteal hemorrhage usually occurs in an elephantoid extremity, and the combination of the two nonspecific findings indicates the correct diagnosis.

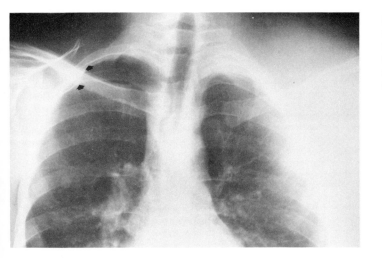

**Fig. 4:** Chest roentgenogram showing soft tissue density and left scapular displacement due to a malignant schwannoma in a 25-year-old man with neurofibromatosis. (Note marginal rib defects seen best at arrows.)

diagnostic feature. They are often the initial abnormality of NF and frequently can be found at birth, usually on the dorsal trunk or buttocks.[2] One or two spots are found in 23% of children less than six years old, while more than two spots are found in less than 1%. A child less than six years old with five or more 0.5 cm spots has neurofibromatosis unless proven otherwise.[3] Six or more 1.5 cm spots in an adult are presumptive evidence of NF.[4] Axillary freckling with numerous small spots is diagnostic, but is always accompanied by other characteristic skin changes. The soft cutaneous nodules of NF have long been called "fibroma molluscum," denoting fibrous tissue, but electron microscopy has demonstrated neural tissue in these nodules, so that actually they are a form of neurofibroma.[1] They usually appear at puberty and are seldom seen at birth. Subcutaneous neurofibromas may be palpable along peripheral nerves. Plexiform neurofibromas cause disfiguring masses and elephantoid soft tissue hypertrophy. They have a definite malignant potential, whereas cutaneous nodules rarely become malignant. The overall incidence of neurofibrosarcoma (Fig. 4) is 3-5%. Giant nevi may develop into malignant melanomas.[1]

Skeletal abnormalities are present in 30 to 70% of patients and include[1,2,6-8]:

Kyphoscoliosis
Overgrowth and undergrowth
Dysplastic deformity and defects
Erosive defects
Macrocranium
Pseudoarthrosis
Subperiosteal hemorrhage
Intraosseous cystic lesions.

Kyphoscoliosis resulting from bone dysplasia is the most common skeletal expression (10-40%) of NF.[9] Conversely, 3% of 3,209 patients with scoliosis had NF.[10] A severe, short, angular curve of the lower thoracic spine involving four to six vertebra is characteristic of NF but occurs in a minority of patients (Figs. 5,6).

Most patients have nonspecific deformity, often identical to idiopathic scoliosis.[9] The deformity tends to be progressive, even after fusion. An interesting but nonspecific finding is posterior vertebral scalloping (Fig. 7). This finding is attributed to dural ectasia demonstrated by myelography. Anterior and lateral scalloping have been reported, so vertebral dysplasia is another factor.[11] Enlarged intervertebral foramina usually are due to erosion by "dumbbell" neurofibromas or lateral meningoceles, but can also be secondary to bone dysplasia with no mass lesion present (Fig. 8).

Bones may be small or enlarged. Enlarged bones usually are associated with soft tissue overgrowth. Curved, thin, and deformed bones (Fig. 3) can be the result of primary dysplasia or secondary to soft tissue overgrowth and adjacent neoplasms.[1] Ribs can have discrete marginal defects (Fig. 4) or a "twisted ribbon" appearance (Fig. 9).

The majority of children with congenital pseudoarthrosis of the leg have NF. Anterolateral tibial bowing precedes the pseudo-arthrosis, which often occurs following spontaneous fracture or osteotomy (Fig. 10).[12,13] Often the tibia is locally constricted and

**Fig. 5:** Spine of a 15-year-old boy who has short segment scoliosis. Computed tomography demonstrated bilateral paraspinal soft tissue masses. Most kyphoscoliosis in NF is due to meso-dermal dysplasia of the spine rather than to neurofibromatous tissue.

**Fig. 6:** Spine and pelvis, showing cuta-neous nodules over the right upper quadrant. The transverse processes of L4,5 are dysplastic. Isolated lumbar scoliosis in NF is rare. Cervical scoliosis in children is highly suggestive of the diagnosis, however.[2]

Figure 5

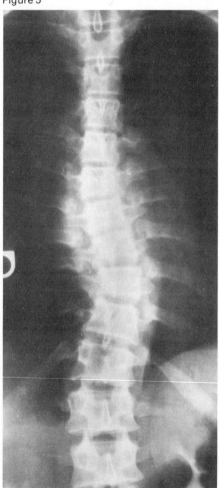

Figure 6

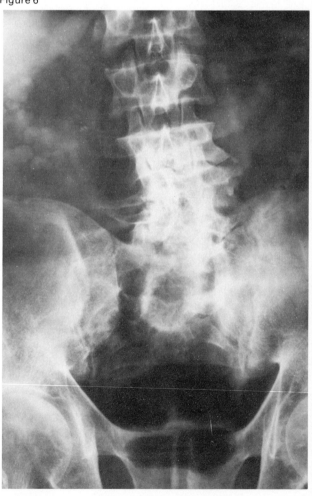

Bone Radiology Case Studies

sclerotic in addition to being bowed prior to fracture. There is no neurofibromatous tissue at the site of the pseudoarthrosis. A congenital pseudoarthrosis present at birth, with accompanying congenital anomalies such as club foot and soft tissue constriction bands, is not associated with NF.[13] NF pseudoarthrosis also may involve the fibula alone or both tibia and fibula. Less often the bones of the forearm are involved. The prognosis for these lesions is poor, and treatment often requires multiple surgical procedures.

Extensive subperiosteal hemorrhage can occur following trivial trauma. Subsequent calcification of the lifted periosteum results in a dramatic lesion (Figs. 1, 2). Most cases have been in a bone of an elephantoid extremity. A loose periosteal attachment has been implicated as a cause of this unusual finding in NF.[14,15]

While erosions are common in NF, intraosseous cystic lesions are rare (Fig. 11). Intraosseous lesions that have been biopsied contained no neural tissue,[2] and probably are coincidental lesions.

In the skull, most defects are the result of bone dysplasia and occur commonly in the posterior superior wall of the orbit (Fig. 12) and along the lambdoid suture. Lambdoidal defects usually are left-sided (Fig. 13), and almost always associated with NF.[16]

Central nervous system problems (19-50%) include:[1,2,6]
  Macrocephaly
  Optic glioma
  Acoustic neuroma

**Fig. 7:** Spine, showing posterior scalloping of the lumbar vertebra. This is a nonspecific finding found with intraspinal pathology and a number of other systemic diseases such as Marfan's disease, acromegaly, pseudoxanthoma elasticum, and cutis laxa.

**Fig. 8:** Cervical spine, showing marked bone erosion and intervertebral foramen widening due to neurofibroma.

Figure 7

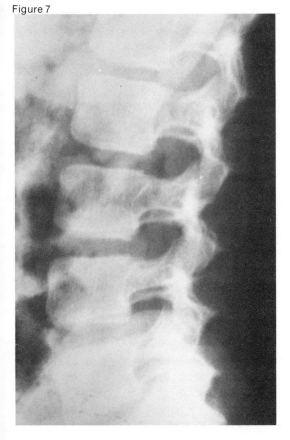

Figure 8

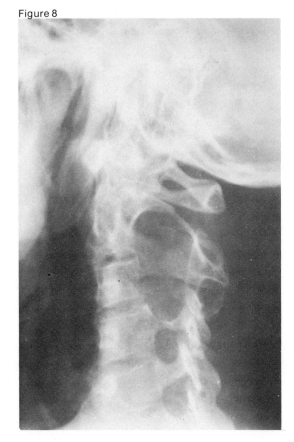

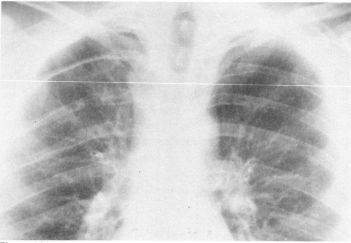

Figure 10

**Fig. 9:** The right 3-6 ribs have a "twisted ribbon" appearance, while the left 3, 4 ribs have inferior marginal defects.

**Fig. 10:** Tibia and fibula, demonstrating congenital pseudoarthrosis due to neurofibromatosis in a 6-year-old boy.

Figure 9

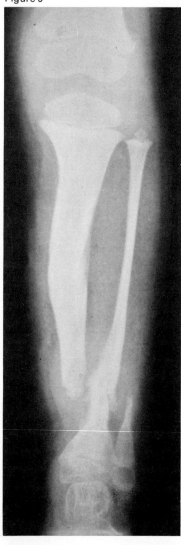

Other neoplasms
Syringomyelia
Lateral meningocele
Obstructive hydrocephalus.

Many patients have large heads due to brain enlargement. Some degree of mental retardation is common. Ophthalmic problems are prominent. Optic gliomas often cause decreased vision before 20 years of age. Exophthalmos can result from dysplastic bony defects of the orbit (Fig. 12), enlargement of the globe, or orbital neoplasm. A characteristic finding is a puffy, drooping, upper eyelid with inferior displacement of the globe, caused by a plexiform neurofibroma, blepharoptosis. Small nodules of the iris are frequent.[1,2]

While most of the patients with optic gliomas (Fig. 14) have NF, bilateral acoustic neuromas are diagnostic of NF.[2] In NF, intracranial and spinal neoplasms tend to be multiple and include meningioma, glioma, ependymoma, hamartoma, and neurofibroma. Hydrocephalus can result from aqueductal stenosis or neoplasm.[17] Syringomyelia occurs in association with other CNS problems. Lateral meningoceles may be seen on chest roentgenographs as posterior mediastinal masses. Differentiation from neural tumors can be made with ultrasound or computed tomography.

Most neurofibromas found in the gastrointestinal tract are unrelated to neurofibromatosis, and symptomatic lesions of the GI tract are rare in NF.

Genitourinary tract involvement is rare. Plexiform neurofibromas of the pelvic autonomic plexus can involve the distal ureters and bladder, with displacement and obstruction. Rarely, neurofibroma originates in the bladder wall.[1]

Cardiovascular lesions include pulmonic valve stenosis, coarctation of the abdominal aorta, stenosis of major arteries, intracranial occlusive disease, and microaneurysms. In a child with NF hypertension usually results from renal artery stenosis. In an adult it is usually due to a pheochromocytoma.[2]

176

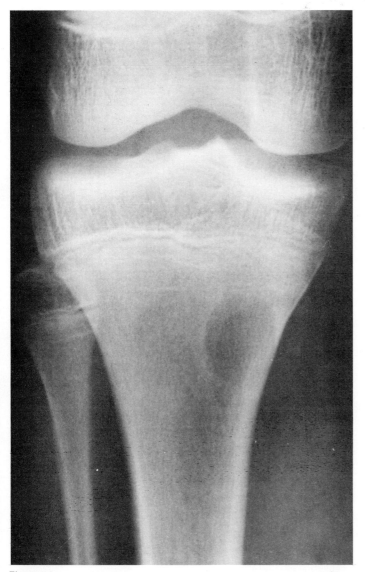

Figure 11

**Fig. 11:** Only a few intraosseous cystic lesions have been reported in NF and are probably incidental findings. This cystic-appearing lesion of the tibia is actually a marginal erosion seen en face and is produced by a posterior neurofibroma.

**Fig. 12:** Waters view of skull. The left orbit is enlarged and a defect in the orbital wall is evidenced by loss of the oblique orbital line (normal oblique line of the right orbit indicated by arrow). The patient had exophthalmos.

Figure 12

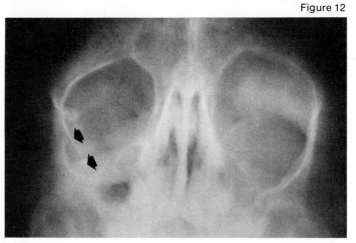

**Fig. 13:** Towne view of skull. A dysplastic calvarial bone defect along the lambdoid suture is usually the result of NF. Most are on the left side as in this patient with NF (contrast material is from a previous myelogram).

**Fig. 14:** An optic canal greater than 7 mm in diameter (large arrow indicates enlarged optic canal; small arrow indicates normal optic canal) is abnormal. This patient with NF had an optic glioma. Enlarged canals can result from bone dysplasia alone.

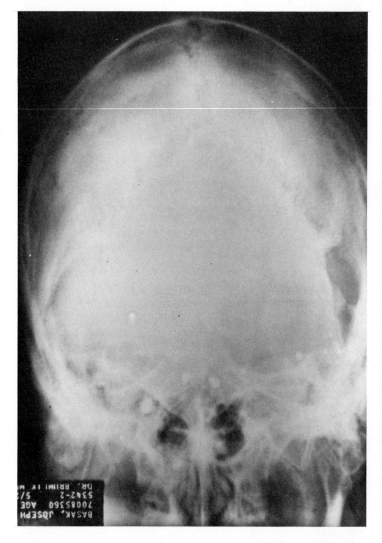

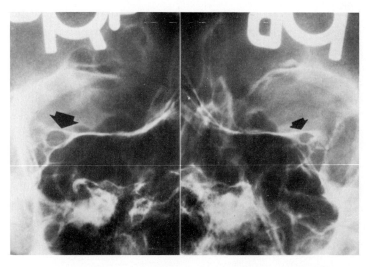

A few patients with NF have interstitial fibrosis of the lung, nonspecific in appearance. A neural neoplasm or lateral meningocele may present as a posterior mediastinal mass. A vagal neurofibroma can present as a superior mediastinal mass.

Endocrine problems associated with NF include[1,2]:

  Pheochromocytoma
  Hyperparathyroidism
  Osteomalacia
  Precocious or late puberty
  Reduced fertility
  Diabetes insipidus.

Pheochromocytoma is best documented. Multiple endocrine adenopathy type IIB (medullary carcinoma of the thyroid, pheochromocytoma, and multiple neuromas with Marfanoid habitus) is not related to neurofibromatosis.[1]

## Discussion

A patient with congenital lower extremity dysplastic bowing or pseudoarthrosis, severe, short angular scoliosis, elephantoid extremity, calvarial bone defects, optic glioma or acoustic neuroma should be examined closely for café au lait spots, which are present in a large majority of patients with this complex neurocutaneous syndrome described by von Recklinghausen.

### References

1. Wander JV, Das Gupta TK: Neurofibromatosis. *Curr Probl Surg* 1977; 14:3.
2. Holt JF: Neurofibromatosis in children. *Am J Roentgenol* 1978; 130:615.
3. Whitehouse D: Diagnostic value of the café-au-lait spot in neurofibromatosis. *Arch Dis Child* 1966; 41:316.
4. Crowe FW, Schull WJ: *A Clinical, Pathological and Genetic Study of Multiple Neurofibromatosis.* Springfield, Charles C. Thomas, 1956.
5. Knight WA, Murphy WK, Gottlieb JA: Neurofibromatosis associated with malignant neurofibromas. *Arch Dermatol* 1973; 107:747.
6. Casselman ES, Miller WT, Lin SR, et al: Von Recklinghausen's disease: Incidence of roentgenographic finding with clinical review of the literature. *CRC Crit Rev Diagn Imaging* 1977; 9:387.
7. Klatte EC, Franken EA, Smith JA: The radiographic spectrum in neurofibromatosis. *Semin Roentgenol* 1976; 11:17.
8. Meszaros WT, Guzzo F, Schorsch H: Neurofibromatosis. *Am J Roentgenol* 1966; 98:557.
9. Chaglassian JM, Riseborough ES, Hall JE: Neurofibromatous scoliosis. *J Bone Joint Surg* 1976; 58A:695.
10. Rezaian SM: The incidence of scoliosis due to neurofibromatosis. *Acta Orthop Scand* 1976; 47:534.
11. Casselman ES, Mandell GA: Vertebral scalloping in neurofibromatosis. *Radiology* 1979; 131:89.
12. Andersen KS: Congenital pseudoarthrosis of the tibia and neurofibromatosis. *Acta Orthop Scand* 1976; 47:108.
13. Andersen KS: Congenital pseudoarthrosis of the leg. *J Bone Joint Surg* 1976; 58A:657.
14. Pitt MJ, Mosher JF, Edeiken J: Abnormal periosteum and bone in neurofibromatosis. *Radiology* 1972; 103:143.
15. Yaghmai I, Tafazoli M: Massive subperiosteal hemorrhage in neurofibromatosis. *Radiology* 1977; 122:439.
16. Gupta SK, Nema HV, Bhatia PL: The radiology of craniofacial neurofibromatosis. *Clin Radiol* 1979; 30:553.
17. Pollnitz R: Neurofibromatosis in childhood: A review of 25 cases. *Med J Aust* 1976; 2:49.

# Study 23

This 77-year-old man has an enlarged right thigh which is painful.
*Your diagnosis?*

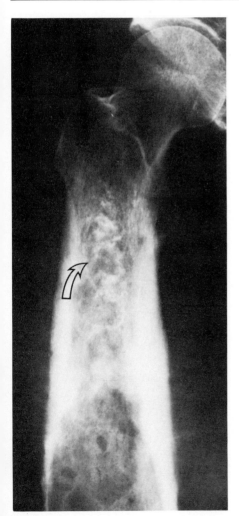

**Fig. 1A:** AP view of right upper femur.

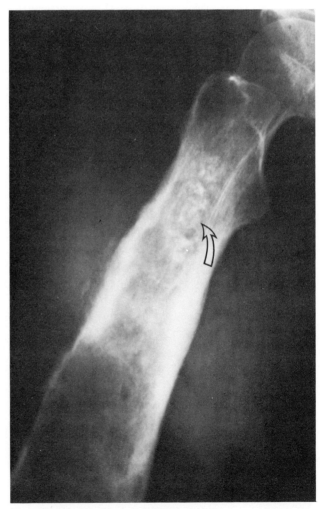

**Fig. 1B:** Lateral view of right upper femur.

# Diagnosis: Sarcomatous Degeneration of an Enchondroma

In Figure 1 there is a calcified enchondroma (arrows) of the proximal femur. The cortex distally is thickened and then thinned and there is spiculated periosteal new bone formation plus a soft tissue mass indicating the presence of sacromatous degeneration.

## Discussion

All enchondromas are secondary to failure of resorption and ossification of the growth plate cartilage. They are therefore cartilagenous hamartomas. Most are located in the metaphyseal region when in a long bone, or in the metaphyseal diaphyseal region of a short bone. The lesions consist of viable cartilage cells within an intercellular matrix composed of hyaline cartilage. The cells are uniformly small and round and the great majority have only single nucleii. The individual lesion in patients with multiple enchondromatosis is often more cellular than a solitary enchondroma.

Over 50% of the solitary lesions occur in the hands and feet. Of these, 90% occur in the hands making enchondroma the most common tumor of the hand.[1] The remainder of the lesions occur most often in the humerus, femur, tibia, fibula and ulna, but they can be found in any bone preformed in cartilage. Rare sites include

**Fig. 2:** Enchondromatosis with expansion of several phalanges and metacarpals and a typical longitudinal linear lucency of the distal ulnar (arrow).

**Fig. 3:** Multiple enchondromatosis involving humerus. Calcified soft tissue hemangioma (arrow) indicates that the patient has the Mafucci syndrome.

Figure 2

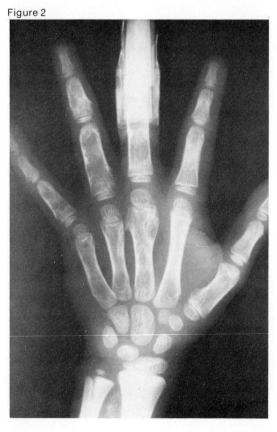

Figure 3

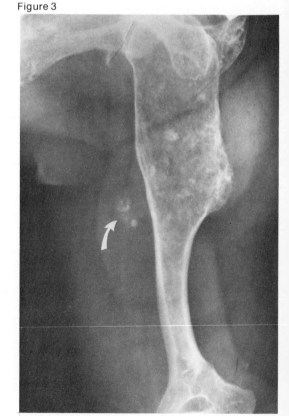

ribs, sternum, pelvis, vertebra, and the patella.

Multiple enchondromas occur as a non-hereditary bone dysplasia (Fig. 2). When the multiple lesions in enchondromatosis are found predominantly on one side of the body the eponym Ollier disease is applied. Maffuci reported the association of enchondromatosis and multiple soft tissue cavernous hemangiomas so that this rare condition is called Mafucci syndrome (Fig. 3).

Multiple enchondromatosis usually presents in early childhood because of fracture, limb bowing, growth abnormality or as swelling of the hand. This is in contrast to solitary enchondromas which usually present in the third or fourth decade and are often discovered after local trauma.[2] Enchondromas usually stop growing when the adjacent growth plate fuses and should not present any new signs or symptoms after puberty. Unless there has been trauma, any pain, swelling or radiographic change after puberty should be suspect for malignancy.[2,3]

The radiographic picture of an enchondroma in the hand is usually characteristic. There is a geographic lytic metaphyseal-diaphyseal lesion with a fairly sharp margin (Fig. 4). There may be bone "expansion" (Fig. 5), cortical thinning, or cortical thickening with endosteal scalloping. Calcification is discrete when present (Fig. 6) and often has a spotty or stippled appearance, characteristic of cartilage tumors.[4]

In long bones an enchondroma usually appears as a cluster of calcifications in the metadiaphysis (Fig. 7). Less often the only

**Fig. 4:** Oval lucent enchrondroma at base of middle finger with thinned but intact medial cortex.

**Fig. 5:** Enchondroma with gross expansion of the middle phalanx and a scalloped appearance of the affected bone.

Figure 4

Figure 5

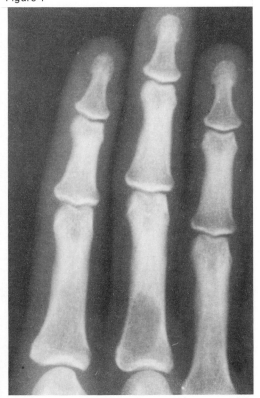

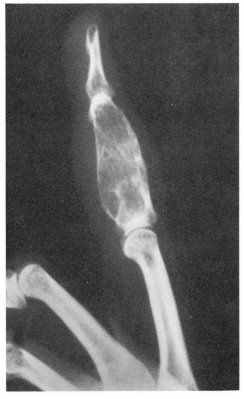

radiographic finding is a non-specific rounded lytic area. Patients with enchondromatosis may have radiolucent longitudinal streaks extending toward the diaphysis from the growth plate (Fig. 2). Periosteal reaction is absent unless a fracture or infarction supervenes.

In long bones an enchondroma must be differentiated from a medullary infarct which generally shows amorphous calcification within a lucent area and often has a thin sclerotic rim (Fig. 8). The calcification in an infarct may have a serpigenous appearance. Infarcts do not expand the bone. Osteochondromas can be confused with enchondromas when viewed in only one projection. Other diseases in the differential diagnosis include fibrous dysplasia, epithelial inclusion cyst, phalangeal sarcoid and chondromyxoid fibroma.[4,5]

Malignant change is extremely rare in solitary lesions in the hands but more frequent, although still rare, in long bones. Lesions closer to the axial skeleton have a higher potential for sarcomatous change.

Enchondromatosis is complicated by malignant degeneration more frequently than single lesions but the reported frequency of malignant change is quite variable.[2,5]

— *Manuel Alonso, MD*

**Fig. 6:** Expanded distal phalanx with thinned cortex and typical sharply defined cartilage calcification in an enchondroma. There is an infarction at the base of the phalanx.

**Fig. 7:** Enchondroma of mid-femur, which took up radioisotope on a bone scan. Note that the cluster of calcifications does not have a sclerotic rim. (Density at right cortex is normal linea aspera.)

Figure 6

Figure 7

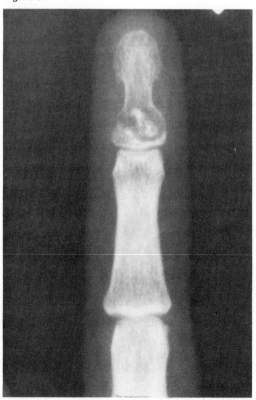

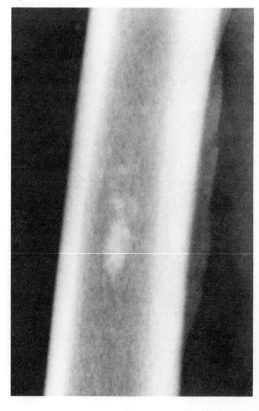

# References

1. Takigawa K: Chondroma of the bones of the hand. A review of 110 cases. *J Bone Joint Surg* 1971; 53A:1591-1600.
2. Aegerter E, Kirkpatrick JA: *Orthopedic Diseases,* ed 3. Philadelphia, WB Saunders, 1968.
3. Roberts PH, Price CHG: Chondrosarcoma of the bones of the hand. *J Bone Joint Surg* 1977; 59B:213-221.
4. Dahlin DC: *Bone Tumors,* Springfield, Charles C Thomas, 1980.
5. Greenfield GB: *Radiology of Bone Diseases,* Philadelphia, JB Lipincott, 1980.

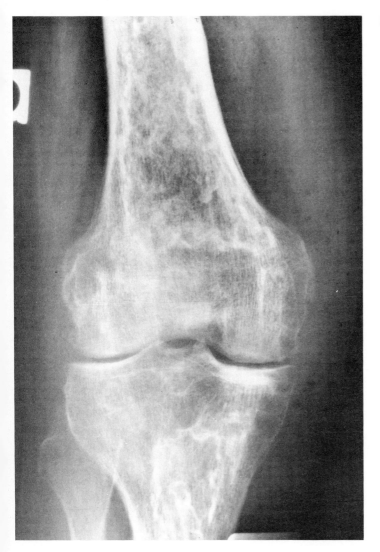

**Fig. 8:** Bone infarcts of femur and tibia. Note well-defined sclerotic rims.

# Study 24

This 56-year-old women has had a painful left foot for five years. She also has asymmetric swelling and stiffness of fingers of both hands. *Your diagnosis?*

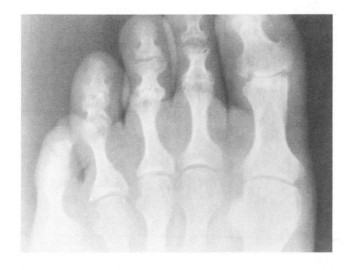

**Fig. 1:** AP roentgenogram. Toes of the left foot.

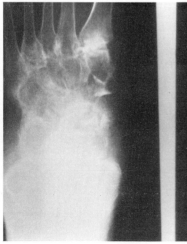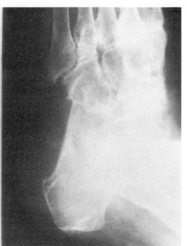

**Fig. 2:** AP and oblique roentgenograms of the left midfoot.

# Diagnosis: Psoriatic Arthritis

The patient has had psoriasis for 30 years and psoriatic arthritis for eight years. Her painful left foot was treated by triple arthrodesis. There is generalized narrowing of the joints of the mid-foot (Fig. 2). There is erosion and narrowing of multiple joints in Figure 1. The widening of several distal joints is characteristic of psoriatic arthritis. In addition, there is bony proliferation at the base of the phalanges of the great toe and several middle phalanges. The tuft of the second toe is eroded.

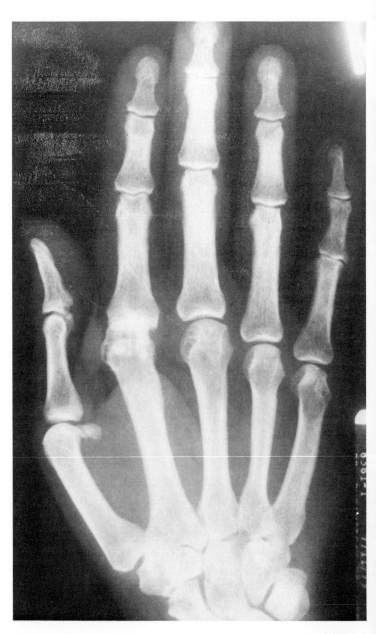

**Fig. 3:** Psoriatic arthritis with isolated involvement of the index finger (Ray pattern).

# Discussion

Psoriatic arthritis is defined as an inflammatory arthritis occurring in a patient with psoriasis who usually has a negative serologic test for rheumatoid factor.[1]

In the past some have felt that psoriatic arthritis was not a distinct entity. They felt that an inflammatory arthritis occurring in a patient with psoriasis simply represented the coincidental occurrence of rheumatoid arthritis. The analysis and follow-up of hundreds of patients, however, indicates that psoriatic arthritis is a distinct entity.[1-5] There are several features that distinguish psoriatic arthritis from rheumatoid arthritis.

1. The incidence of inflammatory arthritis in patients with psoriasis is 5 to 7%.[1] The incidence of rheumatoid arthritis in the general population is 1 to 2%.

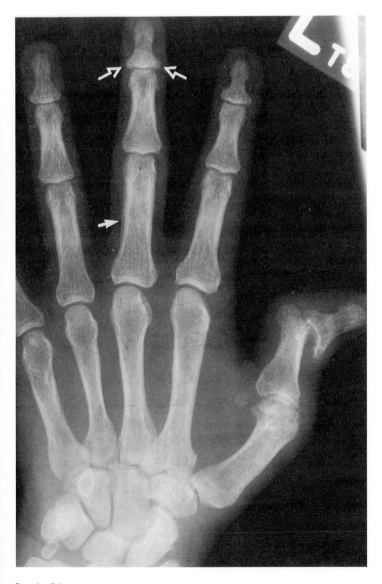

**Fig. 4:** Psoriatic arthritis with isolated severe involvement of the thumb. There is also subtle periosteal reaction (solid arrow), erosion of the tuft of the index finger, and subtle bony proliferation at the base of a phalanx (open arrows).

2. The female to male ratio of psoriatic arthritis is near 1:1. Rheumatoid arthritis has a female to male ratio of at least 3:1.
3. The incidence of positive serologic tests for rheumatoid factor in psoriatic arthritis is near the 5% incidence found in the general population.[2]
4. Rheumatoid nodules, vasculitis and pulmonary fibrosis found in rheumatoid arthritis do not occur in psoriatic arthritis.[1]
5. Sacroiliitis is found in 20 to 50% of patients with psoriatic arthritis but is rare in rheumatoid arthritis.[6]
6. The distribution and radiographic appearance of peripheral arthritis in psoriatic arthritis is sometimes distinctive and usually unlike rheumatoid arthritis.
7. Psoriatic arthritis causes less pain and disability than rheumatoid arthritis.[9]

The type and extent of psoriatic skin involvement is seldom related to the development or fluctuation of arthritis. In fact, some patients with easily identified inflammatory arthritis may have subtle psoriatic lesions confined to hidden areas such as the scalp, perineum, or umbilicus. An even more difficult diagnostic situation is encountered when a patient develops arthritis before any skin lesions appear. Psoriatic arthritis precedes psoriatic skin and nail lesions in 10 to 15% of patients.[2-4] In contrast to skin lesions, nail lesions correlate fairly well with the incidence and progress of arthritis.[1]

The clinical presentation of psoriatic arthritis is usually insidious but is occasionally acute. The most common presentation is asymmetric involvement of scattered joints including distal interphalangeal joints. Uncommonly an acute monoarticular onset may mimic gout. Since some patients with psoriasis have elevated serum uric acid, the only sure way to eliminate the possibility of gout when they present with monoarticular arthritis is to aspirate the joint and examine for urate crystals.

The selective involvement of distal interphalangeal joints in psoriatic arthritis has been emphasized in the literature. This predilection for distal joints is characteristic, when present, but is found in a minority of patients. The clinical presentation of psoriatic arthritis has been divided into several general categories:[7,9]


### Incidence

70%  (1) **Asymmetric arthritis** involving a few joints or a single joint of the hands and feet is most common. Scattered interphlangeal and metacarpophalangeal joints are affected. Distal IP joints may or may not be involved but distal involvement does not predominate. The carpals, tarsals, and large joints may also be involved. A frequent finding in this group of patients is diffuse "sausage" swelling of a single digit of the hand or foot due to joint involvement plus tendon sheath effusion.

15%  (2) **Symmetric arthritis:** This pattern is identical to rheumatoid arthritis. The negative test for rheumatoid factor is helpful in these patients.

5%   (3) **Predominant distal interphalangeal joint involvement of the hands and feet:** This "classic" presentation is not often seen.

5%   (4) **Arthritis mutilans.** There is advanced deformity of the hands and/or feet. The most striking finding is the "opera glass" hand in which the telescoped fingers (or toes) can be pulled in and out.

5%   (5) **Predominant sacroiliitis** with or with-out spondylitis. Peripheral joints may be involved also.

Roentgenograms complement clinical findings by indicating lesion distribution, joint cartilage loss, erosions, bone density, and bony proliferation. Abnormalities of the sacroiliac joints, spine, and calcaneus are often better evaluated by roentgenograms than by clinical findings.

## Roentgenographic Findings

### Distribution

Roentgenograms of the hands and feet reflect the clinical finding of asymmetric, scattered involvement of joints usually found in psoriatic arthritis. Roentgenographic involvement of a single digit is a corollary to the swollen "sausage" digit seen on physical examination (Figs. 3, 4). There may also be unilateral involvement of several joints. That is, multiple joints in only one hand or foot are affected. (These patterns are seldom seen in rheumatoid arthritis but are found in other types of seronegative polyarthritis). In the hands and feet interphalangeal, metacarpophalangeal, and metatarsophalangeal joints are most frequently involved. Involvement of the carpals and tarsals is less frequent (Fig. 2). Predominant distal involvement is characteristic of psoriatic arthritis but is an infrequent occurrence. Asymmetric, scattered joint disease with involvement of several distal joints, however, is very suggestive of psoriatic arthritis (Figs. 1, 5, 6, 7). (Erosive osteoarthritis also causes distal interphalangeal joint disease and will be considered later).

Large joints may also be affected by psoriatic arthritis (Fig. 8). The spine and sacroiliac joints are abnormal in up to 50% of patients.

### Bone Density

The bone density is usually normal but osteoporosis may be present, especially when arthritis is clinically active.

### Joint Space Abnormality

Joint space narrowing is usually uniform as in rheumatoid arthritis. In some patients with psoriatic arthritis, however, there is widening of the joint space. This most commonly occurs in the distal interphalangeal joints and is very suggestive of psoriatic arthritis (Fig. 1, 5, 7). In the big toe, however, a similar appearance is seen in Reiter's syndrome. Bony ankylosis is found in late stages (Fig. 9).

**Fig 5:** Psoriatic arthritis with multiple areas of erosion and joint space narrowing. Notice widening of distal joint spaces (open arrows), lateral "bare area" erosions (solid arrows), and lumpy periosteal reaction producing widening of the bases of multiple phalanges and sclerosis of the proximal phalanges of toes, 3, 4, and 5.

**Fig. 6:** Psoriatic arthritis with subluxations, wide spread joint narrowing, and erosions. Note distal interphalangeal joint erosions (arrows). There is also rotatory subluxation of the navicular.

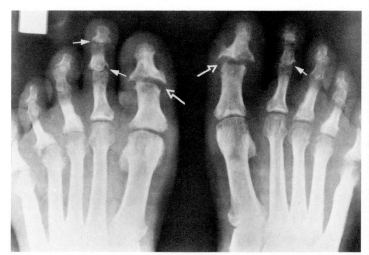

Figure 5

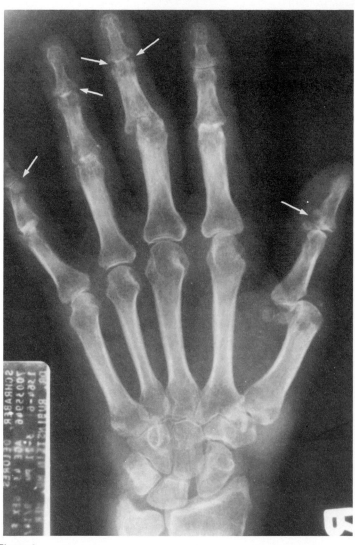

Figure 6

Bone Radiology Case Studies

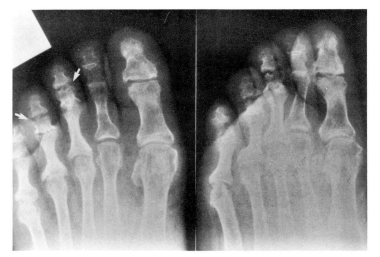

Figure 7

**Fig. 7:** Psoriatic arthritis with multiple narrowed joints and erosions. Note widened distal joints (arrows). Bony proliferation widens the bases of the proximal phalanges of the third, fourth, and fifth toes which are sclerotic.

**Fig. 8:** Psoriatic arthritis with a large erosion of the head of the humerus (arrow).

**Fig. 9:** Psoriatic arthritis with bony ankylosis of both great toes and tuft erosion. There is fluffy periarticular new bone at the bases of the phalanges (arrows) in addition to joint narrowing.

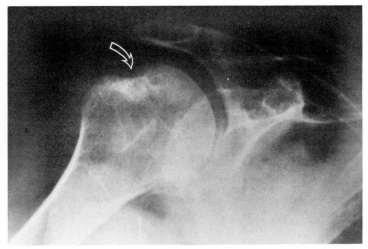

Figure 8

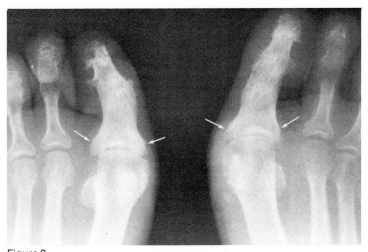

Figure 9

Study 24

193

**Fig. 10:** Psoriatic arthritis with a posterior calcaneal erosion just above the insertion of the achilles tendon (large arrow). Minimal erosion of a planter bone spur is also present (small arrow).

**Fig. 11:** Psoriatic arthritis with abnormalities of the thumb and little finger. The first metacarpophalangeal joint is eroded and subluxed. There is fluffy periosteal reaction of the little finger (arrows), radial styloid, and ulnar styloid.

**Fig. 12:** Psoriatic arthritis with narrowing and erosions of the joints of the great toe. Note fluffy periarticular new bone formation (arrow).

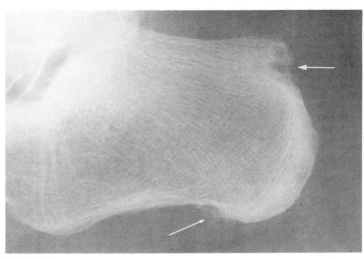

Figure 10

Figure 11

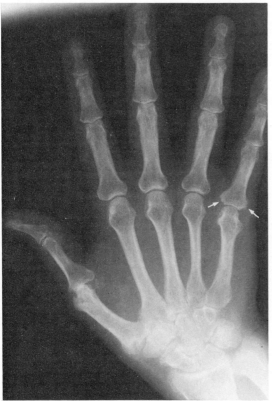

Figure 12

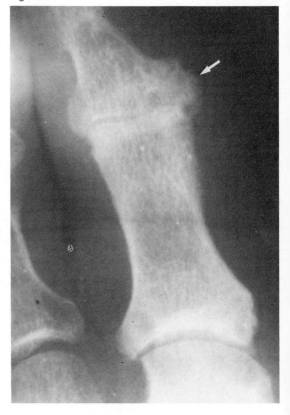

194

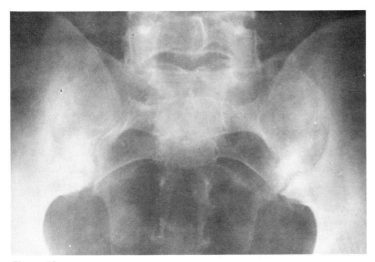

**Fig. 13:** Asymmetric psoriatic sacroiliitis. The right joint is eroded and there is iliac sclerosis. The left joint is less severely involved and there is iliac plus sacral sclerosis.

**Fig 14:** Psoriatic arthritis with a large asymmetric syndesmophyte bridging the L3-L4 interspace (arrows).

**Fig. 15:** Psoriatic arthritis with thin vertical syndesmophytes identical to those found in ankylosing spondylitis (open arrows). The space between the odontoid and the arch of C-1 is abnormally large (closed arrows).

Figure 13

Figure 14

Figure 15

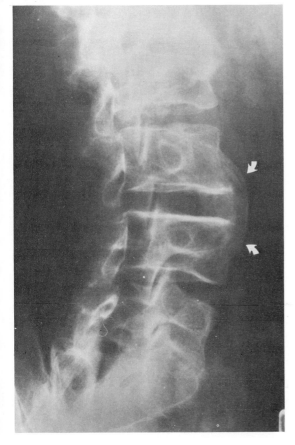

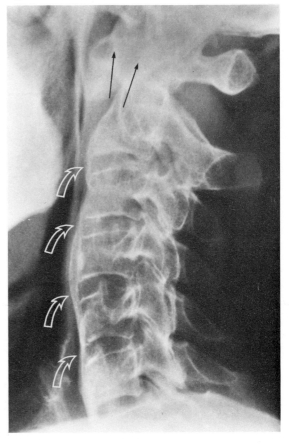

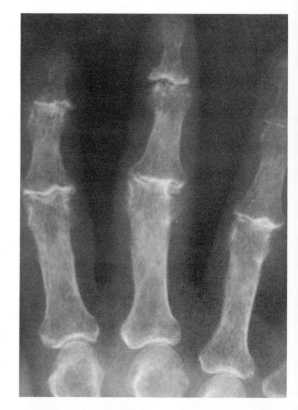

**Fig. 16:** Erosive osteoarthritis. The metacarpophalangeal joints are narrowed but not eroded. The distal joints are eroded but the intact cortical margins indicate that this is not psoriatic arthritis.

**Fig. 17:** Erosive osteoarthritis. Erosion of distal interphalangeal joints plus typical degenerative changes at first metacarpophalangeal joint.

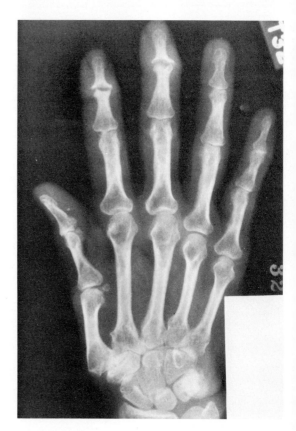

196

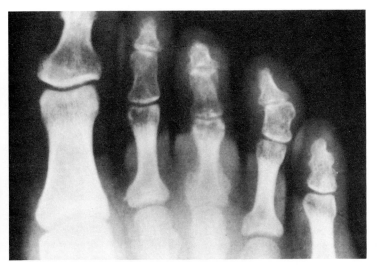

**Fig. 18A:** Reiter's syndrome. Periosteal new bone at base of third toe.

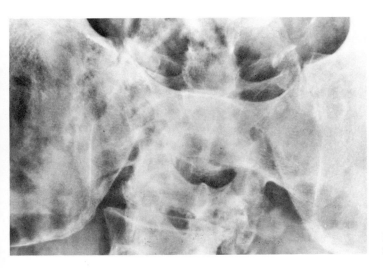

**Fig. 18B:** Bilateral sacroiliitis, worse on the left.

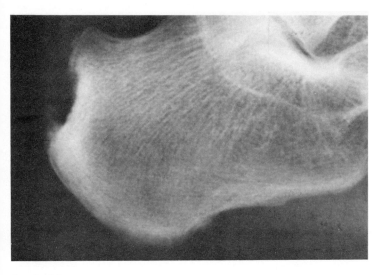

**Fig. 18C:** Erosion of posterior calcaneous with adjacent sclerosis.

### Erosions

Erosions of bone in psoriatic arthritis occur earliest in intra-articular bony "bare areas" which are unprotected by articular cartilage (Figs. 5, 6). They are no different than erosions found in other types of inflammatory arthritis. The calcaneus may be eroded at or near the site of insertion of the achilles tendon or plantar ligament (Fig. 10). This finding is not specific and is found in other types of seronegative polyarthritis and rheumatoid arthritis.[10] Tuft erosion, however, is characteristic of psoriatic arthritis (Figs. 1, 9).

### Bony Proliferation

Periosteal new bone is frequently found in psoriatic arthritis. It may be seen as a thin linear density (Fig. 4) paralleling the cortex of a bone but is much more often a lumpy periarticular density contiguous with the cortex (Figs. 4, 5, 7, 9, 11, 12). In long standing cases the periosteal new bone is incorporated into the cortex which then appears widened. Bony proliferation may also cause increased density of a bone, especially the calcaneus or phalanges (Figs. 5, 7).

### Deformity

In advanced cases subluxation and pencil-like deformity of bone ends occur. Joints may have a pencil in cup appearance. Severe deformity or arthritis mutilans is fortunately unusual.

### Sacroiliacs and Spine

The sacroiliac joints are abnormal in up to 50% of patients. The evidence of sacroiliitis may be symmetric or asymmetric (Fig. 13). Roentgenographic findings range from poorly defined joint margins and clearly eroded joint margins to bony ankylosis. Sclerosis about the joint may be isolated to the iliac side or include the sacral side of the joint.[8] Spine abnormalities are less frequent than sacroiliitis.

A few patients with psoriatic arthritis may have symmetric delicate vertical syndesmophytes bridging vertebrae with an appearance identical to ankylosing spondylitis. Apophyseal fusion, however, is infrequent. Most often the spine does not have the appearance of ankylosing spondylitis. Rather, large asymmetric bridging syndesmophytes are either solitary or separated by normal vertebrae (Fig. 14). Paravertebral bone formation has also been described.

Subluxation of C1 and C2 due to inflammatory changes in the ligaments fixing the odontoid to the axis is often found if a flexion view of the cervical spine is obtained (Fig. 15). This finding is also found in other types of inflammatory arthritis.[6]

Erosive osteoarthritis and Reiter's syndrome may be very difficult to differentiate from psoriatic arthritis. Erosive osteoarthritis is a self limited inflammatory arthritis of the hands and feet. The roentgenographic picture is similar to psoriatic arthritis with distal interphalangeal erosion, periosteal reaction, and bony ankylosis. The metacarpophalangeal joints may be narrowed but are never eroded which is an important differential point[3] (Figs. 16, 17). The vast majority of patients with erosive osteoarthritis are women and most are over 60 years of age, which is in contrast to the equal sex incidence and younger age of onset of psoriatic arthritis.

The roentgen manifestations of Reiter's syndrome may be very similar to those of psoriatic arthritis. Reiter's syndrome affects the lower extremities more often and more severely than psoriatic arthritis. Psoriatic arthritis may severely affect the feet, but severe foot involvement with absent or minimal hand involvement is more frequent in Reiter's syndrome (Figs. 18-20).

Reiter's syndrome does not affect *multiple* distal interphalangeal joints and does not cause tuft erosion. Rieter's syndrome is almost exclusively found in males.

## Summary

The inflammatory arthritis associated with psoriasis is a distinct entity which, in most cases, is separable from other types of arthritis on the basis of differences in clinical findings, serologic tests, and roentgenographic appearances. Psoriatic arthritis is one of the seronegative forms of inflammatory arthritis which are defined by negative serologic tests for rheumatoid factor. It is characterized on roentgenograms by asymmetric and scattered joint involvement. Hand and foot involvement is most frequent and may affect only one digit or may be unilateral. There is a tendency to affect distal interphalangeal joints which may be widened rather than narrowed. Periosteal new bone formation is common. Sacroiliitis is frequent. There may be bony ankylosis of interphalangeal joints and spinal syndesmophytes. Psoriatic arthritis may precede skin lesions. Reiter's syndrome and erosive osteoarthritis can closely resemble psoriatic arthritis.

Psoriatic arthritis is sometimes equated with a hand which is severely deformed by mutilating arthritis. These advanced changes are found, but only in a small minority of patients. Most patients with psoriatic arthritis have milder symptoms and less deformity than those with rheumatoid arthritis.

## References

1. Moll JM, Wright V: Psoriatic arthritis. *Sem Arthritis Rheum* 1973; 3:55.
2. Kammer GM, et al: Psoriatic arthritis: A clinical, immunologic and HLA study of 100 patients. *Sem Arthritis Rheum* 1979; 9:75.
3. Martel W, et al: Erosive osteoarthritis and psoriatic arthritis. *AJR* 1980; 134:125.
4. Roberts ME, et al: Psoriatic arthritis. *Ann Rheum Dis* 1976; 35:206.
5. Eastmond CJ, Woodrow JC: The HLA system and the arthropathies associated with psoriasis. *Ann Rheumatic Diseases* 1977; 6:112.
6. Killebrew K, Gold RH, Shockoff: Psoriatic spondylitis. *Radiology* 1973; 108:9.
7. Wright V: Seronegative polyarthritis. *Arthritis and Rheum* 1978; 21:619.
8. Harvie JN, Lester RS, Little AH: Sacroiliitis in severe psoriasis. *AJR* 1976; 127:579.
9. Moll JM: The clinical spectrum of psoriatic arthritis. *Clin Orthop* 1979; 143:66.
10. Resnick D, et al: Calcaneal abnormalities in articular disorders. *Radiology* 1977; 125:355.
11. Martel W, et al: Radiologic features of Reiter disease. *Radiology* 1979; 132:1.

# SOFT TISSUE

Soft tissue can be calcified, ossified, contain gas, or be increased or decreased locally or generally. Metastatic calcification occurs in normal tissue when the serum calcium-phosphorus (mg/dl) product exceeds 75. Calcium and phosphorus salts produce dystrophic calcification by precipitating in damaged tissue because the tissue has a high pH, in which these salts are less soluble. Calcifications are common in collagen diseases. Formation of cortex and trabeculae indicates soft tissue ossification rather than calcification.

Gas can be due to penetration of the airways or lung, direct trauma, gas-forming organisms, or gas gangrene. Soft tissue masses may be fat, soft tissue, or calcific density. Normal fat planes may be displaced or obliterated, indicating abnormality in the soft tissue or the underlying bone or joint.

Increased and decreased soft tissue and the ratio of muscle to subcutaneous fat can be clues to subtle focal acquired diseases or can accompany obvious widespread congenital diseases. Soft tissue anatomy and pathology is much better demonstrated by computed tomography than radiography.

# Study 25

This 17-year-old girl has had pain of the right hip for five months.
*Your diagnosis?*

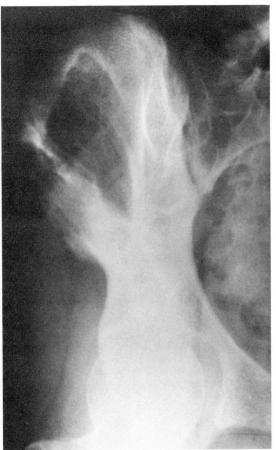

**Fig. 1:** Oblique radiograph of the right iliac bone.

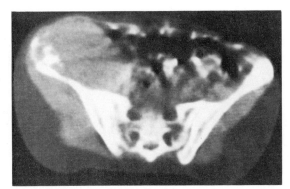

**Fig. 2:** Computed tomography through the level of the anterior superior iliac spine.

Note: Figs. 1, 2 courtesy of Bruce Silver, MD, Chicago, Illinois.

# Diagnosis: Osteosarcoma

In Figure 1 there is a lytic lesion of the iliac bone with sharp and actually sclerotic margins in some areas. Other areas are poorly-marginated, however, indicating more rapid growth at these sites. The computed tomogram in Figure 2 not only demonstrates bone destruction, but also a large soft tissue mass anterior to the right iliac bone which contains tumor bone formation that was difficult to identify on plain films. Up to 10% of osteosarcomas occur in flat bones.

## Definition

Osteosarcoma is a malignant bone-forming neoplasm character-ized by stromal cells with varying degrees of anaplasia, which are directly responsible for the formation of osteoid or primitive bone. The neoplastic cells may be predominantly osteoblastic, cartilag-enous or fibroblastic. Even when small foci of tumor bone are produced by the stromal cells, even if the great bulk of the tumor is cartilagenous or fibrous, it is still, by definition, an osteosarcoma.[1]

## Incidence

Osteosarcomas (OS) comprise about 0.2% of all reported malignancies. The incidence is 0.4 per 100,000 population. Despite its rarity, OS accounts for 20% to 40% of all primary malignant bone neoplasms. It is the second most common primary malignant neoplasm of bone, second only to multiple myeloma. Osteo-sarcoma is twice as common as chondrosarcoma and three times as common as Ewing's sarcoma.

The majority of patients with osteosarcoma are in the second decade of life, but about 10% are under age 10 and 10% over age 40. Peak age is 15 to 20 years. The overall male to female ratio is about 2:1. This may be related to the longer period of skeletal growth and greater volume of bone produced in the male. Osteosarcomas occurring in the older age groups often occur in a diseased bone.[2]

Osteosarcoma may occur in any bone, but a majority occur in long bones. The frequency of occurrence at various sites in long bones correlates well with the rate of growth at those sites. The most common sites, therefore, are the distal femur (40%), proximal tibia (20%), and proximal humerus (10%). Patients are, on the average, taller than their peers. It is of interest that long bone osteosarcomas are also more frequent in large dogs compared to small dogs.[3]

After epiphyseal closure the long and flat bones are more equally affected. Overall about 10% of lesions are found in flat bones. Location in the hand or spine is rare. Rarely OS occurs as a soft tissue primary.

## Classification

Osteosarcoma may be divided into four catagories according to location: (1) intramedullary, (2) parosteal, (3) periosteal (4) soft tissue.

# Intramedullary Type

This type is most common. Most lesions are solitary and occur as a primary lesion in a normal bone. Much less frequently an intramedullary lesion occurs secondarily in a diseased bone. Rarely there are multiple primary lesions.

Two-thirds of primary intramedullary neoplasms occur before age twenty. Secondary OS generally occurs after age 40. It is postulated that many years are required to transform a benign precursor lesion into a malignant neoplasm. Precursor lesions include Paget's disease, bone which has been radiated, and fibrous dysplasia. More rare precursors include bone infarct, osteochondroma, enchondroma, enchondromatosis, and osteoblastoma.[1,3]

Primary OS does occur in older patients. In one institution 24/397 (6%) of patients with primary OS were over age 50. Women were affected more often than men by a 2.4:1 ratio. The lesions had the same radiographic features seen in younger patients. Two lesions which were purely lytic without periosteal reaction resembled metastasis or multiple myeloma (Fig. 3). Sclerotic lesions resembled osteoblastic metastasis but a primary neoplasm was sometimes indicated by tumor bone formation in the soft tissue or a large soft tissue mass.[2]

Patients may rarely have more than one neoplasm. Multiple neoplasms may be synchronous or metachronous.[4] In these patients each neoplasm has the clinical, roentgenographic and pathological features of a primary lesion. Synchronous tumors occur simultaneously and are probably multicentric in origin.

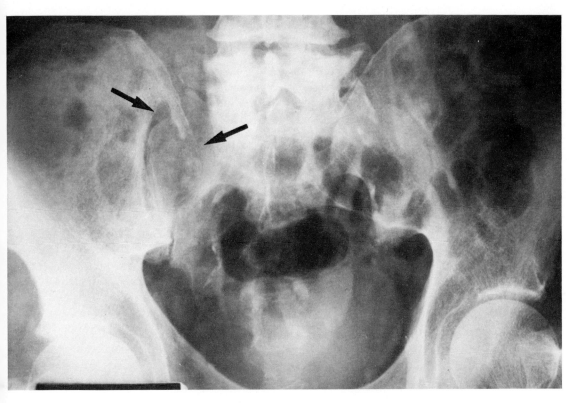

**Fig. 3:** Subtle lytic osteosarcoma of the portion of the right iliac bone extending behind the sacrum (arrows). Compare to left side. The patient is 54 years old and this was initially thought to be a metastasis.

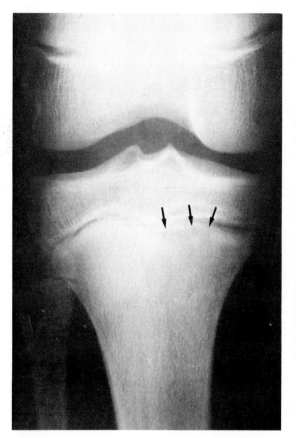

Figure 4

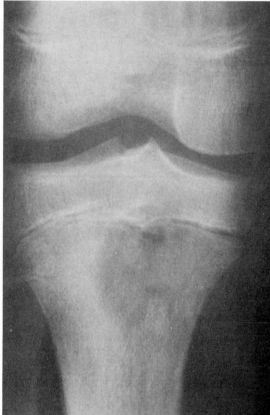

Figure 5

**Fig. 4, 5:** This boy had vague pain for 2 months following an injury. Subtle early lytic metaphyseal osteosarcoma (arrows) in Figure 4 was more evident one month later in Figure 5.

They are symmetric, sclerotic, and metaphyseal. Most of these patients are children and most die in less than one year. Metachronous tumors arise months to years after diagnosis of an initial lesion. They may represent late metastasis or new primaries. The metachronous lesions are sometimes amendable to vigorous therapy aimed at cure.[5]

## Gross Pathology

The gross features of OS are the result of bone and cartilage production, vascularity, degenerative foci, and extent of involvement. Most tumors are white and gritty. Hardness depends on the amount of tumor bone produced. Large lesions usually have eroded the bone cortex in one or more sites, lifted the periosteum, and extended into the soft tissue. There are frequently foci of hemorrhage and small to large islands of translucent bluish cartilage. Rarely the tumor is almost entirely hemorrhagic and cystic (telangiectatic OS).

## Histology

The distinguishing feature of OS is the production of osteoid and/or primitive woven bone by anaplastic stromal cells. When tumor osteoid is not present in a biopsy specimen or the entire

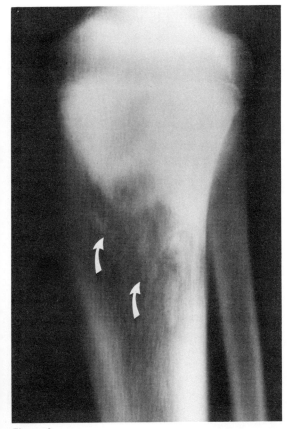

Figure 6

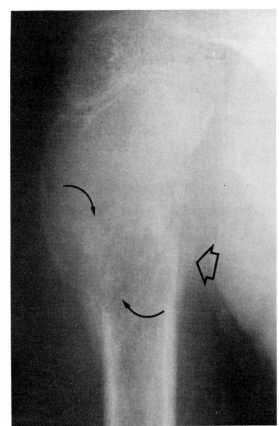

Figure 7

tumor, it cannot be designated as an osteosarcoma. The tumor will be called a fibrosarcoma, chondrosarcoma, unspecified sarcoma, or anaplastic sarcoma, depending on its dominant histology. The demonstration of alkaline phosphatase in the cells by cytochemistry or histochemistry will facilitate the diagnosis of osteosarcoma since alkaline phosphatase is abundantly present in OS and absent or scanty in chondrosarcoma and fibrosarcoma.[6] Other malignant cells found in OS in varying amounts include malignant small and large round cells, malignant giant cells, and spindle cells. Most OS have blatant cellular anaplasia and evident osteoid deposition. Less typical histologic appearances include:[1]

*Sclerotic OS*—Tumor new bone infiltrates the marrow space and replaces it with masses of dense woven bone and osteoid. It may resemble callus, but after 3-4 weeks callus should show a benign osteoblastic rim which is absent in OS. Sclerotic OS may also resemble osteoid osteoma or osteoblastoma.

*Cartilage Predominant*—Obvious malignant cartilage is present in most cases of OS. Those with subtle cartilage anaplasia or excess amounts of cartilage can cause diagnostic difficulty. Tumors with minimal anaplasia may resemble hyperplastic callus cartilage. Almost all patients less than age 30 with chondrosarcomatous tissue in the metaphyseal region have osteosarcoma.

**Fig. 6:** Lateral tomogram of the proximal tibia. Mixed sclerotic and lytic osteosarcoma. Faint fluffy tumor bone production is present in the lytic component (arrows).

**Fig. 7:** Lytic osteosarcoma "expanding" the meta-diaphysis of the humerus. There is cortical destruction medially. There is faint, poorly defined tumor bone production (closed arrows) and a Codman's triangle (open arrow).

*Spindle Cell*—Most cases of OS will show some fields with prominant spindle cell patterns. If there is a predominant spindle cell pattern with anaplastic cells, they resemble fibrosarcoma. If the bundles of cells form pinwheels or a "storiform" pattern, they resemble malignant fibrous histiocytoma. Once again the diagnosis of OS is based on the presence of osteoid or bone production by tumor cells.

*Large Cell Predominant*—If OS is characterized by large cells (greater than 40 microns) with prominent nucleoli there may be confusion with carcinoma, metastatic melanoma, and primary reticulum cell sarcoma. Rarely, these large cells may become phagocytic, enlarge and resemble liposarcoma or malignant fibrous histiocytoma.

*Giant Cell Predominant*—If benign osteoclast-like giant cells predominate, OS may resemble a giant cell tumor. Giant cell tumor is an epiphyseal tumor which almost always occurs after epiphyseal closure, while OS is very rarely located in the epiphysis and often occurs in growing bone.

*Small Cell Predominant*—On rare occasions OS may be largely composed of small bland-appearing to obviously malignant small cells, and mimic chondroblastoma, Ewing's sarcoma, reticulum cell sarcoma, or metastatic tumor. Foci of tumor produced osteoid/bone indicate the proper diagnosis.

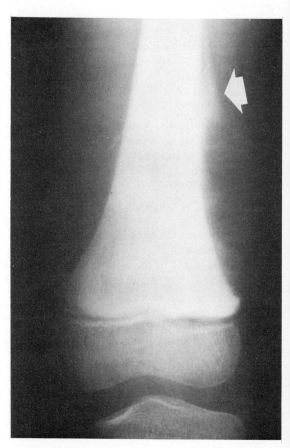

**Fig. 8:** Sclerotic osteosarcoma of the distal femoral shaft with Codman's triangle (arrow) and spiculated periosteal reaction below it.

*Telangiectatic*—This is a rare form of OS and is very difficult to diagnose by radiographic and histologic features. Radiographically there is a predominantly lytic lesion of bone with only minimal sclerosis. The gross specimen is soft and cystic. Histologically there are single or multiple aneurysmally dilated spaces containing blood or degenerated tumor cells. Anaplastic cells and osteoid masses indicate the correct diagnosis.[3]

While knowledge of the varied histology of osteosarcoma is important in arriving at the proper diagnosis, histologic grading is controversial and of limited prognostic value.

## Clinical Features

The most common presenting complaint is local pain (90%) which is often associated with minimal swelling (80%). At first, the pain is slight and intermittant but within a short time it increases in severity and duration. As the swelling becomes more prominent, the overlying skin may become shiny and stretched with prominent superficial veins. Limitation of motion of the adjacent joints with minimal disability or limp is common. Less than 10% of patients have malaise or neurologic symptoms. There is a wide variation in tumor hardness. The sclerosing type may be rock hard, whereas, the osteolytic type may be rubbery firm. Since most lesions occur in the extremities, the patient may think that a blow or some other minor

**Fig. 9, 10:** This 20-year-old girl with Down's syndrome had leg pain two weeks after participating in the Special Olympics. There is a small barely visible soft tissue density (arrow). In Figure 10, six weeks later, fluffy soft tissue tumor bone production is obvious.

Figure 9

Figure 10

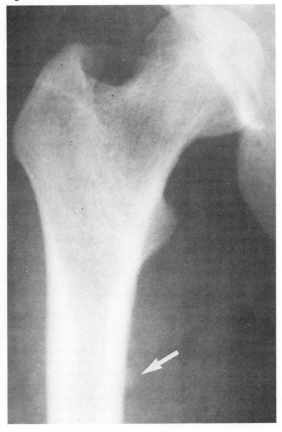
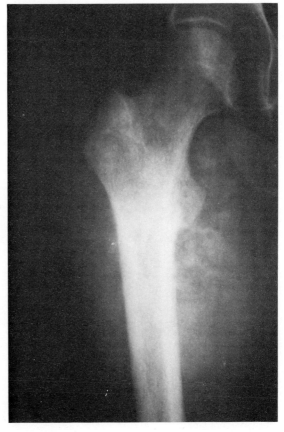

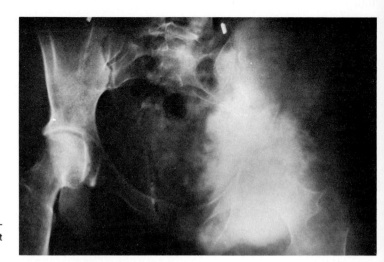

**Fig. 11:** Extensive tumor bone production in pelvic osteosarcoma. Pelvic soft tissue mass displaces bowel gas.

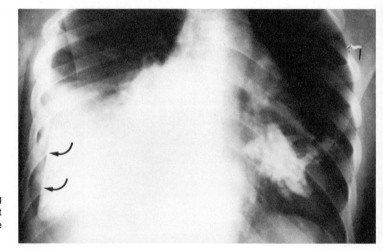

**Fig. 12:** There is a densely ossified lung metastasis in the left lung. There is right hydropneumothorax. Arrows indicate displaced pleural surface.

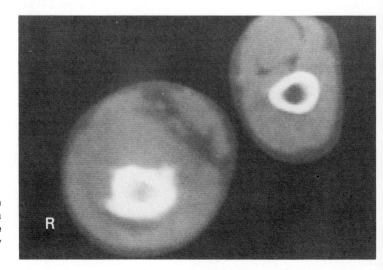

**Fig. 13:** Computed tomography of an osteosarcoma of the right femur with a soft tissue mass, periosteal new bone formation, and an abnormal medullary cavitary (compare to left leg).

208

injury caused the neoplasm. It is felt that the injury only draws the patient's attention to an already existing neoplasm. Symptoms are usually present for 1-8 months. If pain has been present for more than one year, the diagnosis of primary intramedullary osteosarcoma is suspect.[1,3]

The serum alkaline phosphatase is the only helpful laboratory test. It is seldom elevated more than three times normal. The osseous isoenzyme is differentiated from the hepatic isoenzyme by heat incubation. Rising alkaline phosphatase after removal of a neoplasm indicates metastasis or recurrence. A gradual rise in the enzyme may precede obvious clinical reappearance by up to several months.[3,7]

## Radiology

Diagnosis of any bone lesion which is biopsied or removed should be based on careful consideration of clinical, radiographic and pathologic information. The histology of early or hyperplastic callus, osteoid osteoma, osteoblastoma, aneurysmal bone cyst, and healing simple cyst may be mistaken for osteosarcoma, conversely, a sclerotic osteosarcoma may have innocuous features and closely resemble callus, osteoid osteoma, or osteoblastoma.

Radiographic interpretation is sometimes as important as histologic interpretation in arriving at the proper diagnosis, and radiographs should be scrutinized in all patients.[8]

The radiographic features of OS are the result of bone production, bone destruction, and the soft tissue mass present after cortical penetration. These features include:[9]

*Sclerosis:* Increased density may be the result of reactive host produced bone or tumor produced bone. Tumor osteoid/bone present histologically may not be visible on radiographs. Visible tumor bone is present in 90% of lesions while in 10% it is minimal or absent, so that the lesion appears purely osteolytic (Figs. 3, 4, 5,). It may be difficult to differentiate reactive host bone from tumor bone when increased density is confined to the bone. Coalescent, fluffy cloud like density, however, is usually tumor bone (Figs. 6, 7). Lesions may be extremely dense throughout (Fig. 8), moderately dense or have an irregular mixture of density and lucency (Figs. 6, 7).

*Destruction:* Medullary and cortical bone destruction are common. Destruction of compact cortical bone is evident much earlier than destruction of loose medullary bone. Lytic areas almost always have poorly defined margins (Figs. 4, 6, 7) and often consist of coalescent 2 to 10 mm holes producing a moth-eaten appearance or, with a more rapidly growing lesion, innumerable tiny holes permeating the bone. Cortical break through is common on initial examination and is followed by lifting of the periosteum and extension of the neoplastic mass outside the bone.

*Periosteal New Bone:* The rapidly growing tumor lifts the periosteum which then forms new bone. Spiculated periosteal new bone is common in OS and may have a "hair on end" or "sunburst" configuration (Fig. 8). Less commonly slower

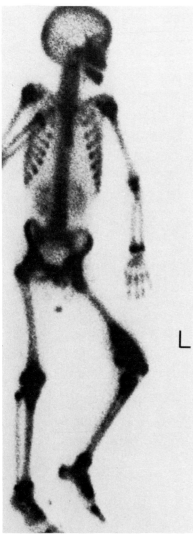

**Fig. 14:** Tc99M diphosphonate bone scan. The osteosarcoma of the distal left femur avidly accumulates the radio-nuclide. There are no other lesions.

growing tumors result in multiple parallel layers of new bone which have an "onion skin" appearance. If the central segment of the lifted periosteum is broken through, the remaining proximal and distal shards make new bone which forms triangles with the cortex of the bone. These Codman's triangles indicate an aggressive process (Figs. 7, 8).

These different patterns indicate rapidity of growth and not malignancy. Most lesions with the spiculated pattern are malignant, but every type of periosteal new bone formation has been reported in benign conditions. No single radiographic sign is pathognomonic of malignancy.

*Soft Tissue Mass:* A soft tissue mass is commonly present in OS. The mass may not be visible in axial lesions except by computed tomography (Fig. 2). When medullary calcification extends into the mass or when the mass contains poorly defined calcifications (Figs. 9, 10, 11) it is certain that this finding does not represent reactive host bone (Fig. 2). This finding usually indicates a malignancy but the early phase of myositis ossificans may look the same. Myositis ossificans, however, will later develop a well defined sclerotic rim. In general, soft tissue edema with osteomyelitis is diffuse compared to the discrete mass found in OS. In osteomyelitis the soft tissue planes are often obliterated, which is not usually the case with OS. Ewing's sarcoma or massive sarcomas compressing vessels, however, may also cause generalized edema.[1]

## Early Osteosarcoma

Up to 10% of lesions present before the tumor has broken through cortex. These early lesions may be difficult to identify as OS.

Early tumors producing bone are characterized by coalescent, fluffy, whitish masses which have been likened to cumulus clouds. There is no rim of host bone reactive sclerosis. The radiographic appearance may resemble a stress fracture, enchondroma, bone infarct, osteoblastoma, or fibrous dysplasia. A stress fracture may have a fracture line or periosteal reaction with an intact cortex. The sclerosis in a stress fracture is often linear. Enchondromas are frequently expansile and can be identified when well defined discrete cartilage type calcifications are present. Infarcts usually have well defined calcifications and a well defined sclerotic rim. Osteoblastomas often have a sclerotic rim and may be expansile. Fibrous dysplasia is often expansile and frequently has a "ground glass" density reflecting the presence of primative woven bone.

Early tumors without visible tumor bone comprise less than 1% of osteosarcomas (Figure 4, 5). They are small (2-4 cm in diameter) and since the cortex is not broken through there is no periosteal new bone or soft tissue mass. The margin of the lesion is poorly defined and there is no sclerotic rim. The radiographic appearance may resemble a solitary bone cyst, aneurysmal bone cyst, or eosinophilic granuloma. Solitary bone cysts most often occur in young children. They are frequently expansile and may have a sclerotic rim. Aneurysmal bone cysts are usually quite expansile and often have a sclerotic rim. Eosinophilic granuloma is most often diaphyseal and usually has a sharp margin.

On rare occasions an early lytic OS may be radiologically indistinguishable from these benign lesions.[1]

*Metastases* –A majority of patients with OS have lung metastases at the time of diagnosis. The metastases may be subclinical. Computed tomography is the best means of detecting lung nodules, but the histology of a nodule cannot be determined. Lung metastases may ossify, cavitate, or be associated with pneumothorax (Fig. 12).

The liver, kidney, bone, and lymph nodes are other metastatic sites. These metastases may also produce radiographically visible tumor bone.[9]

## Computed Tomography

Computed tomography has supplanted angiography if further evaluation of OS is desired prior to therapy.[10,11]

Plain films are still the primary means of diagnosing bone neoplasms including osteosarcoma. No other modality provides such minute detail of the lesion and its interface with normal bone. Computed tomography is more accurate in identifying soft tissue masses and depicting the medullary space and is capable of identifying densities which are not visible on plain films. Experience

**Fig. 15:** Advanced juxtacortical osteosarcoma encircling the distal femur. The outer rim is poorly defined.

**Fig. 16:** Inactive myositis ossificans with characteristic well defined outer rim.

Figure 15

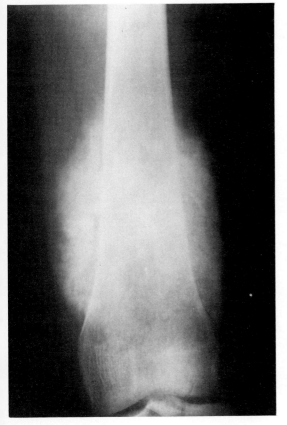

Figure 16

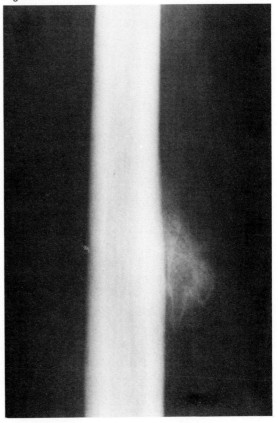

with small numbers of cases so far, however, have shown computed tomography to play only an adjunctive diagnostic role in some patients (Fig. 13).[11]

In this institution, computed tomography has proven to be more valuable in evaluating axial bone lesions, especially those in the lumbar spine and pelvis (Fig. 2).

*Nuclear Medicine*—Prior to the introduction of chemotherapy for the treatment of OS, radionuclide bone scans (Fig. 14) were felt to be of little value since lung metastases almost always occurred before bone metastases. Chemotherapy has now improved the survival rate so that the value of bone scans has increased. In addition in a small number of patients metastases do occur in bone before lung. If additional areas are abnormal they would then be evaluated by plain films and possibly computed tomography.[12]

Bone scans may overestimate the extent of involvement of a bone in planning an amputation. Follow-up bone scans at regular intervals have been advocated, especially during the first 2 years after diagnosis, since the majority of bone metastases are evident by then.[13]

## Prognosis

The overall prognosis for intramedullary OS is poor. The five year survival rate without chemotherapy has been about 20%.

Axial primaries have a poorer prognosis than primaries in the extremities. The more distant the site of the primary the better the prognosis. Facial and jaw primaries have a better prognosis than other lesions in axial sites.

The relationship of survival to duration of symptoms, tumor size, and histologic grading is not reliable.

## Treatment

The treatment of children and young adults with OS of long bones who have no metastases is variable. Major amputation of the limb probably still remains the definitive treatment. Preoperative and postoperative multidrug, multicycle chemotherapy coupled with en-bloc resection of the primary tumor, however, is also done.

Amputation as the sole treatment results in a five year survival of about 20%. Newer treatment modalities are promising and have resulted in longer disease-free survival.[15] Improved survival and even long term cure has also been gained with surgical resection of pulmonary metastases combined with chemotherapy and radiotherapy.[16]

## Juxtacortical (Parosteal) Osteosarcoma

This low grade malignant neoplasm arises in the periosteum of bones and is a distinct clinicopathologic entity. Juxtacortical OS comprise less than 1% of all primary bone tumors. The patients are older than those with osteosarcoma, with peak incidence in the third and fourth decades. There is slight female preponderance. Three-fourths of lesions occur in the distal femur or proximal tibia. The upper humerus is the next most common site. Patients usually have a long history of mild symptoms. A mass is frequently palpable.

On gross examination the tumor is a whitish mass streaked with yellowish flecks of bone. It is sessile and about one-half involve the cortex or invade medullary cavity. Highly malignant lesions are readily diagnosed. Low-grade malignancies are very difficult to differentiate from early myositis ossificans. The peripheral maturation of myositis ossificans which is evolving is a crucial differentiating feature. The surgeon must make certain that biopsies from the center and periphery of a lesion are labeled as such.

The radiographic appearance of juxtacortical OS is characteristic when a large irregularly calcified soft tissue mass is contiguous with the bone (Fig. 15). The calcific masses may seem unattached when they are small. The tumor may be separated from the cortex by the periosteum which appears as a linear lucency except where a pedicle joins the soft tissue tumor to the bone. This feature is not seen unless the x-ray beam is tangential to the pedicle. In addition, myositis ossificans may be separated from underlying cortex.

Myositis ossificans that has matured has a more dense and well defined outer margin (Fig. 16). The outer rim of juxtacortical OS is less dense than the central portion of the lesion and is often poorly defined (Fig. 15). Advanced juxtacortical OS may be indistinguishable from intramedullary OS.[1,3,9]

The prognosis of juxtacortical OS is better than intramedullary OS. Histologic grading is valuable. Grade I lesions have a 90% 10 year survival. Treatment for low grade lesions has included radical or en-bloc resection and cryosurgery combined with en-bloc resection. High grade lesions are more lethal and require the same treatment as intramedullary osteosarcoma.[14]

## Periosteal Osteosarcoma

This uncommon lesion involves the cortex and spares the medullary cavity, just as juxtacortical osteosarcoma often does. Periosteal OS differs in its male preponderance, younger age group, predominant cartilagenous histology and radiographic appearance. A soft tissue mass with spiculations or fine to course tumor bone is usually present. A constant finding is cortical thickening. The soft tissue component is confined to the area overlying the cortical abnormality, which is unlike juxtacortical OS.

The prognosis is better than that of intramedullary OS and treatment is similar to that for low grade parosteal OS.[17]

## Soft Tissue Osteosarcoma

These rare lesions most often occur in the extremities. They have been reported in the face, head, neck, trunk, retroperitoneum, and kidney. Most are clearly malignant histologically. The radiographic appearance may be helpful when calcification is present in the otherwise non-specific soft tissue mass.[9]

*—Philip Ludkowski, MD*

# References

1. Mirra JM: *Bone Tumors.* Philadelphia, J.B. Lipincott, 1980.
2. deSantos LA, Rosengren JE, Wooten WB, et al: Osteogenic sarcoma after the age of 50: Radiographic evaluation. *AJR* 1978; 131:481.
3. Huvos AG: *Bone Tumors.* Philadelphia, W.B. Saunders, 1979.
4. Dahlin DC, Coventry MB: Osteogenic sarcoma: A study of 600 cases. *J Bone Joint Surg* 1967; 49:101.
5. Fitzgerald RH, Dahlin DC, Sim FH: Multiple metachronous osteogenic sarcoma. Report of 12 cases with 2 long term survivors. *J Bone Joint Surg* 1973; 55A:595.
6. Sanerkin NG: Definitions of osteosarcoma, chondrosarcoma, and fibrosarcoma of bone. *Cancer* 1980; 46:178.
7. Rosen G, Suwanisirikul S, Kwon C, et al: High dose methotrexate with citrovorum factor rescue and adriamycin in childhood osteogenic sarcoma. *Cancer* 1974; 33:1151.
8. Dahlin DC: *Bone Tumors.* Springfield, Illinois, Charles C. Thomas, 1980.
9. Edeiken J, Hodes PJ: *Roentgen Diagnosis of Disease of Bone.* Baltimore, Williams and Wilkins, 1981.
10. deSantos LA, Bernardino ME, Murray JA: Computed tomography in the evaluation of osteosarcoma: 25 cases. *AJR* 1979; 132:535.
11. Destovet J, Gilula LA, Marphy WA: Computed tomography of long bone osteosarcoma. *Radiology* 1979; 131:439.
12. Blair RJ, McAfee JG: Radiological detection of skeletal metastases: Radiographs versus scans. *Int J Radiat Oncol Bioc Phys* 1976; 1:1201.
13. Goldstein H, McNeil BJ, Zufall E, et al: Changing indications for bone scintigraphy in patients with osteosarcoma. *Radiology* 1980; 135:177.
14. Krishnan K: Parosteal osteogenic sarcoma. *Cancer* 1976; 37:2466.
15. Glocksman AJ, Maurer HM, Vietti TJ: Overview conference on sarcomas of soft tissue and bone in childhood. *Med Ped Oncolog* 1979; 7:55.
16. Marcove RC, Martini N, Rosen G: The treatment of pulmonary metastasis in osteogenic sarcoma. *Clin Orthop* 1975; 111:65.
17. deSantos L, Murray J, Finkelstein JB, et al: Radiographic spectrum of periosteal osteosarcoma. *Radiology* 1978; 127:123.

# Study 26

This 70-year-old woman has a mass of the medial aspect of the right foot. She discovered the mass about one year ago, and it has enlarged. There is no significant past medical history. The mass is cystic on palpation. It is nontender, and the overlying skin is normal. *Your diagnosis?*

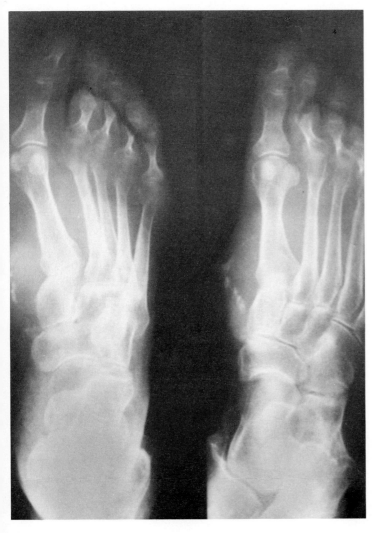

Fig. 1: AP and oblique views of right foot.

# Diagnosis: Soft Tissue Fibrosarcoma

The radiographic appearance of the foot mass is nonspecific, but a soft tissue sarcoma was considered.

At surgery a cystic mass was found. The pathologic diagnosis was fibrosarcoma. The mass infiltrated the anatomy such that it could not be widely excised, and a below-the-knee amputation was performed.

The most common somatic sarcomas in a series of 3,135 were liposarcoma (16.5%) (Fig. 3), rhabdomyosarcoma (16.2%) (Fig. 4), and fibrosarcoma (10.4%).[1] Less frequent are synovial sarcoma, angiosarcoma and malignant fibrous histiocytoma. Rare sarcomas include hemangiopericytoma, osteosarcoma and chondrosarcoma of soft tissue, leiomyosarcoma, epithelioid sarcoma, lymphoma of soft tissue origin and soft tissue plasmacytoma.[2]

**Fig. 2:** Fibrosarcoma of the right foot. There are bundles of fusiform cells with large somewhat pleomorphic oval nuclei. The interlacing fascicles of tumor cells form a "herringbone pattern." There were occasional mitoses. Other sections showed cysts up to 1.2 cm in diameter. Electron microscopy revealed cells with characteristic features of fibroblasts.

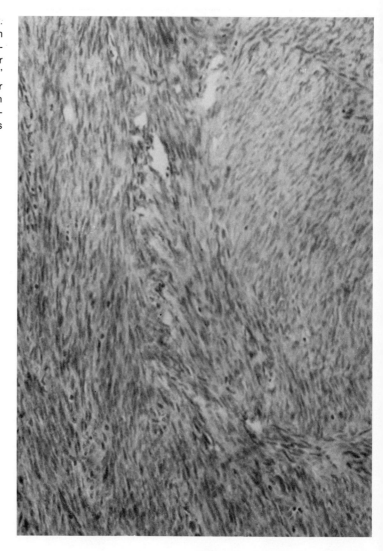

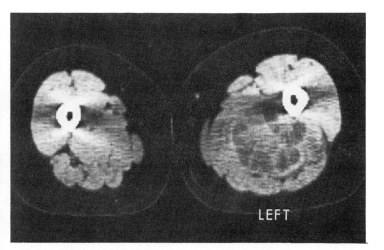

**Fig. 3:** Computed tomography: Liposarcoma of left thigh. The lesion is low density but not fat density.

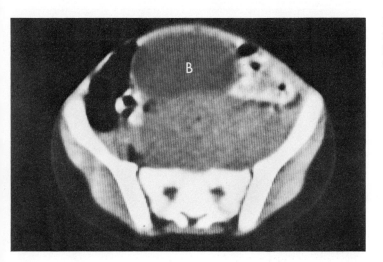

**Fig. 4:** Computed tomography: Large rhabdomyosarcoma of the pelvis displaces intestine and urinary bladder (B) anteriorly.

Fibrosarcoma may arise in any mesenchymal tissue and these neoplasms are found in the trunk and extremities, head and neck, and retroperitoneum. The somatic soft tissues are most frequently involved, and in a series of 199 cases, 60% were in the lower extremities and 30% on the upper extremities.[3] Most are primary, but rarely fibrosarcomas occur in chronic draining infections, scars or tissue which has been radiated. The average age is about 50 years, but fibrosarcomas occur at all ages including childhood, infancy and even as congenital lesions.

Most patients present with a mass. About one-half have pain or tenderness. Occasionally pain or weakness results from pressure on nerves. The average duration of symptoms is about 3.5 years in adults.[1]

Radiology is of little value in the diagnosis of soft tissue sarcomas. When a soft tissue mass is shown, its appearance is nonspecific. Any sarcoma may calcify, but synovial sarcoma (Fig. 5) and fibrosarcoma most commonly calcify. Occasionally there is bony erosion or infiltration. While it is generally agreed that angiography cannot identify lesions as benign or malignant, some advocate vascular studies in preoperative planning. Others feel that computerized tomography can provide the same information as angiography.[1] Technetium polyphosphate bone scans have been used to detect early bone involvement.[4] The most reliable means of evaluating the lungs for metastasis are CT and whole lung tomograms. CT has been shown to be more sensitive then whole lung tomograms in identifying lung nodules, but the additional nodules may be benign rather than metastatic. The CT appearance is nonspecific.[5,6]

Survival has been related to histologic grading and some even advocate less radical surgery with well differentiated tumors.[1] There is a higher incidence of recurrence than metastases with fibrosarcoma. Most metastases are to the lung. Regional lymph

**Fig. 5:** Synovial sarcoma near the base of the fifth metacarpal is calcified. The large majority of these neoplasms are outside the joint space. (Courtesy of Sidney Blair, M.D.)

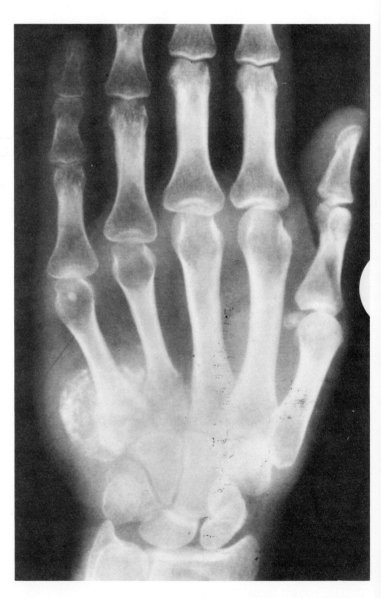

node metastases are uncommon.

Radical local resection is the treatment of choice. Amputation is done only when adequate local resection cannot be done, since there is no increase in survival with amputation as compared to radical local resection. Survival rates up to 60% have been reported in adults.[1,4]

In children it may be difficult to differentiate the histology of fibrosarcoma and the benign juvenile fibromatoses. The prognosis of fibrosarcoma is better in infants and children than in adults. Children less than 5 years of age have a high incidence of recurrence, but five-year survival rates greater than 90% have been reported. Local excision rather than radical resection has been recommended for children less than 5 years. After ago 10, survival is only slightly greater than adults.[7,8]

### References

1. Pritchard DJ, Sim FH, Ivins JC, et al: Fibrosarcoma of bone and soft tissues of the trunk and extremities. *Orthop Clin North Am* 1977; 8:869.
2. delRegato JA, Spjut HJ: *Cancer*. St. Louis, CV Mosby, 1977.
3. Pritchard DJ, Souce EH, Taylor WF, et al: Fibrosarcoma: A clincopathologic and statistical study of 199 tumors of the soft tissues of the extremities and trunk. *Cancer* 1974; 33:888.
4. Simon MA, Enneking WF: The management of soft tissue sarcomas of the extremities. *J Bone Joint Surg* 1976; 58-A:317.
5. Muhm JR, Brown LR, Crowe JK, et al: Comparison of whole lung tomography and computed tomography for detecting pulmonary nodules. *AJR* 1978; 131:981-984.
6. Chang AE, Schaner EG, Conkie DM, et al: Evaluation of computed tomography in the detection of pulmonary metastases. *Cancer* 1979; 43:913-916.
7. Source EH, Pritchard DJ: Fibrosarcoma in infants and children. *Cancer* 1977; 40:1711.
8. Exelby PR, Knapper WH, Huvos AG, et al: Soft tissue fibrosarcoma in children. *J Pediatr Surg* 1973; 8:415.

# Study 27

This 17-year-old boy has a history of low back pain for 7 months. Initially the pain was intermittent but it is now persistent and more severe with radiation to the left buttock and calf. There is tenderness to palpation over the left sacroiliac joint. The sedimentation rate is 68 with normal WBC and no fever. A follow-up radiograph (Fig. 2) was done because his pain did not abate. *Your diagnosis?*

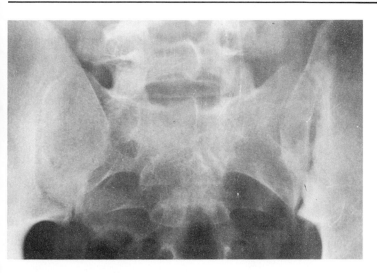

**Fig. 1:** AP pelvis

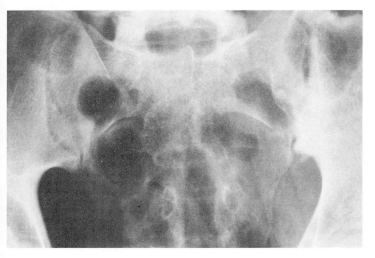

**Fig. 2:** AP pelvis two months after Figure 1.

# Diagnosis: Ewing's Sarcoma

Ewing's sarcoma is a malignant round cell sarcoma of bone characterized by uniform, densely packed small cells with round nuclei and indistinct cytoplasmic borders. The origin of the cells forming the tumor is uncertain but they are most likely derived from the connective tissue framework of the bone marrow.[1] Other "round cell" tumors of bone include primary and metastatic lymphoma, leukemia, myeloma, metastatic neuroblastoma, metastatic oat cell carcinoma of the lung, and eosinophilic granuloma. It is sometimes impossible to differentiate these various "round cell" tumors of bone on the basis of histology alone.[2,3]

Ewing's sarcoma is the most common primary bone neoplasm during the first decade of life and is the third most common primary bone neoplasm overall. In two reported series comprising 3,155 primary bone neoplasms, osteosarcoma was most common (1,208 cases) followed by chondrosarcoma (524 cases), and Ewing's sarcoma (388 cases).[1,2]

Ewing's sarcoma is slightly more common in males and is rare in blacks. Ewing's sarcoma is a tumor of children and adolescents— over ¾ of these tumors occur in the first two decades of life. The diagnosis should be viewed with suspicion in patients under age five years or over age 30 years. (In young children, metastatic neuroblastoma and in older patients histiocytic lymphoma or metastatic oat cell carcinoma of the lung may be histologically identical to Ewing's sarcoma). Rare cases of Ewing's sarcoma have been reported in the extremes of life (5 months to 83 years) and 5 to 10% of patients are over age 30 (Fig. 6).[4,5]

Pain and swelling are the most common presenting complaints in patients with Ewing's sarcoma. The duration of symptoms is usually several months. Symptoms are sometimes intermittent, but pain often becomes more severe and persistent prior to diagnosis. Some patients have systemic manifestations with fever, leukocytosis, anemia, and elevated sedimentation rate. These systemic

**Fig. 3:** IVP done at the same time as Figure 2. There is sclerosis of the left iliac bone adjacent to the sacroiliac joint and a soft tissue mass extending into the pelvis (arrows). The mass is also visible in Figure 2 as density in the left pelvis. In Figure 1 only subtle left iliac sclerosis adjacent to the sacroiliac joint is present.

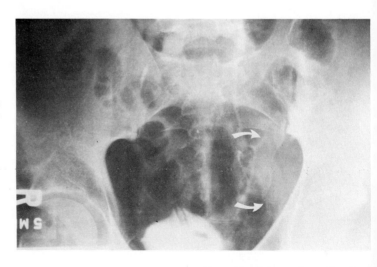

Bone Radiology Case Studies

findings may be the earliest signs of the tumor and can be intermittent also.[1]

The most common physical finding is a tender soft tissue mass. Localized warmth and tenderness associated with the mass, especially when accompanied by fever and leukocytosis, suggest an infectious etiology in some patients. Patients with a rib lesion often have pleural effusion and those with pelvic masses may have neurologic or bladder symptoms related to invasion of nerves by the sarcomatous mass.

The most common locations of Ewing's sarcoma are the femur, pelvis, humerus, and ribs. Table I gives the location of 822 cases of Ewing's sarcoma previously reported.[1,2,6-8]

The "classic" roentgenographic appearance of Ewing's sarcoma

### TABLE I

#### EWING'S SARCOMA — 822 PATIENTS

| | |
|---|---|
| Lower Extremity | |
|    Femur | 193 |
|    Tibia | 72 |
|    Fibula | 67 |
|    Foot | 35 |
| Pelvis | 149 |
| Upper Extremity | |
|    Humerus | 87 |
|    Radius | 15 |
|    Ulna | 13 |
|    Hand | 3 |
|    Ribs | 77 |
|    Scapula | 48 |
|    Spine | 24 |
|    Skull, | |
|       Mandible | 24 |
|    Clavicle | 13 |
|    Sternum | 1 |

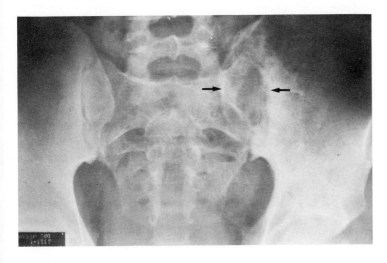

Fig 4: Following radiation therapy the pelvic mass is not visible. There is now destruction of the portion of the iliac bone projected behind (arrows) and above the sacrum.

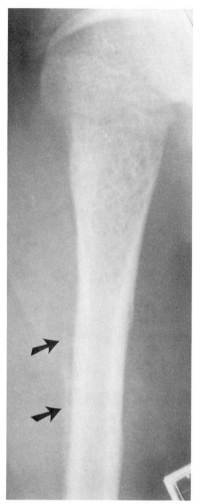

Figure 5

**Fig. 5:** AP view proximal humerus. Ewing's sarcoma causing permeative bone destruction of the meta-diaphysis in a 9-year-old boy. There is linear and spiculated periosteal reaction (arrows).

**Fig. 6:** Lateral tomogram of the proximal fibula. Subtle bone destruction of the proximal fibula in a 55-year-old man with Ewing's sarcoma. There is destruction of the anterior cortex (arrows).

in a long bone is poorly defined destruction of the diaphysis with laminated periosteal reaction and a soft tissue mass. This appearance in a young patient is suggestive but certainly not pathognomonic of Ewing's sarcoma. A similiar appearance may be found in osteomyelitis and other bone neoplasms. Furthermore, the "classic" appearance is seen in slightly less than 50% of cases involving a long bone.[1,7,8] The radiology of Ewing's sarcoma can be considered in terms of location, type of destruction, periosteal reaction, and soft tissue abnormality.

The ends of the long bones are involved as often as the midshaft (Figs. 5, 6). A metaphyseal tumor occasionally crosses the growth plate to involve the epiphysis but rarely is localized solely to the epiphysis. Bone destruction is almost always present. It is usually "permeative" (Fig. 5) with innumerable small areas of destruction or "moth eaten" (Fig. 6) with larger coalescent areas of destruction.

Figure 6

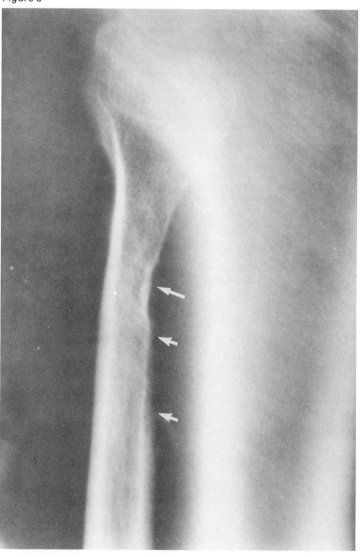

Atypical appearances include destruction localized to the superficial cortex producing a saucerized defect and a solitary lytic area resembling osteosarcoma.[7,8] Ewing's sarcoma does not produce tumor new bone or calcification but there may be reactive bone formation which results in a combination of bone destruction and sclerosis on roentgenograms. Metaphyseal lesions in particular may be very sclerotic and simulate a bone forming neoplasm.[1,7,8]

Cases of Ewing's sarcoma with sequestra have been reported and this finding causes further difficulty in differentiation from osteomyelitis. Periosteal reaction is commonly linear and laminated with multiple layers of periosteal new bone reflecting the episodic growth of the neoplasm. Spiculated or "hair on end" periosteal new bone is also frequent, alone or in combination with the laminated type (Fig. 5). Spiculated periosteal new bone indicates a very rapidly moving process. While spiculated periosteal reaction is very suggestive of a malignant process, it may also rarely be found in florid osteomyelitis.

A soft tissue mass is commonly present in Ewing's sarcoma (rare cases of Ewing's sarcoma primary in soft tissue have been reported).

Figure 7A

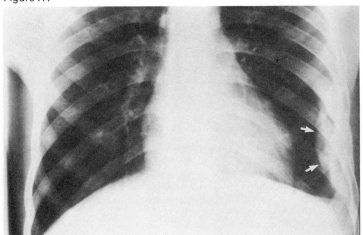

**Fig. 7A:** PA chest of an eleven-year-old boy with vague chest pain. There is a pleural mass (arrows).

**Fig. 7B:** Lower left ribs. There is sclerosis and periosteal reaction of one rib (arrows) with minimal destruction. This rib plus adjacent ribs were excised but the Ewing's sarcoma was confined to the sclerotic rib.

Figure 7B

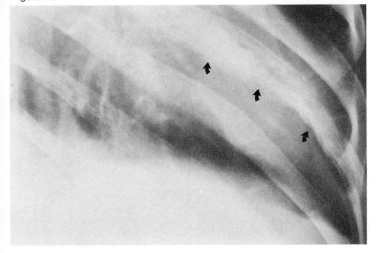

The soft tissue mass is never the site of tumor new bone formation such as that seen in osteosarcoma or chondrosarcoma.

In the flat bones, most commonly the iliac bone, the tumor may be lytic, sclerotic or a mixture of both (Figs. 1-4). Rarely there may be expansion of bone.

The ribs are the site of Ewing's sarcoma in 10% of patients. The most striking radiographic finding is a pleural soft tissue mass seen on a chest roentgenogram (Fig. 7).[9] Bone destruction is common and occasionally sclerosis is also seen. The bone change may be subtle in comparison to the obvious soft tissue mass. Periosteal new bone formation is a later finding. There may be a pleural effusion.

In the past the prognosis of Ewing's sarcoma was dismal. Despite control of the primary lesion by amputation or radiation, the vast majority of patients died with metastatic disease to the lungs and other bones. Currently the outlook is markedly improved with the advent of effective combination chemotherapy. Three year survival of 50 to 75% is now reported.[5,10]

The issue of amputation versus radiotherapy as treatment for the primary lesion is still debated. Radionuclide studies are valuable in demonstrating spread to other bones before radiographic findings are visible.

## References

1. Huvos AG: *Bone Tumors.* Philadelphia, WB Saunders, 1979.
2. Dahlin DC: *Bone Tumors. General Aspects and Data on 6,221 Cases.* Springfield, Illinois, Charles C. Thomas, 1978.
3. Wang CC, Fleischli DJ: Reticulum cell sarcoma of bone. *Cancer* 1974; 34:1131.
4. Lavallee G, Lemarbe L, Bouchard R, et al: Ewing's sarcoma in adults. *J Can Assoc Rad* 1979; 30.223.
5. Sinkovics JG, Plager C, Ayala AG, et al: Ewing's sarcoma: Its course and treatment in 50 adult patients. *Oncology* 1980; 37:114.
6. Netherlands Committee on Bone Tumors. *Radiological Atlas of Bone Tumors.* Baltimore, Williams and Wilkins, 1966.
7. Sherman RS, Soong KT: Ewing's sarcoma: Its roentgen classification and diagnosis. *Radiology* 1956; 66:529.
8. Vohra VG: Roentgen manifestations in Ewing's sarcoma. *Cancer* 1967; 20:727.
9. Branson J: Ewing's tumor of rib. *Aust Radiol* 1976; 20:341.
10. Glicksman AS, Maurer HM, Vietti TJ: Overview of conference on sarcomas of soft tissue and bone in childhood. *Med and Ped Oncology* 1979; 7:55

This man is 64 years old and has never before seen a physician.
*Your diagnosis?*

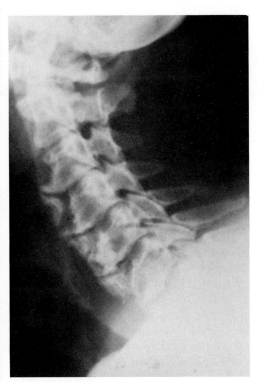

**Fig. 1:** Lateral view of the cervical
spine.

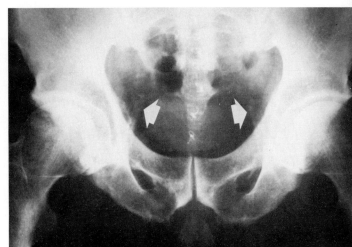

**Fig. 2:** AP view of the pelvis.

# Diagnosis: Diffuse Idiopathic Skeletal Hyperostosis

Ankylosing hyperostosis is an entity of unknown etiology that most often causes few symptoms and little or no disability. Usually it is diagnosed on the basis of a distinctive spinal ankylosis recognized on roentgenograms. Forestier described this peculiar form of spinal ankylosis in 1950 and termed it "senile ankylosing hyperostosis of the spine." Later he omitted the adjective "senile," as young adults with ankylosing hyperostosis were discovered.[1] Other terms that have been applied to this condition include spondylosis hyperostotica, spondylitis ossificans ligamentosa, and physiologic vertebral ligamentous calcification; all of these names refer to the primary finding in this disorder, extensive flowing hyperostosis of the spine. Recently it has been emphasized that this disorder also commonly involves the appendicular skeleton, tendons, and ligaments. These frequent extraspinal manifestations have led to the suggestion that a more accurate name for this disorder is diffuse idiopathic skeletal hyperostosis (DISH).[2]

The incidence of DISH at autopsy has been reported to be as high as 6 to 12%. It is more common in men, and most patients are over 50 years of age. In one report of 254 patients, however, 40 patients were under age 50 and 9 patients were under age 40.[1,2] Most patients are asymptomatic. When symptoms are present they are mild, however, exceptional cases with significant problems have been reported.

The most common symptom is low grade spinal stiffness beginning in late middle age. Spinal range of motion usually is normal. If the lumbar or cervical spines are involved, there may be slight decrease in motion. There may be mild transient aching in large joints. Heel and elbow pain related to spurs also occur. Dysphagia may result from large cervical osteophytes that impinge on the esophagus; there are reports of two patients who had severe progressive dysphagia that was relieved by excision of large anterior cervical bone masses associated with DISH.[4]

Cervical myelopathy has been found in patients with DISH.[5] Sensory deficits, muscle atrophy, and decreased deep tendon reflexes of the upper extremities are related to segmental cord and nerve root compression. Sensory deficits and weakness of the lower extremities, Babinski sign, and urinary tract dysfunction indicate long tract involvement of the cord. Patients with neurologic problems have had extensive calcification or ossification of the posterior longitudinal ligament (PLL) of the spine in addition to cervical hyperostosis. The relationship of DISH, PLL calification, and cervical myelopathy is unclear, since PLL calcification was found in 50% of DISH patients in one retrospective study (Figs. 4, 5).[5] Of interest is the association between PLL calcification and myelopathy in Japan.

Most reports of PLL calcification have come from Japan and have not been associated with DISH. The calcification may or may not be associated with symptoms, but in Japan 2% of patients with cervical myelopathy had associated PLL calcification. The

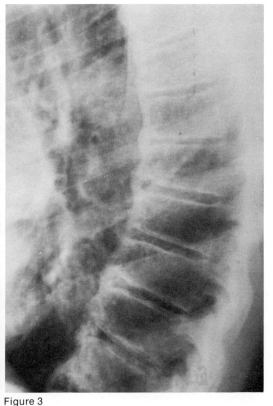

Figure 3

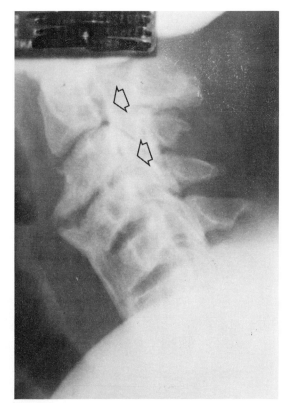

Figure 4

incidence of cervical myelopathy is increased in patients with a narrow spinal canal in addition to cervical spondylosis and PLL calcification. In symptomatic patients with PLL calcification as a sole abnormality there is a high incidence of long tract signs.[6,7] The incidence of cervical myelopathy associated with DISH in the U.S.A. is unknown.

DISH often presents a distinctive roentgenographic picture, with extensive thick, lumpy, flowing anterior spinal hyperostosis (Fig. 3). About 10% of patients with DISH have more delicate spinal changes that may be mistaken for ankylosing spondylitis.[8] Normal sacroiliac joints and apophyseal joints easily differentiate this latter group from patients with ankylosing spondylitis (Figs. 1, 3, 4). Also, patients with ankylosing spondylitis usually are younger, more symptomatic, and have more limitation of motion than those with DISH. HLA-B27 antigen is present in about 95% of patients with ankylosing spondylitis, and the antigen has been reported to be present in up to one third of DISH patients,[9] but recent reports question the association between DISH and HLA-B27. DISH is characterized by excess calcification and ossification involving ligaments and tendons and their insertions, para-articular bone, and the spine. In the spine, calcification and ossification are not confined to the anterior spinal ligament alone, but rather involve a region that includes the peripheral fibers of the annulus fibrosis, the prevertebral connective tissue, and the anterior longitudinal spinal ligament.[1] The low thoracic spine is affected earliest and most

**Fig. 3:** Lateral view of the thoracic spine, showing bony ankylosis with exuberant flowing anterior hyperostosis. In Figure 1 there is extensive anterior bone formation of the cervical spine. The normal intervertebral disc spaces and apophyseal joints found in ankylosing hyperostosis rule out ankylosing spondylitis. In Figure 2, the sacrotuberous ligaments are calcified (arrows) and there is irregular hyperostosis of the ischial tuberosities—both findings are seen in Forestier's disease. The sacroiliac joints are normal.

**Fig. 4:** Lateral view of the cervical spine in a second patient, showing extensive anterior bony bridging with intact disc spaces and apophyseal joints. The posterior longitudinal ligament of the spine is calcified (arrows).

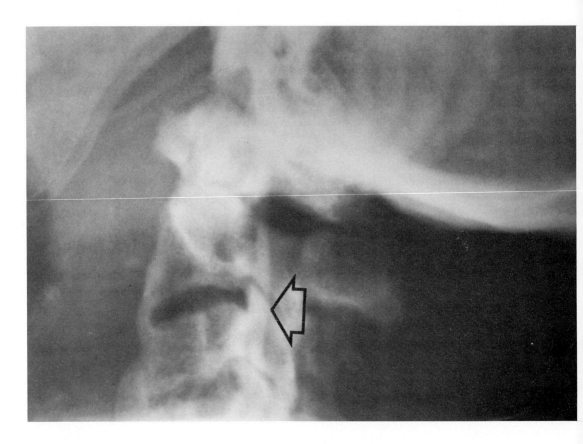

**Fig. 5:** Closeup view of ligament calcification present in Figure 4. The patient
had tingling of the left leg and numb-
ness of the left foot for several years.

commonly. Calcification begins in the prevertebral connective
tissue and adjacent anterior spinal ligament, and progresses later to
the outer fibers of the annulus fibrosis. Calcification extends across
the disc space, and increasing bone deposition leads to a thick,
flowing ankylosis with prominent bumps at the level of discs. Often
there is sclerosis of the anterior vertebral body. Posterior
osteophytes are unusual except in the cervical spine. The
intervertebral disc spaces and apophyseal joints are normal or only
minimally affected.

DISH, ankylosing spondylitis, degenerative disc disease, and
spondylosis deformans of the spine differ in roentgenographic
appearance. Bulky, individual osteophytes at the disc interspace in
DISH are directed first horizontally and then vertically (Fig. 6).
This contrasts with thin, strictly vertical, bridging syndesmophytes
characteristic of *ankylosing spondylitis* (Fig. 7). The osteophytes
found in *degenerative disc disease* are secondary to degeneration of
the nucleus pulposis. These osteophytes usually are small, and disc
space narrowing is marked. There may be gas in the disc, sclerosis of
vertebral endplates, and vertebral defects due to protrusion of disc
material. The spinal ligament is not calcified. *Spondylosis
deformans* results when repeated stress causes tearing of peripheral
fibers of the annulus fibrosis. The disc is no longer attached firmly to
the vertebral body and the intact nucleus pulposis causes prolapse
of the weakly attached annulus, with resultant stretching of the
overlying anterior longitudinal ligament. Osteophytes develop at

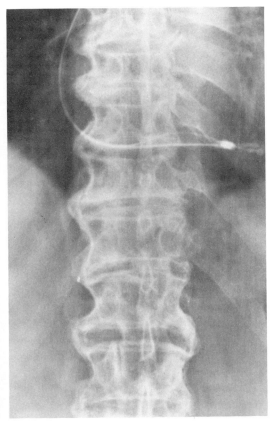

Figure 6

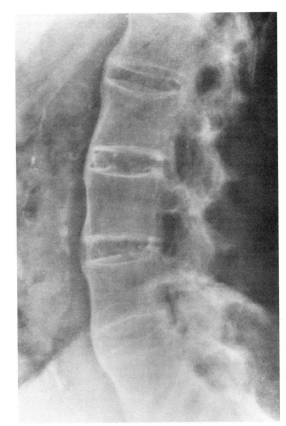

Figure 7

the attachment of the anterior ligament to the vertebral body. These osteophytes may be recognized as distinctive "traction osteophytes" when they originate at a point a few millimeters from the corner of the vertebral body rather than at the corner. Osteophytes in spondylosis deformans, which are *not* the traction type, are identical to those seen in DISH. More extensive hyperostosis, involvement of at least four contiguous vertebrae, and ligamentous calcification distinguish DISH in these cases.

Additional, less common, causes of spinal osteophytosis are: acromegaly, fluorosis, ochronosis, hemochromatosis, hypoparathyroidism, hypophosphatasia, and neurotrophic (Charcot's) spine.

The peripheral skeleton is affected commonly in DISH. Irregular spiculation or "whiskering" is found at bony margins where tendons and ligaments attach, especially the femoral trochanters, lateral iliac bones, and ischial tuberosities (Figs. 8A, 8B). Ligamentous calcification in the pelvis includes the sacrotuberous, sacrospinous (Fig. 2), and iliolumbar ligaments. The patellar and intraosseous ligaments are involved less commonly. Bone spurs are most often calcaneal or at the olecranon. Prominent para-articular osteophytes are most frequent at the inferior sacroiliac joint, lateral acetabulum, and superior pubic symphysis (Fig 9).[1] Roentgenographically the disease is slowly progressive.

Fig. 6: DISH with bulky osteophytes joining multiple vertebral bodies. The osteophytes have an initial horizontal direction.

Fig. 7: Ankylosing spondylitis with more delicate syndesmophytes joining vertebral bodies. The syndesmophytes are vertical and do not have a horizontal component.

DISH disease is common. The spinal ankylosis is characteristic and usually can be differentiated easily from ankylosing
spondylitis. If there is doubt, lack of sacroiliitis assures exclusion of
ankylosing spondylitis. Progressive dysphagia and cervical myelopathy have been reported. The etiology of Forestier's disease is
unknown. It has been suggested that these patients are "bone
formers" and there are reports of cases in which there was extensive
early postoperative heterotropic soft tissue ossification after total
hip arthroplasty.[8]

## References

1. Resnick D, Shaul SR, Robins JM: Diffuse idiopathic skeletal hyperostosis
   (DISH): Forestier's disease with extra spinal manifestations. *Radiology* 1975;
   115:513.
2. Forestier J, Lagier R: Ankylosing hyperostosis of the spine. *Clin Orthop* 1971;
   74:65.
3. Utsinger PD, Resnick D, Shapiro RF: Diffuse skeletal abnormalities in
   Forestier's disease. *Arch Int Med* 1976; 136:763.
4. Meeks LW, Renshaw TS: Vertebral osteophytosis and dysphagia. *J Bone Joint
   Surg* 1973; 55A:197.
5. Resnick D, Guerra J, Robinson CA, et al: Association of diffuse idiopathic
   skeletal hyperostosis (DISH) and calcification and ossification of the posterior
   longitudinal ligament. *Amer J Roentgenol* 1978; 131:1049.
6. Ono K, Ota H, Tada K, et al: Ossified posterior longitudinal ligament: A clinic-
   pathologic study. *Spine* 1977; 2:126.
7. Nakanishi T, Mannen T, Toyokura Y, et al: Symptomatic ossification of the
   posterior longitudinal ligament of the cervical spine. *Neurology* 1974; 24:1139.
8. Resnick D, Niwayama G: Radiographic and pathologic features of spinal
   involvement in diffuse idiopathic skeletal hyperostosis. *Radiology* 1976;
   119:559.
9. Shapiro RF, Utsinger PD, Wiesner KB, et al: The association of HLA-B27
   with Forestier's disease. *J Rheumatol* 1976; 3:4.

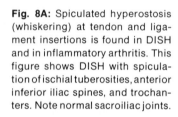

**Fig. 8A:** Spiculated hyperostosis
(whiskering) at tendon and ligament insertions is found in DISH
and in inflammatory arthritis. This
figure shows DISH with spiculation of ischial tuberosities, anterior
inferior iliac spines, and trochanters. Note normal sacroiliac joints.

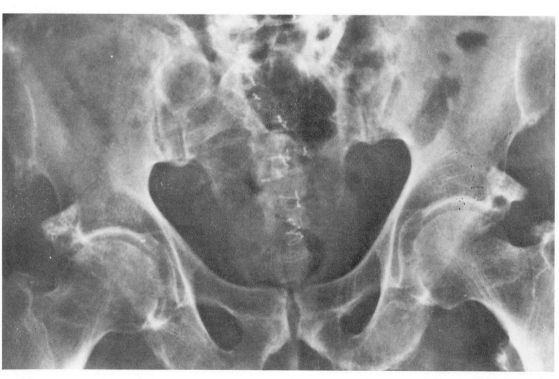

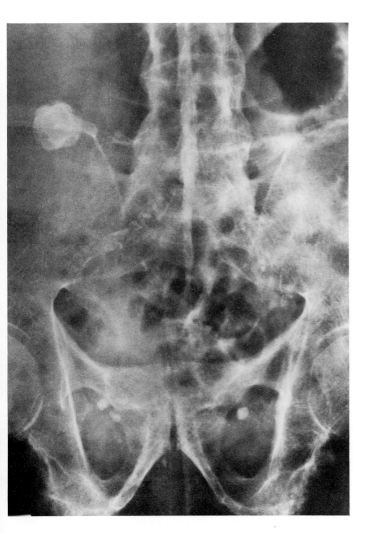

Fig. 8B: Ankylosing spondylitis with exuberant hyperostosis of ischial tuberosities. The sacroiliac joints are obliterated, and the vertebral bodies and their spinous processes are fused.

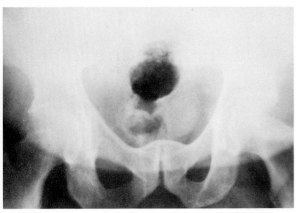

Fig. 9: AP view of the pelvis, showing a periarticular osteophyte bridging the superior pubic symphysis.

# Study 29

This 60-year-old man has had swelling and pain of the left wrist for five days. He has had several similar acute attacks lasting one to two weeks in the past three years. *Your diagnosis?*

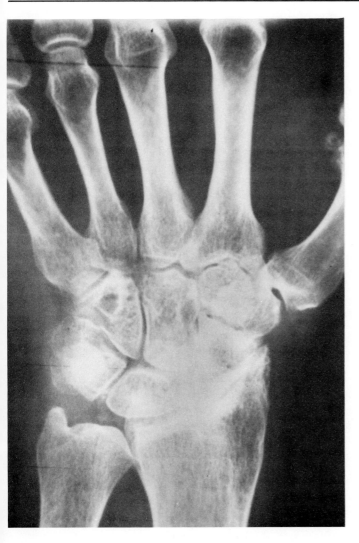

**Fig. 1:** AP Wrist.

# Diagnosis: Calcium Pyrophosphate Dihydrate (CPPD) Deposition Disease

Articular chondrocalcinosis refers to radiographically visible calcification in hyaline and fibrocartilage of joints. Dicalcium orthophosphate dihydrate, hydroxyapatite and calcium pyrophosphate dihydrate (CPPD) crystals all cause detectable calcification.[1] Only CPPD has been well documented as causing arthritis. CPPD deposition disease, especially when presenting as an acute attack, is called pseudogout.

Diagnosis is made by: (1) x-ray diffraction identification of CPPD crystals from biopsy or aspirated fluid or (2) identification of

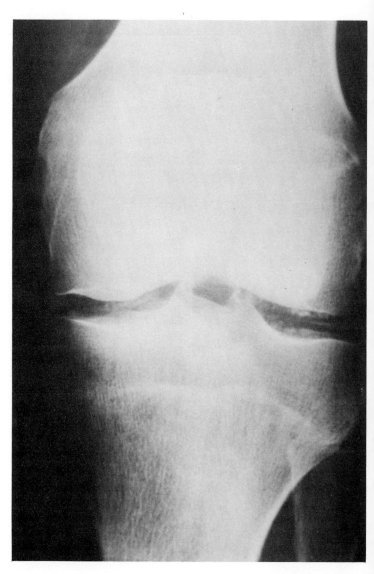

**Fig. 2:** AP Knee. There is cartilage calcification. In Figure 1, there is a small calcification between the ulna and lunate in the triangular ligament. Joint space narrowing and sclerosis is most marked at the radiocarpal joint. This combination strongly suggests CPPD deposition disease.

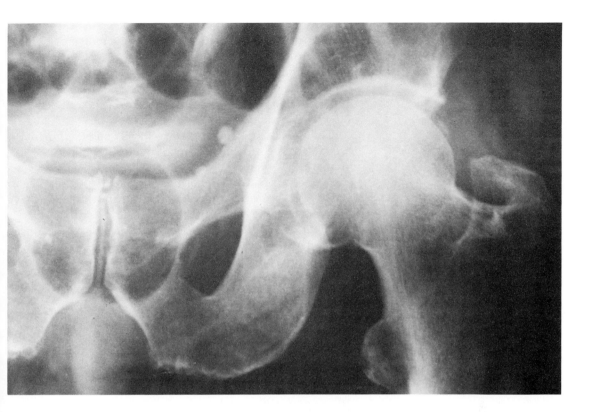

crystals with absent or weakly positive birefringence by compensated polarized light microscopy *plus* radiographic chondrocalcinosis involving more than one set of joints.[2] CPPD deposition disease has occurred without radiographic calcification, however.

Initially CPPD crystals are probably deposited around chondrocyte lacunae, and later occur in tophus-like masses and along clefts in degenerating cartilage. The crystals are in equilibrium with ionized calcium and inorganic pyrophosphate (PPi) in the synovial fluid and serum. Decrease in serum calcium may result in crystal release from cartilage, and attacks have occurred after parathyroid surgery. Crystals may also be released by trauma and altered cartilage matrix. Trauma may cause microfractures and crystal release. Cartilage alteration secondary to other arthritides may allow crystal release. Pseudogout has followed thyroid replacement therapy, probably because metabolic cartilage changes allowed crystal release. The released crystals are coated with IgG and phagocytized by polymorphonuclear leukocytes. Lysosomal discharge and chemotactic factor release by the phagocyte probably causes acute inflammation.[3]

Clinically, patients are often mistaken to have other forms of arthritis. Presentations of CPPD deposition disease include:
1. Pseudogout: acute or subacute attacks lasting one day to four weeks. Most common site is the knee.
2. Pseudorheumatoid arthritis: subacute episodes lasting weeks to months involving multiple joints. Nonspecific inflammatory signs. A few have low titer positive rheumatoid factor.

**Fig. 3:** AP Hip. There is calcification of the symphysis pubis and the articular cartilage of the left hip. The knee and pubis are the commonest sites of calcification in CPPD deposition disease.

3. Pseudo-osteoarthritis: progressive degeneration of multiple joints, usually large joints. Flexion contractures are common. Acute attacks may be superimposed.

4. Asymptomatic: reported incidence of calcification in the knee in the general population (3-25%) is variable depending on the age group and x-ray technique. Many of these patients are asymptomatic.

5. Familial: several families studied. Earlier onset, third, fourth decade, more widespread, progressive arthropathy.

Acute attacks have occurred after surgery, especially post-parathyroid surgery and after orthopedic surgery. Acute vascular disease such as myocardial infarction and cerebral thrombosis have also been followed by acute episodes.[5]

A minority of cases of CPPD deposition disease have been associated with other conditions including:[5]

1. Osteoarthritis*
2. Gout
3. Rheumatoid arthritis
4. Hyperparathyroidism*
5. Hypothyroidism
6. Acromegaly
7. Hemochromatosis*
8. Wilson's disease
9. Ochronosis
10. Hypophosphatasia*
11. Hemophilia
12. Neurotrophic joints*[6]

Radiographic findings include calcifications and arthropathy.[7]

The calcifications occur in hyaline and fibrocartilage of joints and in the synovium, joint capsule, tendons and bursae. Hyaline cartilage calcifications are thin and parallel the articular surface of the bone. Fibrocartilage calcifications are punctate and shaggy and may not be linear. Tendon calcifications are fine and linear, unlike dystrophic calcifications.[8]

Most common sites of calcifications are the knee, pubic symphysis and wrist, followed by the elbow and hip. Almost all cases will be detected by screening the knee and pubic symphysis.[9] Less common sites are shoulder, ankle, metatarsophalangeal, metacarpophalangeal and annulus fibrosis of discs (Fig. 4).

Progressive arthropathy has been documented, especially in the familial form of the disease.[4] The arthropathy is frequently similar to osteoarthritis. Some differing characteristics of CPPD deposition arthropathy are:

1. Frequent wrist, elbow and shoulder and metacarpophalangeal joint involvement. These are uncommon sites for osteo-arthritis.

2. Isolated radiocarpal and patellofemoral compartment changes are common. Osteoarthritis often involves the first metacarpocarpal joint, but seldom involves the radiocarpal

---

*Best documented.*

joint. Osteoarthritis isolated to the patellofemoral joint is uncommon (Fig. 5).

3. Neurotrophic changes may be present.[6]
4. The CPPD arthropathy tends to numerous subchondral cysts and fewer osteophytes than osteoarthritis.

The arthropathy can suggest the proper diagnosis, even when it is not accompanied by chondrocalcinosis. This is especially so in the wrist when isolated radiocarpal disease is present.[10]

## References

1. McCarty DJ: Studies on pathological calcifications in human cartilage. *J Bone Joint Surg* 1966; 48A:309.
2. McCarty DJ: Pseudogout, Articular Chondrocalcinosis, Arthritis, and Allied Conditions, ed 7. *In:* Hollander JL (ed), Philadelphia, Lea & Febiger, 1966, pp 947-963.
3. McCarty DJ: Calcium pyrophosphate dihydrate crystal deposition disease— 1975. *Arthritis Rheum* 1976; 19:275.
4. Zitnan O, Sitaj S: Natural course of articular chondrocalcinosis. *Arthritis Rheum* 1976; 19:363.
5. Hamilton EB: Disease associated with CPPD deposition disease. *Arthritis Rheum* 1976; 19:353.
6. Menkes CJ, Simon F, Delriev F, et al: Destructive arthropathy in chondrocalcinosis articularis. *Arthritis Rheum* 1976; 19:329.
7. Genant HK: Roentgenographic aspects of calcium pyrophosphate dihydrate crystal deposition disease. *Arthritis Rheum* 1976; 19:307.
8. Gerster JC, Bavd CA, Lagier R, et al: Tendon calcifications in chondrocalcinosis. *Arthritis Rheum* 1977; 20:717.
9. Resnik D, Niwayama G, Georgen TG, et al: Clinical radiographic and pathologic abnormalities in calcium pyrophosphate dihydrate deposition disease: Pseudogout. *Radiology* 1977; 122:1.
10. Resnik D, Utsinger PD: The wrist arthropathy of "Pseudogout" occurring with and without chondrocalcinosis. *Radiology* 1974; 113:633.

**Fig. 4:** AP view of the shoulder. Chondrocalcinosis (arrows). The patient had hyperparathyroidism.

**Fig. 5:** Isolated patellofemoral joint space narrowing in a patient with CPPD deposition disease.

Figure 4

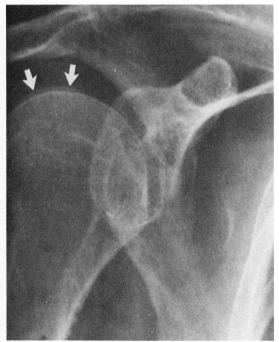

Figure 5

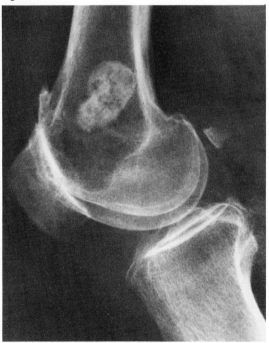

This 28-year-old man was found to have a subcapsular hematoma of the liver following minor abdominal trauma. *Your Diagnosis?*

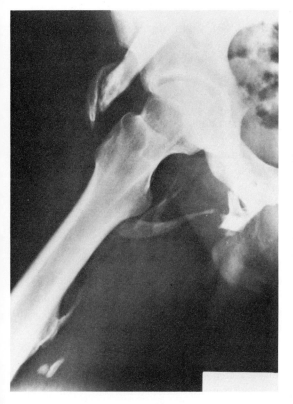 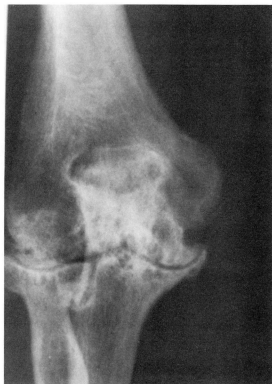

**Fig. 1A:** Lateral view of hip.

**Fig. 1B:** AP view of elbow.

# Diagnosis: Hemophilia

In Figure 1A there are multiple elongated areas of myositis ossificans. In Figure 1B there are joint space narrowing, slight eburnation, and numerous small cysts indicating hemophilic joint disease.

## Hemophilia and Myeloproliferative Diseases

The *hemophilias* are a group of diseases that result from coagulation factor deficiencies.[1] The two most common are hemophilia A, in which Factor VIII is deficient, and hemophilia B (Christmas), in which Factor IX is deficient. Both are X-linked and therefore are almost exclusively male diseases. There are a few reports of females with the disease. The manifestations range from bleeding only during surgery to spontaneous hemorrhage. Bone changes are seen secondary to hemarthrosis, intraosseous and soft tissue bleeding.

The knee, elbow (Fig. 1B), ankle, hip and shoulder are the most common joints affected.[2,3] Acute hemarthrosis is usually secondary to minor trauma, and only a joint effusion is seen. With recurrent bleeding, synovial inflammation, hypertrophy, fibrosis, and hemosiderin deposition occur. Radiographic changes range from soft tissue swelling, decreased bone density (Fig. 2), epiphyseal overgrowth (Fig. 3), periarticular subchondral cysts (Figs. 4,5) and joint space narrowing (Fig. 3) to complete joint space obliteration.

In the knee the common changes include overgrowth of the femoral and tibial epiphyses, a widened intercondylar femoral notch, and subchondral cysts (Figs. 2,3,4,5).[4] In the ankle, erosions, joint space narrowing and tibiotalar slant can be seen.

In addition to joint space disease, avascular necrosis (Fig. 3), myositis ossificans from soft tissue hemorrhage (Fig. 1A), frequent fractures and pseudotumors can occur.[5] Pseudotumors result from intravascular or subperiosteal hemorrhage. They can resemble Ewing's or osteogenic sarcoma, and are found in the bones of the lower extremity, pelvis (Fig. 6), and small hand and foot bones. They are often large lytic lesions with periosteal reaction and a soft tissue component.[6]

The major differential of hemophilic articular changes is juvenile chronic arthritis (JRA). In hemophilia, the knee, ankle and elbow are most commonly affected, while in JRA the wrist and hands are affected along with the knee and ankle. At times differentiation is impossible. Tuberculosis and synovial hemangioma can also cause a similar appearance.

The *myeloproliferative diseases* are those disorders characterized by abnormal proliferation of granulocytes, erythrocytes, and platelets or their precursors. In this category are the acute and chronic granulocytic leukemias, polycythemia vera, myelofibrosis, primary thrombocythemia and erthroleukemia.

*Myelofibrosis* is an end-stage bone marrow process characterized by replacement of the normal marrow cellular components by fibrous tissue.[7] A precise etiology has not been found, but the process can be seen in end-stage chronic granulocytic leukemia, polycythemia vera, primary thrombocythermia, and in response to benzene exposure. Generally patients are over 40 years of age and present with nonspecific constitutional complaints. Some have localized bone pain and most, but not all, have hepatosplenomegaly. Portal hypertension may be the result of liver involvement (Fig. 7). There is mild anemia with increased numbers of reticulocytes and the abnormal presence of nucleated red blood cells. The white blood cell count early is usually increased, as are the platelets. As the disease progresses, cell lines decrease in number and blast transformation can occur. The diagnosis is made by bone marrow biopsy. The disease is ultimately fatal but the course is variable.

Bone changes occur as a result of pathologic fibrous tissue replacement of the marrow spaces.[8,9] In general this is seen as sclerosis, but decreased bone density can be seen also. The spine (Fig. 7), pelvis (Fig. 8), ribs, skull and proximal humerus (Fig. 9) and femur (Fig. 10) are most commonly affected. These are the adult sites of hematopoiesis. Cortical thickening (Fig. 9) and periosteal new bone formation (Fig. 11) can be seen in long bones. As a result of extramedullary hematopoiesis, paravertebral soft

**Fig. 2:** Hemophilia: Decreased bone density and widened intracondylar notch.

**Fig. 3:** Hemophilia: Decreased bone density, severe joint space narrowing, widened intracondylar notch, and avascular necrosis. There is also overgrowth of the medial femoral condyle.

Figure 2

Figure 3

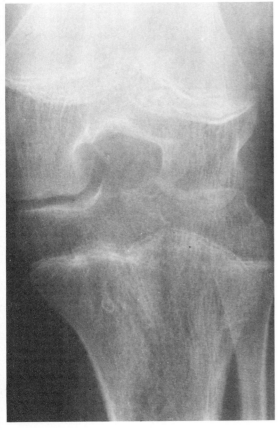

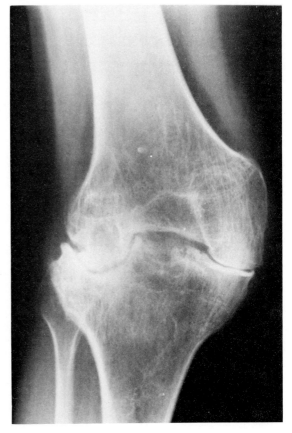

tissue masses (Fig. 12) and renomegaly occur. Hematomas may be the result of abnormal platelet number and function. Finally, because of increased cellular turnover, uric acid levels increase and gout may result.

*Acute myelogenous (granulocytic) leukemia* (AML) is a progressive neoplastic process involving the abnormal proliferation of an immature cell line of the myelogenous series, resulting in markedly elevated numbers of blast cells.[10] It accounts for 80% of acute leukemia in adults and less than 20% of acute leukemia in children. Symptoms range from constitutional complaints to serious infections secondary to granulocytopenia, and uncontrolled bleeding secondary to thrombocytopenia. The diagnosis is made on the peripheral smear and with bone marrow examination.

The reported incidence of bone changes in adult leukemia is low.[11] Unfortunately none of the studies have stated what type of leukemia is present. If we assume that most acute leukemia in adults is of the myelogenous line, then bone changes in AML are uncommon. Decreased bone density and lytic lesions are the most common changes when found. Metaphyseal lucency is very uncommon (7%).

*Chronic granulocytic leukemia* is a disease of adulthood characterized by excessive proliferation of granulocytes with an abnormal chromosome (the Philadelphia chromosome).[12] Most patients are in their middle years, present with constitutional complaints, and have hepatosplenomegaly. Generally a mild anemia is associated with markedly elevated white and platelet

**Fig. 4:** Hemophilia: Trabecular coarsening and irregularity of the articular surfaces of the knee. Growth arrest lines indicate episodic nature of the disease.

**Fig. 5:** Hemophilia: Articular surface irregularity and small to large subchondral cysts.

Figure 4

Figure 5

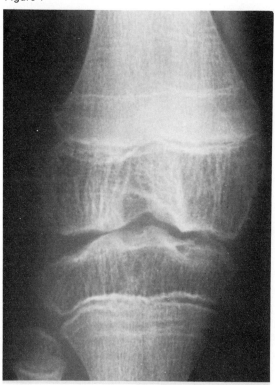

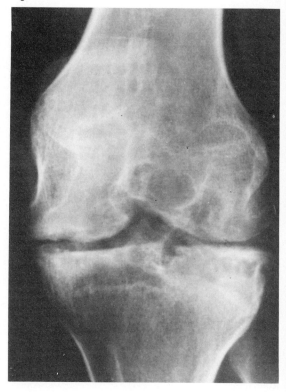

Bone Radiology Case Studies

counts. The course is far more benign than AML, but blast transformation can occur. Decreased bone density is the most common skeletal change with lytic lesions found in less than 3%.[13] A polyarticular arthritis (either migratory or simultaneous) can occur in the knees, shoulder and ankles. This is secondary to leukemic infiltration of the synovium. As in all the myeloproliferative diseases with high nucleoprotein turnover, secondary gout can occur.

*Systemic mastocytosis* is a rare, multiorgan-system disease resulting from mast cell proliferation and infiltration.[14] Onset is generally postpubertal and is characterized by skin lesions resembling juvenile urticaria pigmentosa. Symptoms include periodic urticaria accompanied by a variable degree of flushing, diarrhea and hypotension. Manifestations vary from a mild course to severe hepatosplenomegaly, pancytopenia, lymphadenopathy and small nodules of the intestine (Fig. 13). Bone changes are common and result from mast cell infiltration.[15] Both lytic and sclerotic lesions occur, sometimes simultaneously. Lytic lesions when generalized simulate osteoporosis and are most frequent in the skull, pelvis, spine and ribs. Focal lytic lesions are generally surrounded by a sclerotic rim. Sclerotic lesions may be focal or generalized, and can be indistinguishable from changes secondary to myelofibrosis, Paget's disease, metastasis, tuberous sclerosis, and sickle cell disease (Fig. 14).

—*Mark Baker, MD*

**Fig. 6:** Hemophilia: Large hemorrhagic pseudotumor has destroyed most of the left iliac bone. Note the large soft tissue mass superior and lateral to the iliac bone. (Illustration courtesy of Rogelio Moncada, MD.)

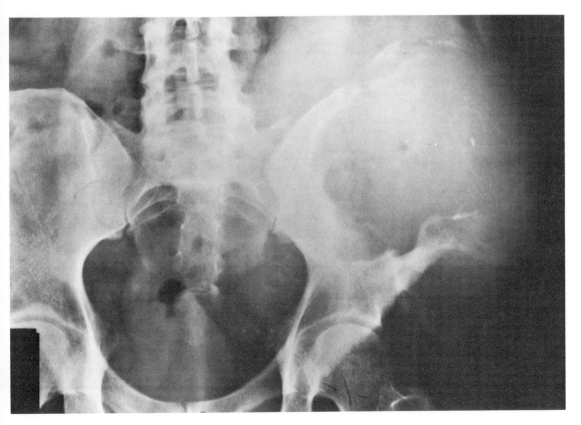

**Fig. 7:** Idiopathic myeloid metaplasia: Enlarged spleen impresses the greater curvature of the stomach. There are esophageal varices. The vertebrae are sclerotic in this 64-year-old man.

**Fig. 8:** Idiopathic myeloid metaplasia: Sclerosis of the pelvis and upper femurs.

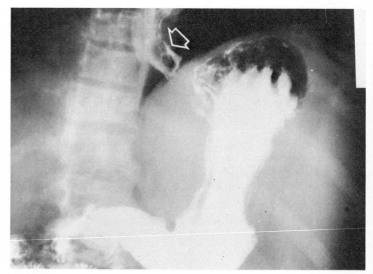

Figure 7

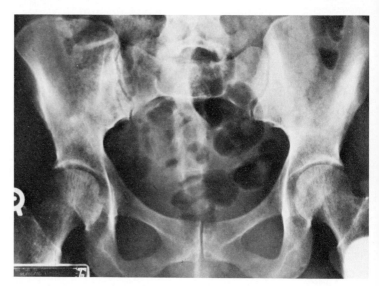

Figure 8

# References

1. Hougie C: Hemophilia and related conditions, in Williams W (ed); *Hematology*, ed 2. New York, McGraw-Hill 1977, p 1404.
2. Arnold WD, Hilgartrer MW: Hemophilic arthropathy. Current concepts of pathogenesis and management. *J Bone Joint Surg* 1977; 59 A:287.
3. Webb JB, Dixon AS: Haemophilia and haemophilic arthropathy. An historical review and a clinical study of 42 cases. *Ann Rheum Dis* 1960; 19:143.
4. Handelsman JE: The knee joint in hemophilia. *Orthop Clin North Am* 1979; 10:139.
5. Gilbert MS: Musculoskeletal manifestations of hemophilia. *Mt Sinai J Med* 1977; 44:339.
6. Brant EE, Jordan HH: Radiographic aspects of hemophilic pseudotumors in bone. *Am J Roentgenol* 1972; 115-525.
7. Gunz FW. Myelofibrosis, in Williams W (ed): *Hematology*, ed 2. New York, McGraw-Hill 1977, p 797.

Figure 9

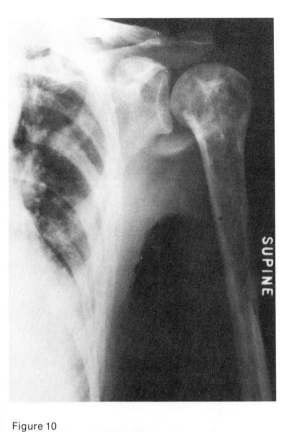

SUPINE

**Fig. 9:** Idiopathic myeloid metaplasia: Cortical thickening and patchy sclerosis of the head of the humerus. The ribs and scapula are also abnormally dense.

**Fig. 10:** Idiopathic myeloid metaplasia: Sclerosis of the pelvic and upper femurs.

Figure 10

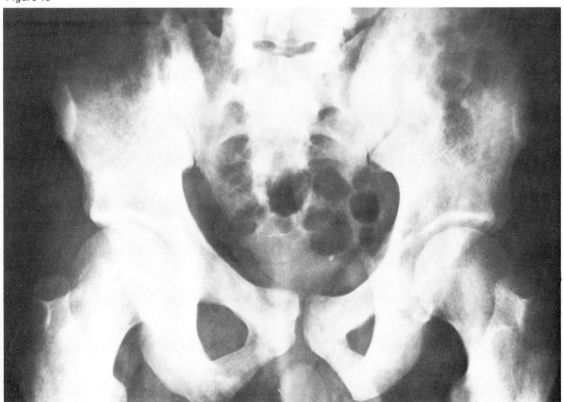

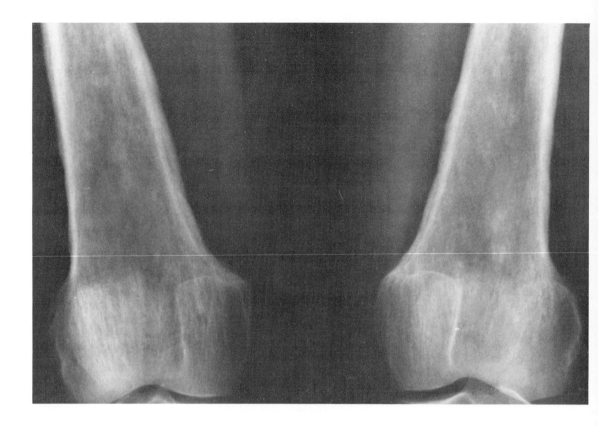

**Fig. 11:** Idiopathic myeloid metaplasia:
Solid periosteal new bone of the distal
femurs.

8. Leigh TF, Corley CC Jr, Huguley CM Jr, et al: Myelofibrosis. The general and radiographic findings in 25 proven cases. *Am J Roentgenol* 1959; 82:183.

9. Pettigrew JD, Ward AP: Correlation of radiologic, histologic and clinical findings in agnogenic myeloid metaplasia. *Radiology* 1969; 93:541.

10. Henderson ES: Acute myelogenous leukemia, in Williams W (ed): *Hematology*, ed 2. New York, McGraw-Hill, 1977, p 830.

11. Thomas LB, Forkner CE Jr, Frei E, et al: The skeletal lesions of acute leukemia. *Cancer* 1961; 14:608.

12. Rundles RW: Chronic granulocytic leukemia, in Williams W (ed): *Hematology,* ed 2. New York, McGraw-Hill, 1977, p 777.

13. Chabner BA, Haskell CM, Canellos GP: Destructive bone lesions in chronic granulocytic leukemia. *Medicine* 1969; 48:401.

14. Clinicopathologic conference: Systemic mastocytosis. *Am J Med* 1976; 61:671.

15. Poppel MH, Gruber WF, Silber R, et al: The roentgen manifestations of urticaria pigmentosa (mastocytosis). *Am J Roentgenol* 1959; 82:239.

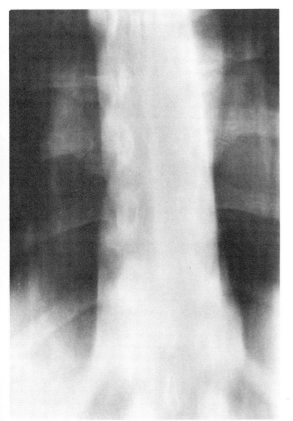

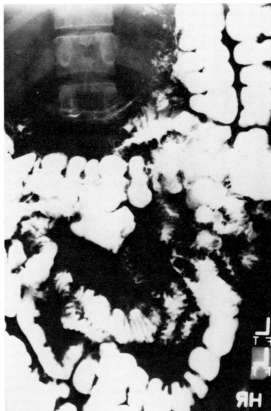

Figure 12                                    Figure 13

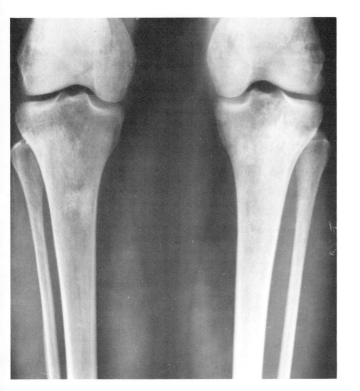

**Fig. 12:** Idiopathic myeloid metaplasia: Extramedullary hematopoiesis in the paraspinal areas at the level of the diaphragm demonstrated by tomography.

**Fig. 13:** Systemic mastocytosis (urticaria pigmentosa): Small bowel nodules cause thickened valvulae conniventes in several loops of small bowel.

**Fig. 14:** Systemic mastocytosis (urticaria pigmentosa): Sclerosis of the distal femurs and proximal tibias. Sclerosis was generalized but other radiographs are not shown. (Courtesy of Miguel Garces, MD.)

# Study 31

This 48-year-old man has limited motion of the left shoulder because of pain. He has had several painful episodes involving the shoulder and other joints in the past years. There is a firm, nontender, fluctuant mass of the distal middle finger of his right hand. *Your diagnosis?*

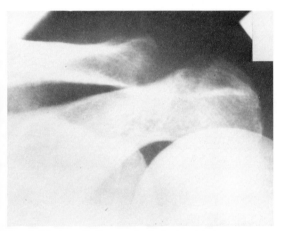

**Fig. 1:** AP view of left acromioclavicular joint.

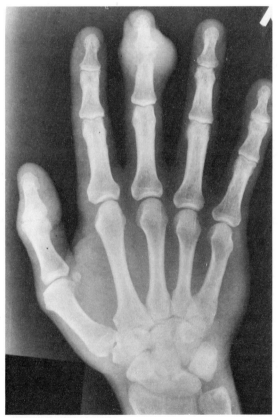

**Fig. 2:** AP view of right hand.

# Diagnosis: Gout

Gout is characterized by:

1. Acute episodes of crystal-induced arthritis
2. Chronic deposition of monosodium urate monohydrate crystals in tophi of cartilage, synovia, tendon sheaths, epiphyseal bone, subcutaneous tissue and the interstitium of the kidney
3. Uric acid renal stones.[1]

The incidence of gout in this country is about 3/1000. Gout is 20 times more common in men. Ninety-five percent of gouty patients have elevated serum uric acid (greater than 7 mg/100 ml using a uricase method).

**Fig. 3:** The first metatarsophalangeal joint is narrow with eburnation and an erosion of the distal MT. (An adjacent tophus cannot be seen here.) This is the most common joint affected in gout. The hand (Fig. 2—erosion and tophus) is less commonly involved, and the acromioclavicular joint (Fig. 1—wide irregular joint space due to erosion) is uncommonly involved.

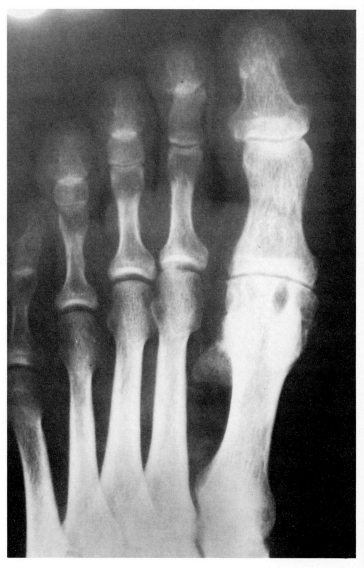

Bone Radiology Case Studies

Most with hyperuricemia never develop gout, but the higher the serum UA level the greater the possibility of developing gout with the passage of years.[2] Asymptomatic patients with primary hyperuricemia are usually not treated unless the serum uric acid exceeds 9 mg/100 ml. Since many patients with hyperuricemia do not have gout and since a few patients with gout have normal serum UA values, the diagnosis of gouty arthritis is only definite when sodium urate crystals are identified in synovial fluid. These needle-shaped crystals are characterized by strong negative birefringence with compensated polarizing light microscopy.

If synovial fluid is negative or not obtained, presence of six of the following provides a probable (not definite) diagnosis of gout:

1. More than one attack of arthritis.
2. Maximum inflammation within one day.
3. Oligoarthritic attack.
4. Redness over joint.
5. Swollen or painful first metatarsophalangeal joint.
6. Unilateral attack, first metatarsophalangeal joint.
7. Unilateral attack, tarsal joint.
8. Suspected or proven tophus.
9. Hyperuricemia.
10. Asymmetric joint swelling.
11. Complete termination of attack.[3]

In primary gout the hyperuricemia is hereditary, either idiopathic or less often due to known metabolic errors. In secondary gout, hyperuricemia is the result of identifiable, usually acquired disorders. Hyperuricemia in either case can be the result of overproduction or underexcretion of uric acid. Patients on a purine free diet who excrete greater than 600 mg of UA in 24 hours are overproducers, and those excreting less than 600 mg of UA are underexcretors. About one-third of patients with primary gout overproduce, one-third underexcrete and one-third have combined defects.

Some disorders associated with secondary hyperuricemia due to uric acid overproduction and underexcretion are:

**UA Overproduction**
Myeloproliferative diseases
Lymphoproliferative diseases
Sickle hemoglobinopathies
Hemolytic anemia
Sarcoidosis
Psoriasis
Diet

**UA Underexcretion**
Renal failure
Lactic acidosis
Starvation and ketosis
Lead poisoning
Alcohol
Low dose salicylates
Diuretics

One-half of patients with secondary gout are women.

Primary gout can be divided into three stages: early (asymptomatic), intermediate (recurrent arthritis) and chronic (tophaceous). Acute arthritis is caused by precipitation of sodium urate crystals in synovial fluid. The crystals are phagocytized by polymorphonuclear leukocytes and synovial lining cells. The crystals fuse with

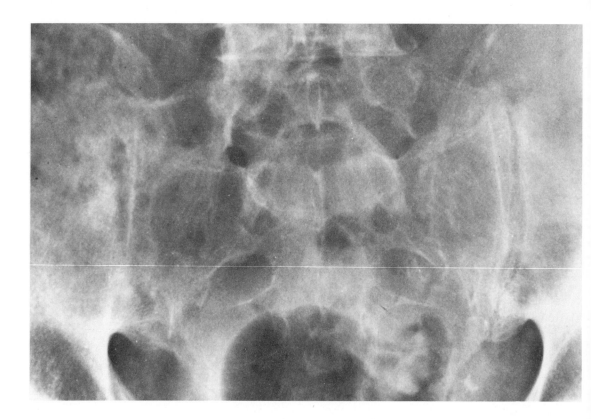

**Fig. 4:** Gouty involvement of right sacroiliac joint with loss of cortical margins.

lysosomes. Enzymes formed result in lysis of the leukocyte and release of the lysosomal enzymes, causing inflammation.[6] Acute attacks are known to follow trauma, surgery, dietary excess, alcohol and drugs. Multiple mechanisms affecting urate crystal formation are known (protein binding, proteoglycans, temperature, pH, trauma, resorption of effusions), but precise pathogenesis remains unproven. Repeated attacks result in synovial proliferation and tophi of synovia, cartilage and bone causing progressive joint damage.

The initial attack is in a single joint about 85% of the time. The majority of first attacks are in the big toe (podagra). Joint involvement is usually asymmetric and pauciarticular with a predilection for the lower extremities. Sites of involvement in order of frequency are the tarsals, ankles, heels, knees, wrists, fingers and elbows.[7] The high incidence in the distal extremities may be related to the lower temperature distally since urate is less soluble at lower temperatures. The shoulders, hips, sternoclavicular, acromioclavicular, spine and sacroiliac joints are uncommonly involved (Fig. 4). Symmetric polyarthritis simulating rheumatoid arthritis occurs in up to 5% of patients.[8] Gout and rheumatoid arthritis rarely coexist.

Radiographic findings are not found in most patients until they have had symptomatic gout for many years. The primary abnormalities are tophi and bone erosions.

Tophaceous nodules consist of urate crystals, matrix, inflammatory reaction and foreign body granulomas. They appear as

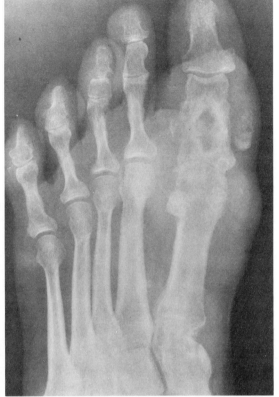

Figure 5

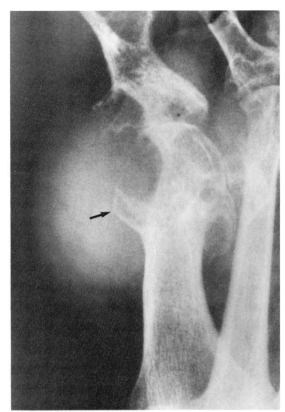

Figure 6

eccentric soft tissue masses. Occasionally they are calcified and rarely ossified (Fig. 5). Bony erosions occur in the joint, para-articular area and away from the joint. They are often located beneath tophi. Most are sharply defined and may have sclerotic margins. Many of these erosions have a marginal, thin bony projection extending outward along a part of the adjacent tophus. This overhanging edge is characteristic of gout (Fig. 6). End-stage disease may produce a mutilating arthritis.

Bone density is usually normal or only slightly decreased except for disuse osteoporosis in advanced cases. The joint spaces are preserved until late in the course of the disease. Late symmetric narrowing can be followed by fibrous ankylosis or rarely bony ankylosis.[9] Secondary osteoarthritis is common.

Some reports indicate a relationship between gout and chondrocalcinosis. The incidence of chondrocalcinosis in gout is probably no higher than that in the general population according to more recent studies. Quadriceps tendon rupture, giant popliteal synovial cysts and nerve compression syndromes including carpal tunnel syndrome have been reported with gout.

**Fig. 5:** Advanced gouty changes with calcified soft tissue tophi adjacent to big toe.

**Fig. 6:** Large, dense tophus erodes the distal first metatarsal, producing a characteristic overhanging edge (arrow).

### References

1. Boss GR, Seegmiller JE: Hyperuricemia and gout. *N Engl J Med* 1979; 300:1459.
2. Liang MH, Fries JF: Asymptomatic hyperuricemia: The case for conservative management. *Ann Intern Med* 1978; 88:666.

3. Wallace SI, Robinson H, Masi A, et al: Preliminary criteria for the classification of the acute arthritis of primary gout. *Arthritis Rheum* 1977; 20:895.
4. Smyth CJ: Disorders associated with hyperuricemia. *Arthritis Rheum* 1975; 18:173.
5. Wyngaarden JB, Kelley WN: *Hyperuricemia and Gout.* New York, Grune and Stratton, 1977.
6. Scott JT: New knowledge of the pathogenesis of gout. *J Clin Pathol* 1978; 31(suppl 12):205.
7. Talbott JM, Yu T: *Gout and Uric Acid Metabolism.* New York, Stratton Intercontinental Medical Book Corp, 1976.
8. Talbott JH, Altman RD, Yu TF: Gouty arthritis masquerading as rheumatoid arthritis or vice-versa. *Semin Arthritis Rheum* 1978; 8:77.
9. Resnick D: The radiographic manifestations of gouty arthritis. *Diag Radiol* 1977; 9:265.

# VII

# *JOINTS*

A joint can be narrowed or widened, and it can be the site of calcification, effusion, or erosion. The radiographic joint space indicates the thickness of articular cartilage. Narrowing can be symmetric, as in inflammatory arthritis, or asymmetric, as in degenerative joint disease. Widening of the joint space is found with joint effusion, extensive joint erosion, and acromegaly. Calcification of articular and para-articular structures can be the result of the same disorders which cause calcification of other soft tissues. Chondrocalcinosis may be due to calcium pyrophosphate dihydrate deposition disease or hydroxyapatite, and it may indicate the etiology of arthritis or lead to a diagnosis of a systemic disease, especially hyperparathyroidism.

Joint effusions may be clues indicating trauma or inflammation. A fat-fluid level usually indicates the presence of a fracture but is not visible unless the x-ray beam is horizontal.

Erosions are an important feature of inflammatory and crystal-induced arthritides. Early erosions of inflammatory arthritides are located peripherally on the intra-articular bone surfaces unprotected by cartilage. Larger cysts or geodes can occur in all types of arthritis and are attributed to granulation tissue growing into the bone or to the action of joint fluid under increased pressure in association with cartilage defects.

# Study 32

This 57-year-old man with rheumatoid arthritis acutely developed right calf pain. The right calf is erythematous and tender, and there is a positive Homan's sign. The right calf is 7 cm larger than the left. Film from bilateral venogram is shown. *Your diagnosis?*

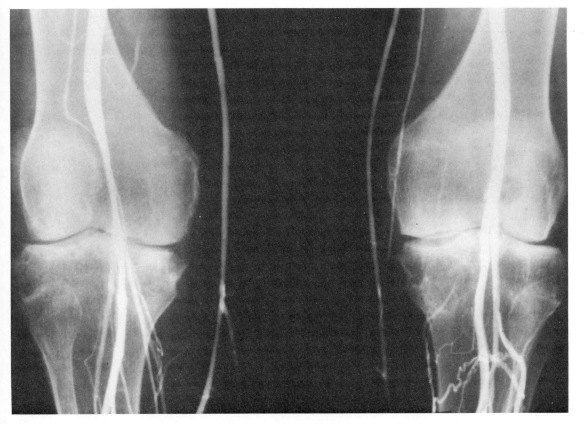

**Fig. 1:** Bilateral lower leg venograms.

# Diagnosis: Giant Synovial Cyst

Synovial cysts commonly occur in rheumatoid arthritis. Occasionally, a popliteal cyst may masquerade as thrombophlebitis. In a series of 45 patients with rheumatoid arthritis, 12 had popliteal cysts and six of these presented with signs and symptoms mistakenly diagnosed as thrombophlebitis.[1] This was the reason a venogram was ordered in the case presented here. When venograms are obtained, they show vascular narrowing and displacement only (Fig. 1).

When the proper diagnosis is considered, ultrasound is an accurate, rapid, noninvasive means of confirming the cystic nature of a mass or leg enlargement caused by a mass[2] (Fig. 2). Intra-articular radioisotopes have also been successful.[3] Arthrography (Figs. 3, 4) is definitive and has the advantage of demonstrating joint pathology. Rarely, a noncommunicating cyst or multilocular cyst results in nonfilling on arthrography.[4] Nonfilling has also been reported when films in 90° flexion were not obtained.

**Fig. 2:** Longitudinal (top) and transverse (bottom) ultrasonograms. Cystic mass communicating with joint space accounts for displacement and narrowed popliteal vein in Figure 1.

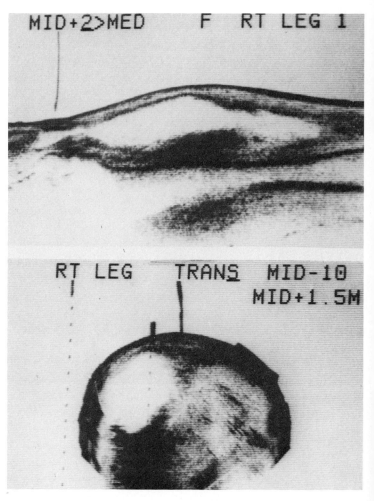

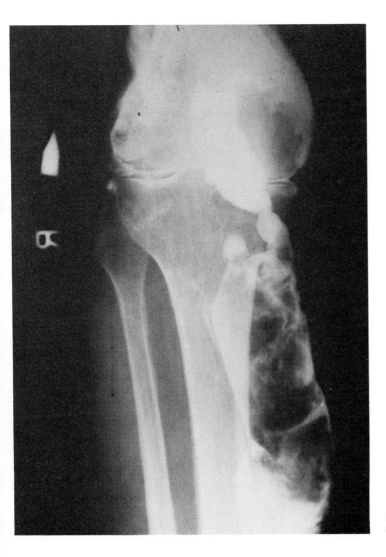

**Fig. 3:** Arthrogram confirms the presence of a large popliteal cyst.

**Fig. 4:** Giant synovial cyst of shoulder is demonstrated by arthrography in this patient with rheumatoid arthritis.

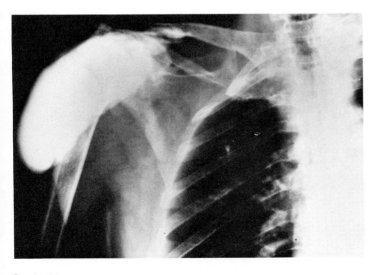

The majority of adults with popliteal cysts have intra-articular pathology including Reiter's syndrome, rheumatoid arthritis and other collagen diseases, osteoarthritis, meniscal tears, septic arthritis, gout, villonodular synovitis and osteochondrosis dessicans.[5] Giant popliteal cysts and cysts associated with "pseudo-thrombophlebitis" are most commonly seen in patients with rheumatoid arthritis, however.

Rare complications of popliteal cysts include the posterior compartment syndrome,[6] popliteal artery occlusion[7] and infection with external drainage.[8]

## References

1. Good AE: Rheumatoid arthritis, Baker's cyst and "thrombophelbitis." *Arthritis Rheum* 1964; 7:56-64.
2. McDonald DG, Leopold GR: Ultrasound B-scanning in the differentiation of Baker's cyst and thrombophlebitis. *Br J Radiol* 1972; 45:729-732.
3. Watkins AE, Poulose KP, Reba RC: Arthroscintigraphy with technetium albumin in diagnosis of pseudophlebitis (Baker's) cyst. *Br Med J* 1975; 11:86.
4. Bryan RS, DiMichele JD, Ford GL: Popliteal cysts. *Clin Orthop* 1967; 50:203-208.
5. Schmidt MC, Workman JB, Barth WF: Dissection or rupture of a popliteal cyst. *Arch Intern Med* 1974; 134:694-698.
6. Scott WN, Jacobs B, Lockshin MD: Posterior compartment syndrome resulting from a dissecting popliteal cyst. *Clin Orthop* 1977; 122:189-192.
7. Schlenker JD, Johnston K, Wolkoff JS: Occlusion of popliteal artery caused by popliteal cysts. *Surgery* 1974; 76:833-836.
8. Williams P: Spontaneous external rupture of an infected popliteal cyst in rheumatoid arthritis. *Proc R Soc Med* 1972; 65:1015-1016.

# Study 33

This 34-year-old man has had knee pain for two months. He had knee surgery two years ago but doesn't know what was done. *Your diagnosis?*

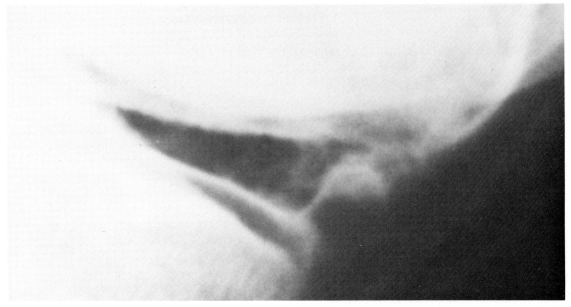

**Fig. 1:** Double contrast arthrography.
Medial aspect of left knee joint.

# Diagnosis: Partial Menisectomy with Torn Remnant

Complaints regarding pain and function of the knee constitute common orthopedic problems. Meniscal tears are often included in the differential diagnosis of these complaints and knee arthrography is a safe procedure that may provide a definitive diagnosis. Levinsohn[1] has evaluated prearthrotomy, arthrography and arthroscopy and found arthrography superior in the diagnosis of peripheral and mid-body tears. Arthrography was also superior in the diagnosis of posterior horn tears in either meniscus; however, the arthroscoper in this study used an anterolateral approach. Tegtmeyer[2] found arthrography to be between 93% to 97% accurate in assessing meniscal tears. Ireland,[3] Gillies[4] and Gillquist[5] all report lesser degrees of accuracy but all conclude that arthrography and arthroscopy are complementary procedures in the evaluation of meniscal lesions.

Knee arthrography may diagnose not only torn menisci but other meniscal and extrameniscal lesions as well.

## Technique

The only contraindication to arthrography is a previous severe reaction to iodinated contrast material. If this has not occurred, the procedure may begin.

First, scout films (AP, lateral and oblique) of the knee are taken to evaluate for an unexpected diagnosis such as tumor, osteochondritis dissecans, arthritis or fracture. These preliminary radiographs also warn of chondrocalcinosis (Fig. 3) which could make evaluation of a meniscal tear most difficult.

The patient then lies supine and the knee is prepped. A 21-gauge 1½ inch needle is placed directly posterior to the patella into the knee joint. A lateral approach is most common but not necessary. Local anesthetic is not used as the needle puncture and burning of the anesthetic appears to be more painful than the single puncture. Any joint fluid is removed and, in order to bring the fluid to the needle tip, it is often necessary to compress down on the patella and

**Fig. 2:** The patient had a menisectomy two years ago. The joint space (asterisk) is empty; the vertical line (arrowhead) is the coating of the inner margin of the meniscal remnant. The contrast-filled defect (arrow) is a new tear.

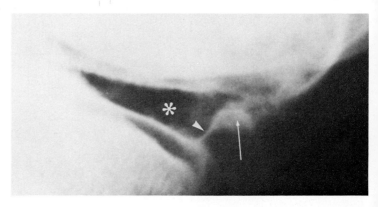

suprapatellar pouch while withdrawing on the plunger. Also, rotating the leg or angling the needle may result in aspiration of additional fluid. The fluid may be sent for analysis or discarded. If no fluid was withdrawn from the joint, a test injection of 0.5 cc of lidocaine is then done to confirm intra-articular position of the needle tip. If the needle is in the joint space, there should be very little resistance to the plunger. Lidocaine is used instead of contrast material in order to avoid staining the soft tissue in the event of an extra-articular injection. A drop or two of contrast material is now

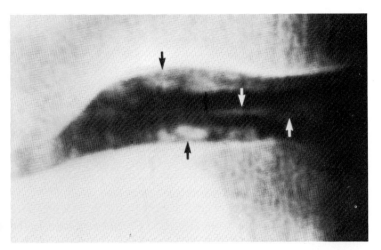

**Fig. 3:** 75-year-old female with chondrocalcinosis involving both articular cartilages (black arrows) and meniscus (white arrows) etiology unknown.

**Fig. 4A:** Normal arthrogram done with contrast material only—and drawing.

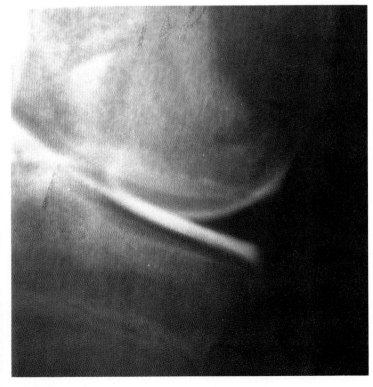

injected under flouroscopic control and, if in the joint space, it will flow freely away from the needle tip. Once this is seen, approximately 5 cc of contrast agent and 30 cc of air are injected. Hall[6] and Spataro[7] have shown that the addition of epinephrine into the knee joint delays the resorption of contrast material and, so, results in enhancement and prolongation of good radiographic quality. This promotes superior radiographs over enough time to allow for repeat films to be taken, so 0.3 cc of 1:1000 epinephrine solution is added to the syringe containing contrast agent.

The patient then walks several steps and flexes the knee two times in order to distribute the contrast and air throughout the joint space. The patient then lies prone on the flouroscopic table and multiple films are taken with the x-ray beam perpendicular to the long axis of the leg. The leg must be rotated about 360° during examination so that all of the medial and lateral meniscus is seen. The knee is placed against some kind of restraining device (the shoulder brace used during cervical myelograms works nicely) so that lateral distraction can be applied during filming.

In order to evaluate the cruciate ligaments, two lateral films are taken with the knee flexed 60° to 70°, the foot stabilized by any restraining device and traction put on the proximal tibia to bring it forward. One film is done with the patient lying on his side and the other with the patient sitting on the edge of the table. It is best if these films are slightly overpenetrated.

Finally the patient flexes the knee 90° and a lateral film is taken to evaluate the presence of a Baker's cyst. Clark[8] has shown that flexion causes compression of the anterior joint space and relaxation posteriorly so that this technique yielded a 24% increase in the diagnosis of Baker's cyst. Unfortunately, the significance of the presence of a cyst is not always clear.

## Normal Anatomy

The fibrocartilaginous medial meniscus (Drawing I) is a C-shaped structure slightly wider posteriorly than anteriorly. The

**Drawing 1:** Coronal section through knee.

**Drawing 2:** Coronal section through

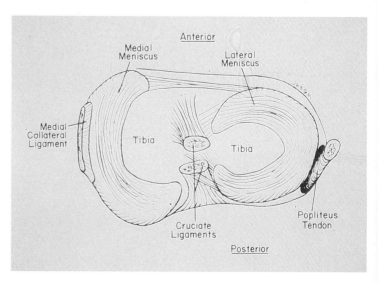

fibrocartilaginous lateral meniscus is more curved, almost making a complete circle but leaving a gap at its farthest internal extension. Both menisci are tall peripherally, and slope to a thin internal edge so that in vertical cross-section (and on the radiographs) the meniscus appears as a wedge (Figs. 4A, B).

The medial meniscus is attached to the capsule throughout its periphery while there is a defect in the capsular attachment of the lateral meniscus. This defect (Fig. 5) is located slightly posterior to the midline of the meniscus and is due to the bursa, which houses the popliteus tendon, traversing the peripheral aspect of the meniscus at a slight angle heading posteriorly as it goes inferiorly.

## Meniscal Lesions

The most common meniscal abnormality is a tear. The normal meniscus (Fig. 4A) appears as a wedge-shaped tissue coated by

**Drawing 4:** Coronal section through knee.

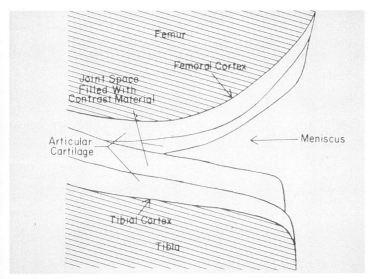

Drawing 2A

Drawing 2B

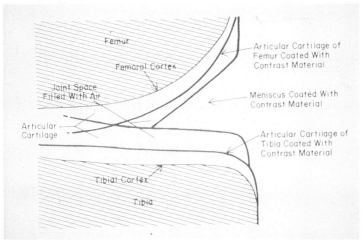

contrast agent and partially surrounded by air. The contrast material should stay on the surface of the meniscus; if it is seen within the meniscal substance, there must be a defect (tear) in the integrity of the meniscus allowing the contrast to enter. Tears may be vertical (Fig. 6), horizontal (Fig. 7), oblique (Fig. 8A), peripheral (Fig. 9) or at the free margin (apex of the radiologic wedge) (Fig. 10). They may be filled with contrast material (Fig. 11), air (Fig. 12), or both (Fig. 13). The meniscus fragment may be shattered (Fig. 14). A meniscal fragment may be visible (Fig. 15) or it may not be seen, as it has migrated to the area of the intercondylar eminences (Fig. 16). The previously described defect caused by the popliteus tendon bursa (Fig. 5) must not be mistaken for a tear in the posterior aspect of the lateral meniscus.

After meniscectomy, a piece of the posterior horn often remains. The remnant should be intact (Fig. 17) but may show a tear (Fig. 18) in the same manner as does a whole meniscus. A remnant, torn or intact, is usually removed in a symptomatic patient.

It is the lateral meniscus that almost exclusively exhibits the discoid deformity. The discoid shape is represented by extension of the meniscus far into the center of the joint; thickening of the apex of the wedge may or may not occur (Fig. 19). Like postmeniscectomy remnants, a discoid meniscus is usually removed if the patient is symptomatic, regardless of whether or not it is torn.[9]

Meniscal cysts[10] are located in the periphery of the meniscus; usually the lateral. If a tear bridges the joint space to the cyst then all three spaces can be visualized (Fig. 20).

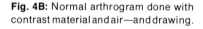

**Fig. 4B:** Normal arthrogram done with contrast material and air—and drawing.

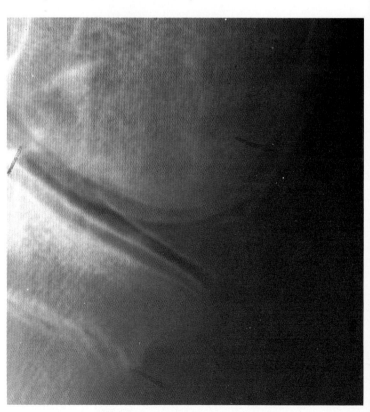

## Extrameniscal Lesions

Baker's cysts are enlarged gastrocnemius-semi-membranosus bursae which may be associated with a variety of entities. As stated earlier, they are commonly found using Clark's[8] flexed knee technique (Fig. 21) but are of dubious significance.[11]

A narrow channel is often seen extending from the joint space to the cyst (Fig. 22) and this lends some support to the Bunsen-valve mechanism[12] of cyst formation.

Baker's cyst may dissect down the calf mimicking the signs of symptoms of thrombophlebitis.[13-16] Arthrography will diagnose the extension of the cyst (Fig. 23) and allow appropriate therapy while sparing the patient the administration and dangers of anticoagulants. Cysts may also dissect superiorly (Fig. 24) and recently reported[17] are five antefemoral dissecting synovial cysts in patients with rheumatoid arthritis. Also reported[18] are five cases of entrapment neuropathy resulting from Baker's cysts.

Tear of the anterior cruciate ligament is a common entity which can often be seen using the film technique previously described.

In normal studies (Fig. 25) the anterior and posterior cruciates are seen as straight surfaces; and, if one is demonstrated, the other should be seen as well.

If the posterior cruciate is well displayed but there is pooling of contrast material (Fig. 26) where the anterior cruciate should be, then the anterior cruciate is torn. A stretched and attenuated

**Fig. 5:** Posterior horn of lateral meniscus showing popliteus tendon bursa (arrows).

**Fig. 6:** Contrast material filling wide vertical tear (arrow).

**Fig. 7:** Horizontal tear (arrow).

**Fig. 8:** Oblique tear (arrow).

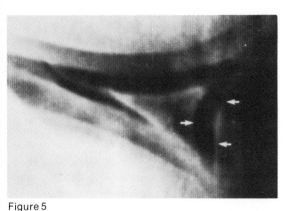

Figure 5

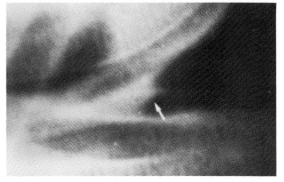

Figure 6

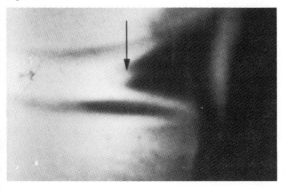

Figure 7

Figure 8

anterior cruciate is manifest by the surface being bowed rather than taut. These radiographic criteria also apply to the less frequently involved posterior cruciate ligament.

The integrity of the medical collateral ligament can also be evaluated arthrographically. Because the deep fibers of the medial collateral ligament are attached to the joint capsule, tearing of these fibers also tears the capsule allowing contrast material to escape the joint (Fig. 27). However, "the arthrogram should be performed within 48 hours of the injury because later the capsule may become air- and watertight, preventing leakage of contrast agent even when the ligament is torn and the knee is unstable."[19]

Osteochondritis dissecans often presents the problem of whether the osteochondral body is free in the joint space requiring surgery or covered by articular cartilage. An arthrogram can demonstrate air or contrast agent surrounding the fragment (Fig. 28) thus indicating that the fragment is loose. However, if the arthrogram (Fig. 29) shows overlying intact articular cartilage preventing contast material from entering the lesion then conservative therapy is instituted. Arthrotomography is often helpful in this evaluation (Fig. 30).

Irregularity, thinning, or disappearance of the articular cartilage is seen in osteoarthritis. Fraying and irregularity of the meniscus often accompanies this (Fig.31).

A suprapatellar plica is a congenital synovial fold which may cause generalized symptoms of internal derangement of the knee. These symptoms present when the plica becomes thickened and fibrotic secondary to synovitis caused by a variety of conditions such as torn ligaments, torn menisci, effusion or hemorrhage. The postulated mechanisms of symptom production are reviewed by Blatz.[20] While some doubt exists as to the significance of the plica, Blatz studied 380 knee procedures including 58 cases in which plicectomy was done and concluded that "based on this series, findings and results, we feel the plica is a significant contributing factor to internal derangement problems of the knee, and should be thought of, sought, and sectioned by arthroscopy, or removed by

**Fig. 9:** Air-filled peripheral tear (arrows).

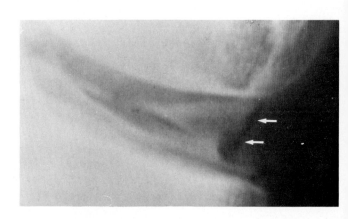

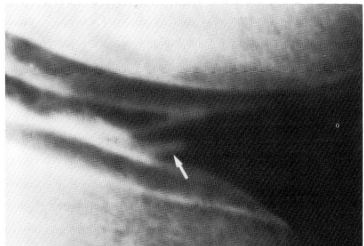

Figure 10

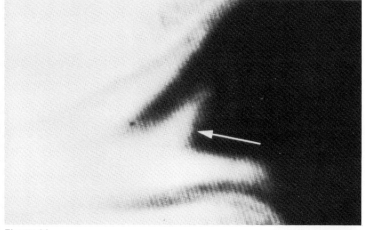

Figure 11

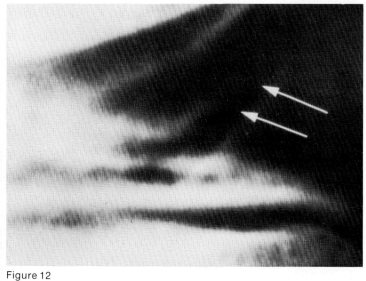

Figure 12

**Fig. 10:** Tear (arrow) at free margin.

**Fig. 11:** Oblique tear (arrow) filled with contrast material.

**Fig. 12:** Oblique tear (arrows) filled with air.

Study 33

arthrotomy."[20] The suprapatellar plica may be sought by arthrography (Fig. 32).

Knee arthrography has also been used in the evaluation of adhesive capsulitis, rheumatoid arthritis, foreign bodies, pigmented villonodular synovitis and synovial tumors.

*—Richard Cooper, MD*

## References

1. Levinsohn EM, Baker BE: Prearthrotomy diagnostic evaluation of the knee.

**Fig. 13:** Horizontal tear containing both contrast material (white arrows) and air (black arrow).

**Fig. 14:** Inner half of meniscus is irregularly invaded by air and contrast material.

**Fig. 15:** Large meniscal fragment (asterisk) is seen coated by contrast material and almost entirely surrounded by air.

**Fig. 16:** Apex of mensicus had avulsed and cannot be seen. The meniscus now terminates with a triangular defect.

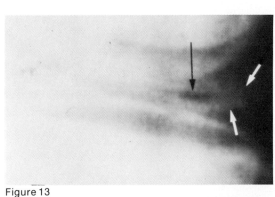

Figure 13

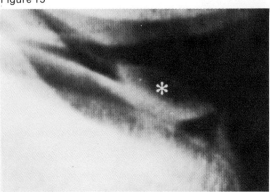

Figure 15

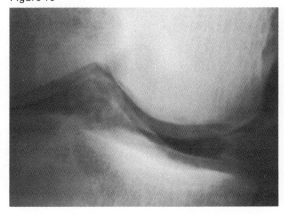

Figure 14

Figure 16

*AJR* 1980; 134:107-111.

2. Tegtmeyer CJ, McCue III FC, Higgins SM, et al: Arthrography of the knee: a comparative study of the accuracy of single double contrast techniques. *Radiology* 1979; 132:37-41.

3. Ireland J, Trickey EL, Stoker DJ: Arthroscopy and arthrography of the knee: A critical review. *J Bone Joint Surg (Br)* 1980; 62B:3-6.

4. Gillies H, Seligson D: Precision in the diagnosis of meniscal lesions: A comparison of clinical evaluation, arthrography and arthroscopy. *J Bone Joint Surg AM* 1979; 61:343-346.

5. Gillquist J, Hagberg G: Findings at arthroscopy and arthrography in knee injuries. *Acta Orthop Scand* 1978; 49:398-402.

6. Hall FM: Epinephrine-enhanced knee arthrography. *Radiology* 1974; 111:215.

7. Spataro RF, Katzberg RW, Burgener FA, et al: Epinephrine enhanced knee arthrography. *Investigative Radiology* 1978; 13:286-290.

8. Clark JM: Arthrography diagnosis of synovial cysts of the knee. *Radiology* 1975; 115:480-481.

9. Lovell WW, Winter RB: *Pediatric Orthopedics*. ed 1. Philadelphia, Toronto, JB Lippincott Co., 1978, 903.

10. Schuldt DR, Wolfe RD: Clinical and arthrographic findings in meniscal cysts. *Radiology* 1980; 134:49-52.

11. Pulich JJ: Asymptomatic popliteal cysts. *Journal AOA* 1975; 75:319-323.

**Fig. 17:** Small, intact, post-meniscectomy remnant (arrows).

**Fig. 18:** Post-meniscectomy remnant with irregular contrast-filled superior aspect (arrow).

**Fig. 19A:** Discoid lateral meniscus seen to extend far into the joint space.

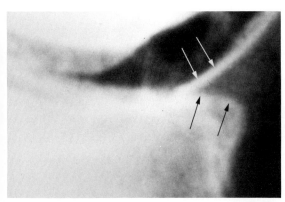

Figure 17

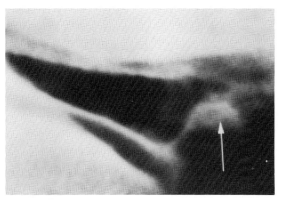

Figure 18

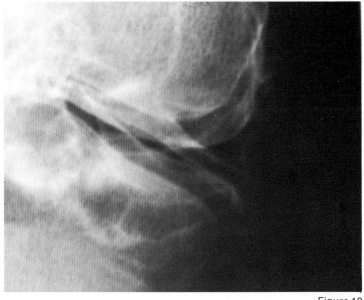

Figure 19

12. Jayson MIV, Dixon A ST J: Valvular mechanism in juxta-articular cysts. *Ann Rheum Dis* 1970; 29:415-420.
13. Cooper RA: Computerized tomography (body scan) of Baker's cyst. *J Rheumatol* 1978; 5:184-189.
14. Schmidt MC, Workman JB, Barth WF: Dissection or rupture of a popliteal cyst. *Arch Intern Med* 1974; 134:694-698.
15. Rudikoff JC, Lynch JJ, Philipps E, et al: Ultrasound diagnosis of Baker's cyst. *JAMA* 1976; 235:1054.
16. Eyanson S, Macfarlane JD, Brandt KD: Popliteal cyst mimicking thrombophlebitis as the first indication of knee disease. *Clin Orthop* 1979; 144:215-219.
17. Seidl G, Scherak O, Hofner W: Antefemoral dissecting cysts in rheumatoid arthritis. *Radiology* 1979; 133:343-347.
18. Nakano KK: Entrapment neuropathy from Baker's cyst. *JAMA* 1978; 239:135.
19. Freiberger RH, Kaye JJ: *Arthrography*. New York. Appleton-Century-Crofts, 1979, p 112.
20. Blatz DJ, Fleming R, McCarroll J: Suprapatellar plica: A study of their occurrence and role in internal derangement of the knee in active duty personnel. *Orthopedics* 1981; 4:181-185.

**Fig. 19B:** Surgical Specimen. Anterior (A), Posterior (P), Lateral (L) and note the loss of concavity on the medial (M) aspect of the meniscus. Note, also, its medial thickness as indicated by the linear glare of light.

**Fig. 20:** A horizontal tear (arrows) provides communication allowing air from the joint space to fill the meniscal cyst (asterisk).

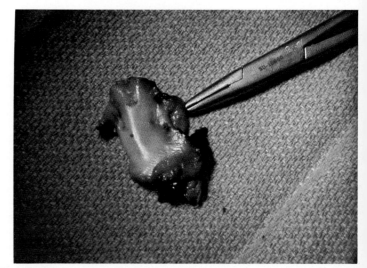

Figure 19B

Figure 20

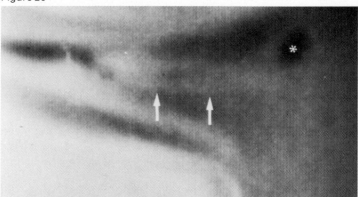

Bone Radiology Case Studies

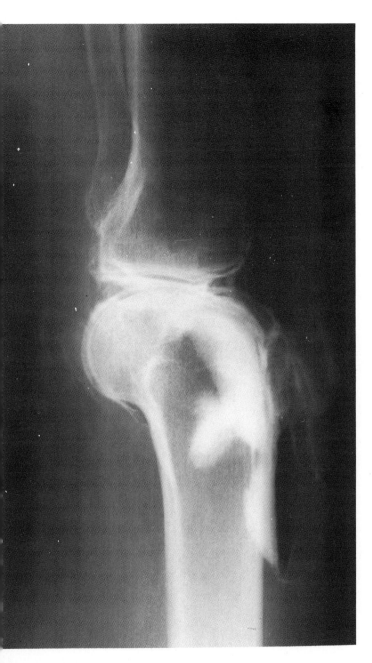

**Figure 21B:** With leg flexed, the posterior knee is relaxed and a Baker's cyst (asterisk) is seen to fill with air.

**Fig. 22:** Channel (arrows) leading to Baker's cyst.

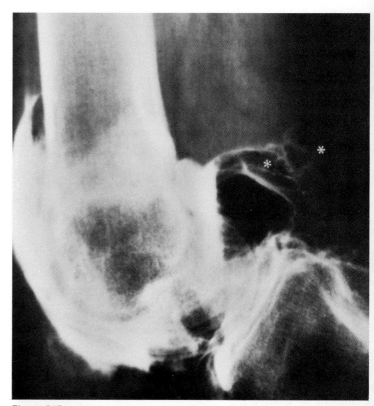

Figure 21B

Figure 22

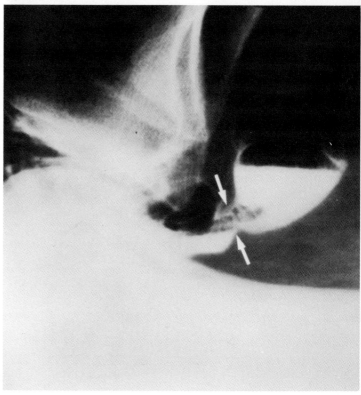

Bone Radiology Case Studies

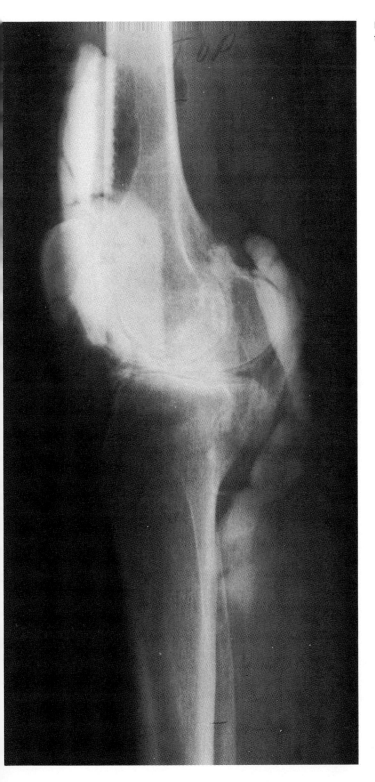

**Fig. 23:** Baker's cyst dissecting down the calf mimicking thrombophlebitis.

**Fig. 24:** Cyst extending superiorly into thigh.

**Fig. 25:** Straight edge of the anterior (white arrows) and posterior (black arrows) cruciate ligaments are seen in the film taken with the patient lying on his side.

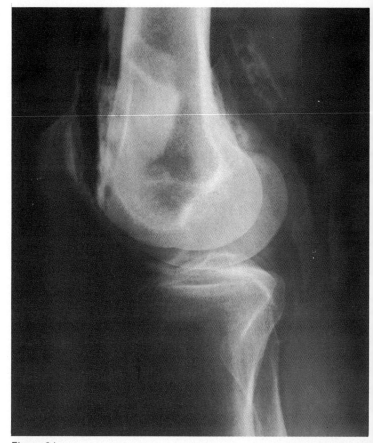

Figure 24

Figure 25

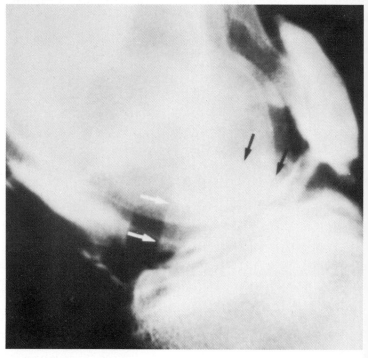

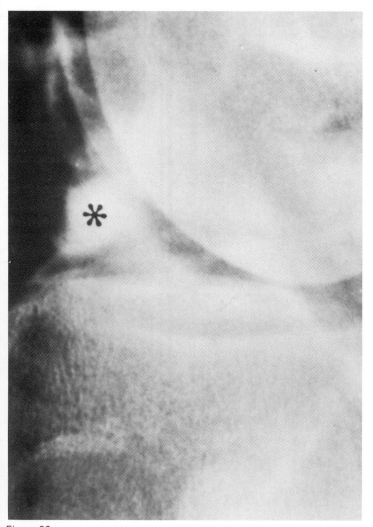

Figure 26

**Fig. 26:** There is pooling of contrast material (asterisk) where the straight anterior surface of the anterior cruciate should be—this indicates a torn anterior cruciate ligament.

**Figs. 27A, B:** Two examples of contrast material (arrows) escaping from the medial aspect of the joint in patients with torn medial collateral ligaments.

Figures 27A

Figure 27B

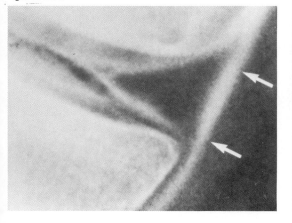

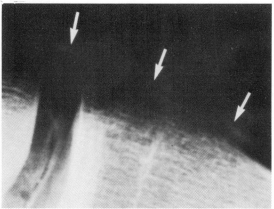

**Fig. 28A:** Plain film showing osteo-chondritis dissecans of the medial femoral condyle.

**Fig. 28B:** Arthrogram showing bony fragment (arrows) completely sur-rounded by air and, therefore, loose.

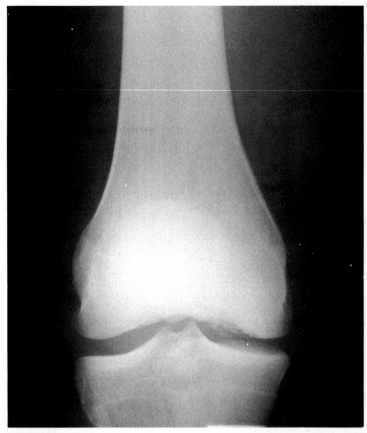

Figure 28A

Figure 28B

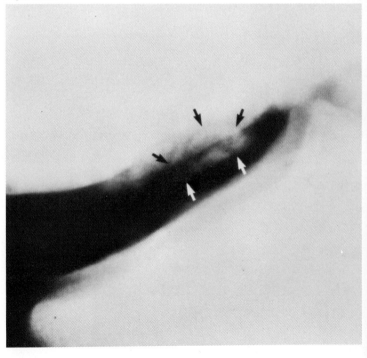

Bone Radiology Case Studies

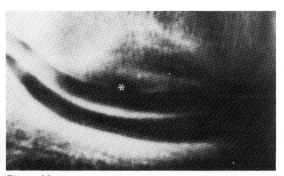

Figure 29

**Fig. 29:** Femoral defect (asterisk) is completely covered by contrast-coated articular cartilage.

**Fig. 30:** Tomogram showing osseous body covered by articular cartilage. The cartilage keeps the contrast material below the fragment and does not allow wit to enter the femoral defect.

**Fig. 31:** Absence of femoral articular cartilage and waviness of the superior surface (arrows) of the postero-medial meniscus indicating degenerative joint disease.

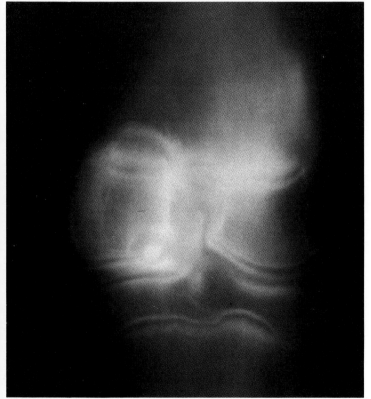

Figure 30

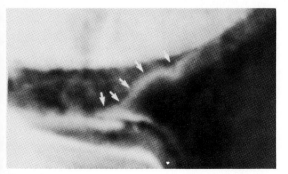

Figure 31

Study 33

**Fig. 32A, B:** Frontal and lateral view of contrast material-coated plica (arrows) in a symptomatic patient. The symptoms abated after plicectomy and repair of a torn anterior cruciate ligament.

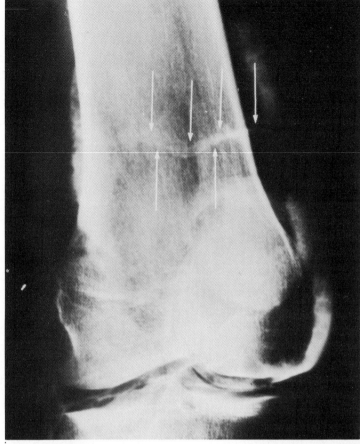

Figure 32A

Figure 32B

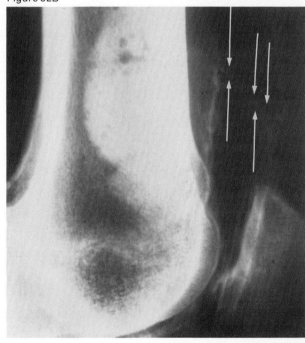

# Study 34

This 29-year-old man was sideswiped by a car while riding a motorcycle. He was thrown off, and suffered multiple abrasions and contusions. His right ankle was swollen with pain on movement. Initial roentgenograms were negative. Although his ankle symptoms improved in two days, he could not bear full weight, and the repeat films shown above were done. *Your diagnosis?*

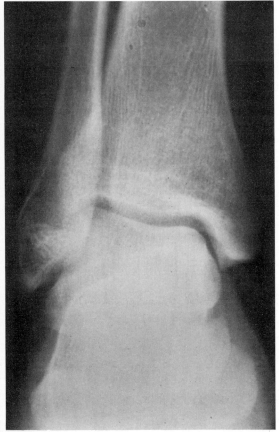

**Fig. 1:** AP right ankle.

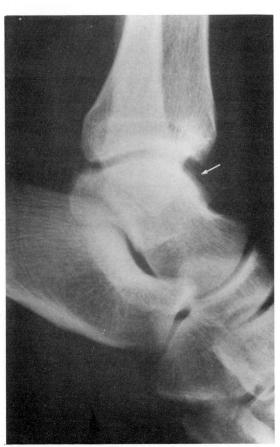

**Fig. 2:** Lateral right ankle.

# Diagnosis: Osteochondral Fracture

Osteochondral fractures are frequently missed or present problems in diagnosis. These fractures result from shearing, rotational or impaction forces produced by abnormal joint motion. If the fragment is cartilage alone, it will not be seen in roentgenograms. Even when the fragment is osteochondral, the bony portion is often small and difficult to detect. In the case presented here, initial films of the ankle were not optimum, and a slightly obliqued lateral film caused the fracture fragment to be obscured by normal bone. Later films done on the basis of clinical suspicion showed the pathology.

The most common sites of osteochondral fractures are the knee and elbow. (Figs. 4, 5) Much less common locations are the ankle, shoulder and hips. The fractures are usually tangential, and through subchondral bone, uncalcified cartilage or the histologic zone between calcified and uncalcified cartilage termed the tidemark.[1] Most fracture fragments are probably resorbed after becoming attached to the synovium. A fragment maintaining some attachment to its origin may revascularize with subsequent trabecular bone formation. Loose fragments that are not resorbed may grow by forming cartilage and bone, or they may undergo degenerative calcification.[1]

In the ankle, most osteochondral fractures involve the talar dome on its lateral side. Clinically the patients present with swelling,

**Fig. 3:** Lateral laminogram right ankle. A thin linear bone fragment adjacent to the anterior superior talus is shown inside the joint space on this laminogram. It is the bone part of a 1.5 cm × 1 cm x$^2$mm osteochondral fragment off the lateral talus which was removed surgically. Figure 2 showed the fragment, plus a fracture of the tip of the lateral malleolus.

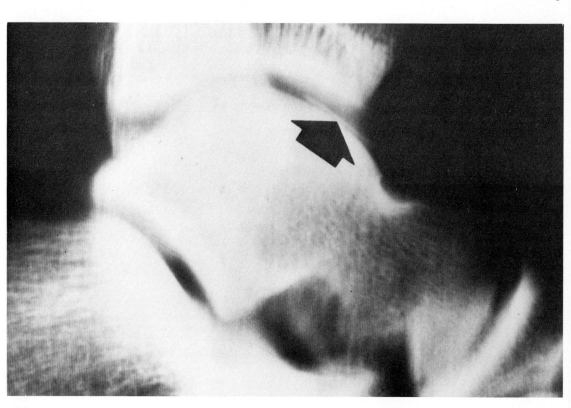

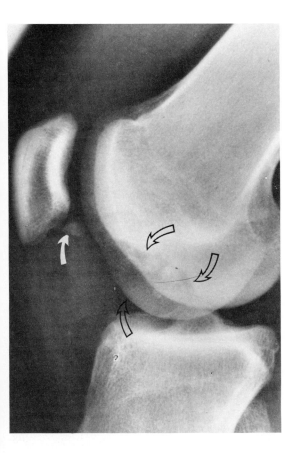

**Fig. 4:** "Osteochondrosis Dissecans" of the knee is usually located in the *medial* femoral condyle (open arrows) and may result in a loose body (closed arrow). These lesions are usually residuals of old, undiagnosed osteochondral fractures.

ecchymosis, limited motion and tenderness. Symptoms are usually due to soft tissue injury, since subchondral bone is insensitive. When routine ankle views are called normal, the patient is considered to have a sprain. If the fragment is discovered at a later date, it may be considered to be osteochondrosis dissecans (Fig. 6). Loose bodies may result in degenerative changes or joint locking.[2,3]

In the ankle, an osteochondral fracture is usually caused by an inversion injury, with the superior medial talar dome striking the tibia and the superior lateral dome contacting the fibula. Degree of flexion or extension of the ankle determines the specific site of the dome which is fractured.[4] The fractures have been classified as stages 1 to 4: (1) minimal subchondral compression deformity; (2) partially detached osteochondral fragment; (3) detached, undisplaced fragment; and (4) displaced osteochondral fragment.[5]

Radiographs must be scrutinized to identify these subtle fractures. Multiple projections and repeat views should be obtained if clinical suspicion is strong, or roentgenograms are equivocal or technically deficient. Most fractures involve the lateral or medial corners of the talar dome, and are seen on AP views. The dome is better seen on an AP film with 10° to 15° internal rotation. Only minimal cortical irregularity, sclerosis or lucency may be present. Tomograms can define and confirm questionable findings. Tomographic localization also helps decide the surgical approach (Fig. 7). Arthrography can identify a loose body, even if it is composed of cartilage alone.

Treatment depends on the fragment size, the amount of bone in the fragment and degree of displacement. Small displaced fragments are excised. Small undisplaced fragments may unite with conservative treatment. Open reduction and fixation are reserved for large fragments with a large segment of bone which then may heal as a free bone graft.[3,4,6]

### References

1. Milgram JW, Rogers LF, Miller JW: Osteochondral fractures: Mechanisms of injury and fate of fragments. *Am J Roentgenol* 1978; 130:651.
2. Smith GR, Winquist RA, Allan NK, et al: Subtle transchondral fractures of the talar dome. *Radiology* 1977; 124:667.
3. Davidson AM, Steele HD, MacKenzie DA, et al: A review of twenty-one cases of transchondral fractures of the talus. *J Trauma* 1967; 7:379.
4. Mukherjee SK, Young AB: Dome fracture of the talus. *J Bone Joint Surg* 1973; 55B:319.
5. Berndt AL, Harty M: Transchondral fractures of the talus. *J Bone Joint Surg* 1959; 41A:988.
6. Yvars MF: Osteochondral fractures of the dome of the talus. *Clin Orthop* 1976; 114:185.

**Fig. 5A:** Normal distal femoral lucencies in children may be mistaken for "osteochondrosis dissecans." This normal variant (arrow) is typically located in the *lateral* femoral condyle.

**Fig. 5B:** Normal variant (arrows) in another patient with typical posterior location in lateral condyle.

Figure 5A

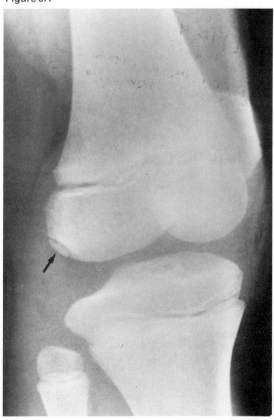

Figure 5B

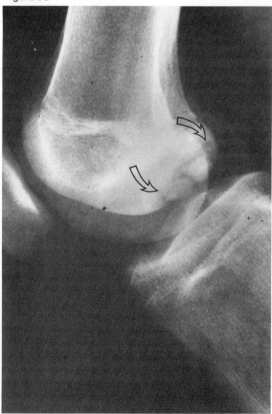

**Fig. 6:** Residual of osteochondral fracture of medial side of talar dome (arrow).

**Fig. 7:** Computed tomography may be useful in problem cases. Osteochondral fragment (arrow) of the posterior talus was only equivocally demonstrated by plain radiographs.

Figure 6

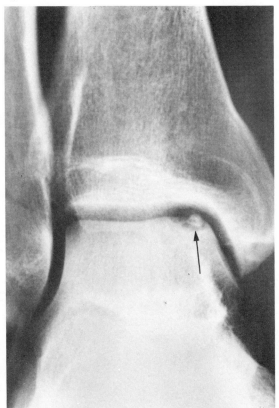

Figure 7

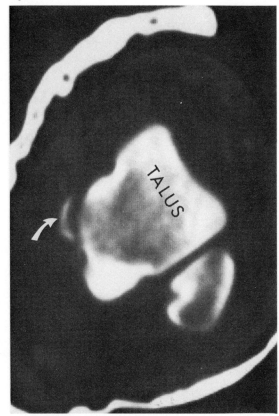

# Study 35

This 12-year-old boy fell on his outstretched left arm. He resists passive supination or pronation. *Your diagnosis?*

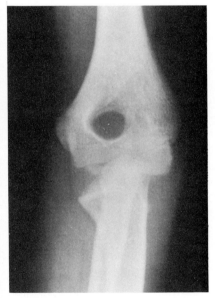

**Fig. 1:** AP left elbow.

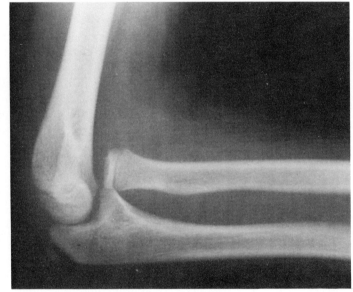

**Fig. 2:** Lateral left elbow.

# Diagnosis: Isolated Traumatic Dislocation of Radial Head

Traumatic dislocation of the radial head is almost always accompanied by a fracture of the ulna—Monteggia's fracture (Fig. 4). Rarely, dislocation of the radial head is an isolated injury. Isolated dislocation can also be nontraumatic. This nontraumatic congenital form is rare and can occur alone or in association with one of several syndromes.

Most traumatic dislocations occur in children. The child usually falls on an outstretched arm with the forearm pronated. The mechanism of injury is similar to that producing a Monteggia's fracture, but in children the elasticity of the ulna may spare it from fracture when the radial head is dislocated.

The radial head is maintained in the radial notch of the ulna by the annular ligament, the interosseous membrane, the elbow joint capsule which extends distally to blend with the annular ligament, the quadrate ligament extending from the radial neck to the inferior radial notch and the supinator muscle with its deep fascia.[1] The annular ligament and interosseous membrane are most important in fixing the radial head, but the interosseous membrane is lax in pronation, in keeping with the fact that isolated dislocation is usually a pronation injury. The annular ligament ruptures anterolaterally or laterally, and the radial head dislocates anteriorly, laterally, or, uncommonly, posteriorly, depending on positioning of the arm following injury.[1] The patient presents with a painful elbow with minimal distortion. There is guarding against movement, especially pronation and supination.[2]

Dislocation may be obvious on radiographs. To detect lesser degrees of displacement, it is important to note the relationship of the long axis of the radius to the capitellum. In all projections the long axis of the radius should extend through the capitellum. A single exception to this relationship is in the child prior to ossification of the epiphysis of the radial head. In this age group, on the frontal view, the radius appears to point laterally. This is a normal finding prior to ossification of the radial head, and alignment on the lateral view will be normal.[3,4]

Closed reduction of the acutely dislocated radius is usually successful. Some children, however, have few symptoms and little disability, and are not brought to a physician. They may present months or years following dislocation. These patients may be mistaken as having congenital dislocation.[5]

The existence of unilateral congenital dislocated radial head is contested. Some feel these cases represent unrecognized, long-standing traumatic dislocations. A convex radial head, dysplastic capitellum, concave posterior proximal ulna and soft tissue calcification have been said to indicate a congenital lesion, but all these findings have been found with long-standing traumatic dislocation.[5,6] Bilateral dislocations are more easily accepted as congenital.

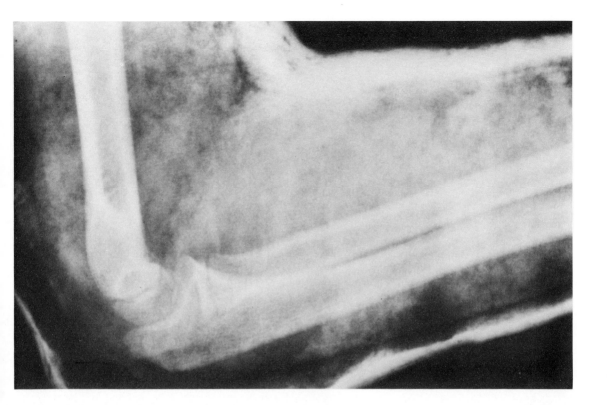

Congenital dislocations can be posterior, anterior or lateral. A posterior position is common (Fig. 5). Most are isolated anomalies, but some are one facet of a syndrome. Syndromes associated with congenital radial head dislocation include: (1) nail-patella syndrome, (2) Ehlers-Danlos syndrome, (3) Klinefelter's syndrome, (4) Silver's syndrome, (5) Cornelia de Lange's syndrome, (6) arthrogryposis, (7) auriculo-osteodysplasia, (8) epiphyseal dysplasia, (9) hereditary osteochondritis dissecans, (10) hereditary multiple exostoses, (11) congenital web-elbow, (12) tibiofibular synostosis, (13) hemimelia, (14) Madelung's deformity, (15) familial tarsal and carpal synostosis and (16) cerebral palsy.[7]

The dislocation is probably caused by a developmental defect in some syndromes (Klinefelter's) and mechanical forces in others (cerebral palsy). These patients have little pain. Functional impairment is small, mostly related to supination-pronation. Children with established dislocations who have increasing deformity have been treated surgically with late open reduction and annular ligament reconstruction.[5,6]

**Fig. 3:** Lateral left elbow with cast following closed reduction of anteriorly dislocated proximal radius. The long axis of the radius was not aligned with the capitellum in Figures 1 and 2, indicating dislocation. The extension of the longitudinal axis of the radius now bisects the capitellum in a normal manner.

### References

1. Wiley JJ, Pegington J, Horwich, JP: Traumatic dislocation of the radius at the elbow. *J Bone Joint Surg* 1974; 56B:501.
2. Vesley DG: Isolated traumatic dislocations of the radial head in children. *Clin Orthop* 1967; 50:31.
3. Rogers LF: Fractures and dislocations of the elbow. *Semin Roentgenol* 1978; 13:97.

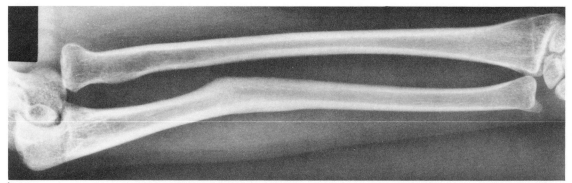

Figure 4

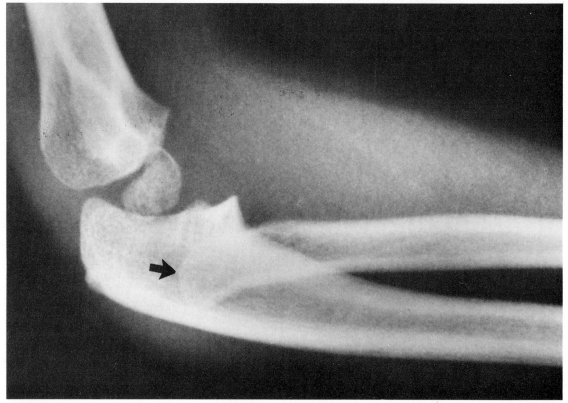

Figure 5

**Fig. 4:** Healed fracture of the ulna. The long axis of radius no longer aligned with the capitellum indicates persistent dislocation of the radial head.

**Fig. 5:** Congenital dislocation of the radial head (arrow), which is convex and in a posterior position.

4. Silberstein MJ, Brodeur AE, Graviss ER: Some vagaries of the capitellum. *J Bone Joint Surg* 1979; 61A:244.
5. Lloyd-Roberts GC, Bucknill TM: Anterior dislocation of the radial head in children. *J Bone Joint Surg* 1977; 59B:402.
6. Bucknill TM: Anterior dislocation of the radial head in children. *Proc Roy Soc Med* 1977; 70:620.
7. Almquist EE, Gordon LH, Blue AI: Congenital dislocation of the head of the radius. *J Bone Joint Surg* 1969; 51A:1118.

# Study 36

This 17-year-boy fell and injured his left forearm. *Your diagnosis?*

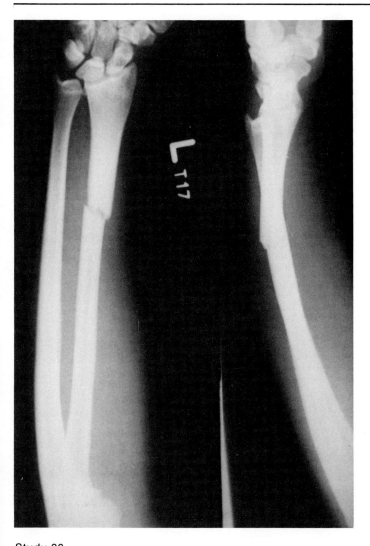

**Fig. 1:** AP and lateral view of left forearm.

# Diagnosis: Galeazzi Fracture Dislocation

Fracture of the distal radius can be divided into two groups: articular and nonarticular.[1]

## Articular

1. Marginal fracture of the dorsal radius with dorsal dislocation of the fracture fragment, wrist and hand: *Dorsal Barton's Fracture.*
2. Metaphyseal fracture of the radius with volar displacement of the fracture fragment, wrist and hand: *Volar Barton's Fracture.*
3. Displaced fracture of the radial styloid: *Chauffeur's Fracture.*

## Nonarticular

1. Metaphyseal fracture with dorsal tilting of the distal fragment: *Colles' Fracture.*
2. Metaphyseal fracture with volar tilting of distal fragment: *Smith's Fracture (Reverse Colles').*
3. Distal radial shaft fracture with radioulnar dislocation: *Galeazzi Fracture.*

Fracture of the distal radial shaft with disruption of the radioulnar joint has been called the Galeazzi fracture, Piedmont fracture, Darrach-Hughston-Milch fracture, and reverse Monteggia fracture. This uncommon injury is often misdiagnosed because disruption of the radioulnar joint is not identified. Proper diagnosis is important since this is an unstable fracture-dislocation associated with a high incidence of poor results if not treated by open reduction and internal fixation.[2-5]

There is lack of agreement concerning the mechanism of this injury. Most often it results from a fall on the outstretched hand with the forearm in extreme pronation. Force is transmitted across the radiocarpal articulation, dislocating and foreshortening the radius. With further radial displacement the ulnar head is dislocated, causing tearing of the triangular cartilage. A less common mechanism of injury is a direct blow to the dorsoradial aspect of the forearm.[2,5]

The distal radioulnar joint is fixed by anterior and posterior radioulnar ligaments, the ulnar collateral ligament, the pronator quadratus, and the triangular cartilage. The triangular cartilage covers the articular surface of the distal ulna, with its base attached to the medial articular margin of the radius and its apex to the base of the ulnar styloid. The triangular cartilage is by far the most important stabilizing structure. Distal radioulnar dislocation does not occur without rupture of this cartilage. Avulsion fracture of the ulnar styloid is equivalent to triangular cartilage rupture.[2,6,7]

The shaft of the radius is defined as the portion extending from the bicipital tuberosity to a point about 4 cm proximal to its distal end. The radial shaft component of the Galeazzi fracture usually occurs at the junction of the middle and distal third, and less often in the middle third, of the bone. The radioulnar dislocation usually is evident clinically and radiographically. In about 20% of cases, however, the ulna is only subluxed. In these cases the roentgenogram may not demonstrate the abnormality clearly. The diagnosis of radioulnar subluxation must be made on the basis of clinical findings in these cases.[2]

The clinical findings of the Galeazzi fracture are: (1) angular, concave deformity of the radial side of the forearm, with apparent shortening of the forearm; and (2) a swollen, painful radioulnar joint with a prominent, mobile ulnar head when there is dorsal displacement of the head. With volar displacement, the normal ulnar prominence is lost and the ulna may appear as a mass proximal to the pisiform. In either case the wrist may appear narrowed transversely. When swelling is marked, anatomic landmarks are obliterated. In this case, inability to pronate or supine may be the only manifestation of the injury.[8]

The radial shaft fracture is evident on roentgenograms. When an isolated fracture of the radius is present, the examination should include the elbow and wrist. Positioning of the wrist for a lateral view is often inexact, and variations in alignment of the radius and ulna frequently are ignored. In this situation, however, the lateral view should be scrutinized. The fidelity of the view can be judged by

**Fig. 2:** Close-up lateral view of left wrist. There is dorsal displacement of the distal ulna in addition to the fracture at the junction of the middle and distal thirds of the radius. The patient was treated with open reduction and internal fixation. The radial fracture was fixed with a plate. The radioulnar joint was dislocated in mid-pronation. The joint was reduced by supination and the arm casted in supination.

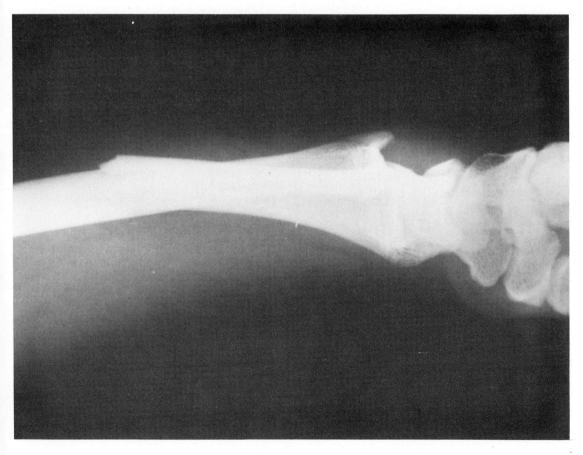

noting the position of the carpals (particularly the radius, lunate, and capitate axis) and the metacarpals. If the patient can cooperate in moving the arm, a proper lateral view should be obtained. A comparison lateral view of the opposite wrist can help if there is questionable deviation of the ulna.[8]

In problem cases, wrist arthrography has been used to detect distal radioulnar joint disruption. A contrast medium is injected into the radiocarpal joint. Contrast extending into the radioulnar joint indicates rupture of the triangular cartilage. Unfortunately false positive studies are common, due to normally occurring fenestration of the triangular cartilage. This normal variation is less often a problem in a young patient. Fenestration of the cartilage is rare under age 20 and increases progressively with age to an incidence of 50% in the sixth decade.[2]

The distal radioulnar joint can be disrupted as an isolated injury.[7,8] Other fractures associated with disruption of this joint include Colles' fracture, Smith's fracture, Essex-Lopresti's fracture (radial head fracture with distal radioulnar dislocation), fracture of both bones of the forearm, and isolated ulnar fracture.[2,6]

Subluxation of the joint has been reported without rupture of cartilage or ligament.[9] In cases without associated fractures, the patients had pain and limited motion but no deformity. Lateral roentgenograms did not show ulnar displacement. PA films of the wrist (in pronation) with elbow flexed to 90° showed abnormal positioning of the ulnar styloid. Normally in the pronated PA position the ulnar styloid is on the medial side of the ulna. With subluxation the styloid was projected from the center or radial side of the ulna.

## References

1. Cautilli RA, Joyce MF, Gordon E, et al: Classifications of fractures of the distal radius. *Clin Orthop* 1974; 103:163.
2. Mizic Z, Sad N: Galeazzi fracture-dislocation. *J Bone Joint Surg* 1975; 57A:1071.
3. Rockwood CA, Green DP: *Fractures*. Philadelphia, J.B. Lippincott, 1975.
4. Reckling FW, Cordell LD: Unstable fracture-dislocations of the forearm. *Arch Surg* 1968; 96:999.
5. Hughston JC: Fracture of the distal radial shaft. *J Bone Joint Surg* 1957; 39A:249.
6. Vesely DG: The distal radioulnar joint. *Clin Orthop* 1967; 51:75.
7. Rose-Inns AP: Anterior dislocation of the ulna at the inferior radio-ulnar joint. *J Bone Joint Surg* 1960; 42B:515.
8. Kingsbury G, Heiple MD, Freehafer AA, et al: Isolated traumatic dislocation of the distal end of the ulna or distal radioulnar joint. *J Bone Joint Surg* 1962; 44A:1387.
9. Snook GA, Chrisman OD, Wilson TC, et al: Subluxation of the distal radio-ulnar joint by hyperpronation. *J Bone Joint Surg* 1969; 51A:1315.

# Section VIII

# *BONE IMAGING*

Recent articles and books on bone imaging by nuclear medicine and computed tomography are listed below.

*Nuclear Medicine*

Bassett LW, Gold RH, Webber MM: Radionuclide bone imaging. *Radiologic Clinics of North America* 1981; 19:675-702.

Fordham EW, Ali A, Turner A, et al. *Atlas of radionuclide imaging.* New York, Harper and Row, 1982.

*Computed Tomography*

Genant HK, Cann CE, Chafetz NI, et al: Advances in computed tomography of the musculoskeletal system. *Radiologic Clinics of North America* 1981; 19:645-674.

Lee JKT, Sagel S, Stanley R. *Computed body tomography.* New York, Raven Press, 1983, pp 415-515.

# Study 37

This 25-year-old man presented with pain below the right knee which had been present for one week. He played rugby regularly, but could not recall any direct trauma to the leg. His pain improved with rest and after aspirin. The pain worsened with physical activity. He limped and was tender to palpation below the patella. *What other studies would you order? Your diagnosis?*

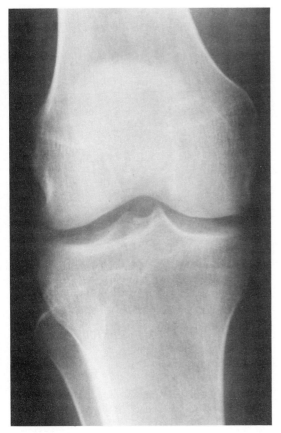

**Fig. 1:** AP right knee.

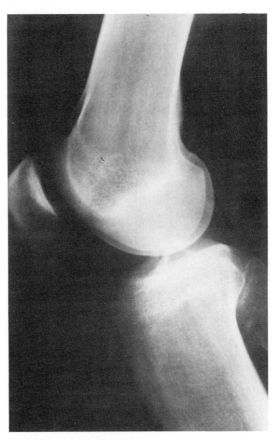

**Fig. 2:** Lateral right knee.

# Diagnosis: Stress Fracture

The radiographs (Figs. 1, 2) are normal, but the bone scan done the same day is positive (Figs. 3, 4 arrows), with a localized area of increased activity in the upper, anterior tibia. X-rays later became positive, confirming a stress fracture. The patient's symptoms resolved after limitation of physical activity.

Stress fractures in military recruits and athletes are well known, and several large series have been assembled.[1,2] These injuries, however, may occur in any individual with the highest frequency in adolescents and young adults. These injuries usually result from repeated mechanical insults which are associated with occupational or athletic activity. The incidence is currently increasing as a result of the popularity of jogging and other means of physical conditioning.

Stress fractures have also been reported following orthopedic surgical procedures including femoral and tibial osteotomies,[3] Keller bunionectomies,[4] bone plates and hip prostheses. Stress fractures have been reported in almost every bone in the body. The most common bone involved is the metatarsal (Fig. 5), and next in order of frequency are the calcaneous and tibia (Figs. 6, 7). Rare

**Fig. 3:** AP view right knee, $^{99}$Tc MDP.

**Fig. 4:** Lateral view right knee, $^{99m}$TcMDP.

Figure 3

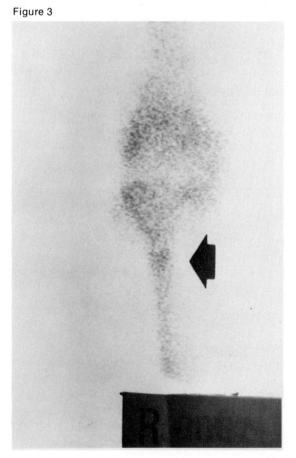

Figure 4

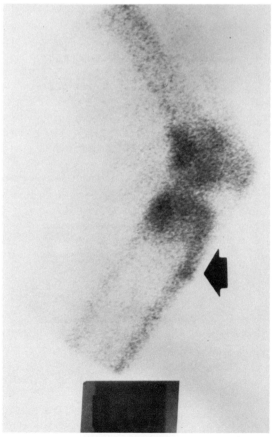

locations include the base of the coracoid process and the tarsal navicular.

Most stress fractures are not associated with extended disability or deformity, but a small percentage may go on to complete fracture if not recognized and treated. Femoral neck stress fractures have the highest complication rate and may progress to frank fracture with displacement requiring surgery. (Fig. 8).[6]

Stress fractures may occasionally present diagnostic problems. They have been mistaken clinically and radiographically for primary bone tumors and biopsied.[7] In rare cases, there have been amputations when the histology was interpreted as malignancy. Most of these problems have been in children, probably due to delayed clinical presentation and florid x-ray changes.

When stress fractures occur in normal bone, they are termed *fatigue fractures;* those occurring in abnormal bone, which is less resistant to stress, are termed *insufficiency fractures.*

Prolonged or unusual activity for the individual results in accelerated osteonal resorption (tunneling) of the cortex. Laying down the new bone is not as rapid as resorption, and when stress continues, microfractures occur in the weakened area.[8] These early changes are not visible on radiographs. Radiographs become positive after one to three weeks when an actual infarction of bone and/or changes of bony repair are identified.

Clinically the common presentation is localized pain which is

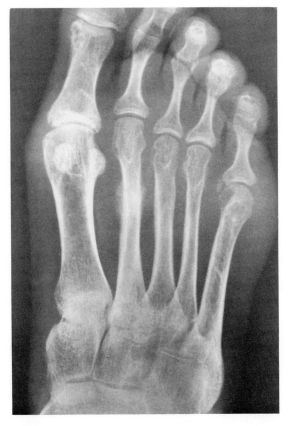

**Fig. 5:** Insufficiency type stress fracture occurring in osteoporotic second metatarsal of a patient with rhematoid arthritis. There is hazy callus formation.

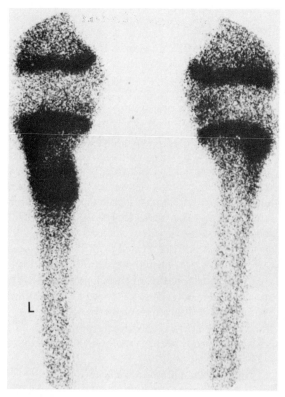

**Fig. 6A:** Fatigue type stress fracture of upper tibia, the most common site in children. Uptake in upper left tibia on bone scan.

**Fig. 6B:** Frontal view of tibia with solid periosteal new bone.

**Fig. 6C:** Lateral view shows typical (in child) posterior location of linear fracture (arrow) surrounded by sclerosis.

Figure 6B

Figure 6C

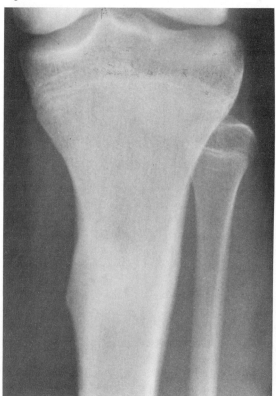

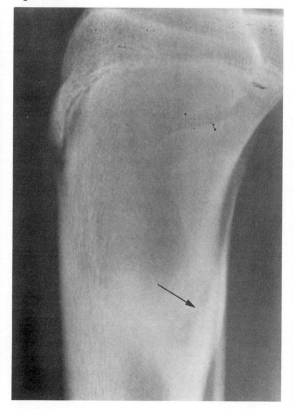

variable in intensity. The pain may be mild, or occasionally even absent, with incidental demonstration of the stress fracture. The pain is characteristically partially or completely relieved with rest and/or aspirin, and is often increased with further activity. There is often local tenderness.

The radiographic signs include: (1) fracture line; (2) a zone of sclerosis; (3) periosteal reaction; and (4) callus. In stress fractures at the ends of long bones and in short bones such as the calcaneus, there is usually only a zone of sclerosis. In the diaphysis of long bones, a unilateral cortical break and periosteal reaction are frequently seen.[9]

When a stress fracture is clinically suspected but the radiographs are normal, a bone scan almost invariably demonstrates the lesion.[10] The bone scan is positive early (1-2 days) while again, radiographs are positive late (1-3 weeks). While the scan is extremely sensitive, it is not specific. In the proper clinical setting, however, the diagnosis has been quite accurate.[11]

### References

1. Morris JM, Blickenstaff LD: *Fatigue Fractures, A Clinical Study,* Springfield, Illinois, Charles C. Thomas, 1967.
2. Wilson ES, Katz N: Stress fractures: An analysis of 250 consecutive cases. *Radiology* 1969; 92:481.

**Fig. 7:** Insufficiency type stress fracture with sclerotic band crossing distal tibia in a patient with osteomalacia.

**Fig. 8:** Fatigue type stress fracture of the femoral neck (arrow).

Figure 7

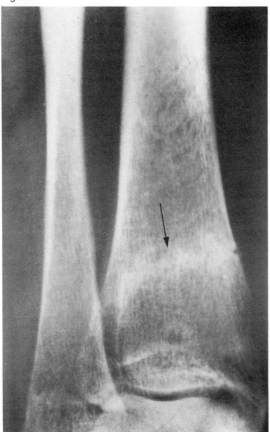

Figure 8

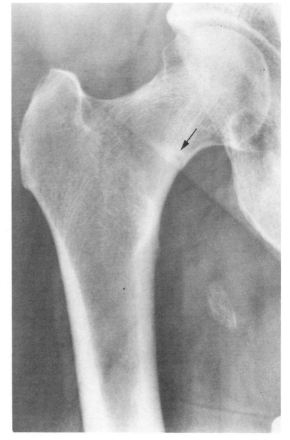

3. Korhonen BJ, Grogono BJ: Fatigue fractures complicating osteotomy. *Clin Orthop* 1971; 79:32.
4. Ford LT, Gilula LA: Stress fractures of the middle metatarsals following the Keller operation. *J Bone Joint Surg* 1977; 59A:117.
5. Miller AJ: Late fracture of the acetabulum after total hip replacement. *J Bone Joint Surg* 1972; 54B:600.
6. Blickenstaff LD, Morris JM: Fatigue fracture of the femoral neck. *J Bone Joint Surg* 1966; 48A:1031.
7. Engh CA, Robinson RA, Milgram J: Stress fractures in children. *J Trauma* 1970; 10:532.
8. Johnson LC, Stradford MT, Geis RW: Histiogenesis of stress fracture. *J Bone Joint Surg* 1963; 45A:1542.
9. Savoca CJ: Stress fractures: A classification of the earliest radiographic signs. *Radiology* 1971; 100:519.
10. Geslein GE, Thrall JH, Espinosa JL, et al: Early detection of stress fractures using 99mm Tc-polyphosphate. *Radiology* 1976; 118:115.
11. Wilcox JR, Monlot AC, Green JP: Bone scanning in the evaluation of excessive related stress injuries. *Radiology* 1977; 123:699.

This 15-year-old boy is a high school wrestler. He has had back pain for several months. *Your diagnosis?*

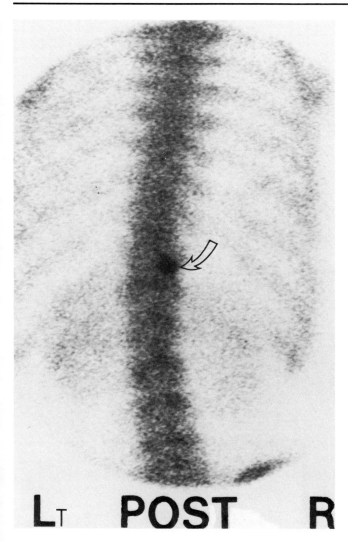

**Fig. 1:** $^{99m}$ Tc MDP bone scan of the thoraco-lumbar spine. Focal avid uptake (arrow).

# Diagnosis: Vertebral Column Osteoid Osteoma

The scintigram in Figure 1 shows a focal area of increased activity at the midconcavity of a thoracolumbar scoliosis. The appearance is typical of an osteoid osteoma but is not specific. An osteoblastoma or spondylolysis could also cause focal increased uptake. The vascular osteoid osteoma would also be visible during the early blood-pool stage of imaging soon after isotope injection, but spondylolysis would not be visible during the blood-pool stage.

## Radionuclide Bone Imaging

The ability of radionuclide bone imaging to detect bone metastases when radiographs are normal has been recognized for many years. The more recent development of technetium 99m radiopharmaceuticals has resulted in the application of bone scintigraphy to an increasingly wide variety of bone and joint problems including infection, primary neoplasms, trauma, and osteonecrosis. In most situations the advantage of scintigraphy is still the discovery of bone abnormalities while radiographs are normal. Another basic principle which remains true is that radionuclide bone imaging is remarkably sensitive but nonspecific, especially for single lesions. In the evaluation of most patients, sites of abnormality identified by scintigraphy are correlated with recent radiographs or radiographs are obtained for correlation. These images are, of course, always considered along with pertinent clinical and laboratory findings.

## Radiopharmaceuticals

The first bone seeking radionuclides, strontium-85 and strontium-87m, were ionic substitutions for calcium. Strontium-85 examinations were limited to patients with proven malignant disease because of the high radiation dose. The isotope necessitated a one week interval between injection and scanning to allow for a maximal lesion to nonlesion ratio. It was also excreted through the bowel, which sometimes obscured portion of the bone scan. Strontium-87m was a considerably better imaging agent. It had a shorter half life (2.8 hours) and, therefore, a lower radiation dose to the patient. The lesion to nonlesion ratio was considerably lower than strontium-85, however, sometimes making interpretation of the images difficult.

Fluorine 18, a cationic substitute for phosphate, subsequently proved to be a valuable agent in bone scintigraphy. Fluorine 18, which decays by positron emission, permitted more precise spatial localization than previous isotopes. Fluorine 18, however, is a cyclotron produced product with a very short half life of 1.8 hours. As a result, the isotope was limited to nuclear medicine laboratories near cyclotron facilities.

The agents currently used in nuclear medicine laboratories are phosphate inorganic complexes labeled to reduce technetium 99m. These technetium tagged agents have physical properties suitable for imaging with modern gamma camera equipment and give a considerably lower radiation dose than earlier isotopes. Phosphate and phosphonate compounds such as methylene diphosphonate (MDP) and hydroxyethylidene diphosphonate (HEDP) are most frequently used (Fig. 2).

The exact mechanism by which bones take up these isotopes is unknown. It is believed that the compounds are taken up via chemisorption onto the calcium hydroxyapatite crystals in bone. A prerequisite for uptake within the bone is an intact osseous blood supply to allow delivery of the isotope to the bone. The technetium labeled compounds are taken up more avidly by metabolically active bone. This is believed to be related to increased osteoblastic activity.

## Benign Bone Diseases

There are two basic reasons for the use of bone scintigraphy in the

**Fig. 2A:** Normal bone scintigram. *Adult:* there is uniform symmetric bone activity and widespread symmetric joint activity including intense sacroiliac joint activity, which is normal. Note symmetric kidney uptake (arrows) and bladder (b) activity.

**Fig. 2B:** *Child:* Note avid uptake at joints of growing bones.

Figure 2A

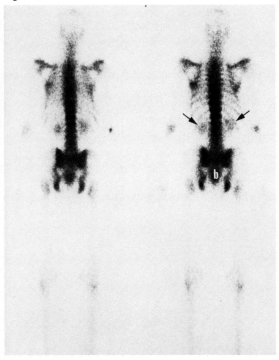

Figure 2B

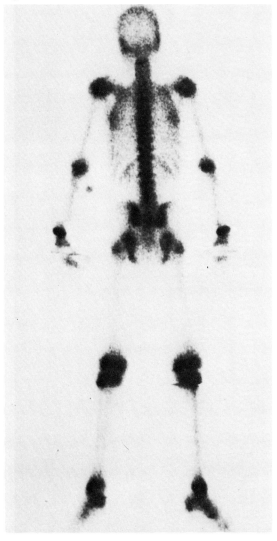

evaluation of benign bone disease. The first is to identify a process causing bone pain when it is not evident radiographically (e.g., osteoid osteoma or stress fracture). The second is to determine the extent of progression of known bone disease (e.g., fibrous dysplasia, Paget's disease, osteochondromatosis).

### Osteoid Osteoma

Patients with osteoid osteomas usually have pain. The nuclear medicine laboratory is called upon to determine if there is an osseous abnormality at the site of that pain. Scintigraphy is particularly helpful in identifying osteoid osteomas in the hands, feet, and spine.

Radiographic evaluation of the spine for osteoid osteoma is difficult, especially when the lesion is located in the posterior elements of the spine. Even with tomography, the characteristic nidus of an osteoid osteoma may not be evident. The scintigram is characteristic, displaying a focal area of increased uptake with associated scoliosis (Fig. 1). Spondylolysis can also result in focal uptake, but lack of uptake in the blood-pool image early after injection differentiates it from osteoid osteoma. The small bones of the hands and feet as well as the femoral neck are other areas that are difficult to evaluate radiographically. Scintigraphy in these cases will demonstrate a focal area of increased uptake which will direct the surgeon to an appropriate biopsy site.

### Bone Cyst

The bone scan offers little help in the evaluation of bone cysts. These lesions do not demonstrate abnormal uptake unless there is an insufficiency fracture.

**Fig. 3:** Hereditary multiple exostosis: There is focal increased activity in multiple bones in this child. Note the osteochondromas of the knees which project away from the joint (arrows).

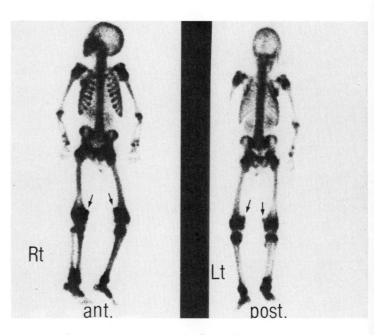

Bone Radiology Case Studies

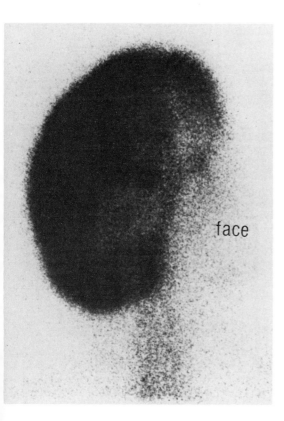

**Fig. 4A:** Paget's disease. Intense uptake in the calvarium.

face

**Fig. 4B:** Intense uptake in the right innominate bone typical of Paget's disease.

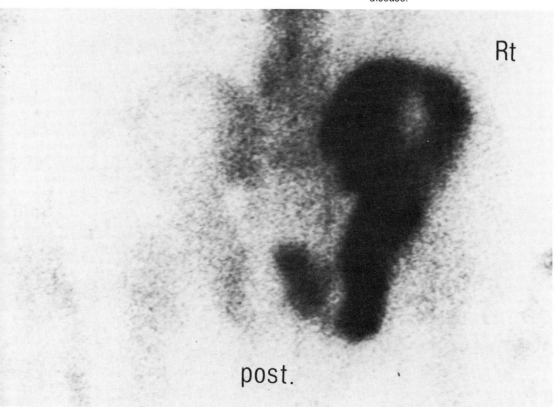

Rt

post.

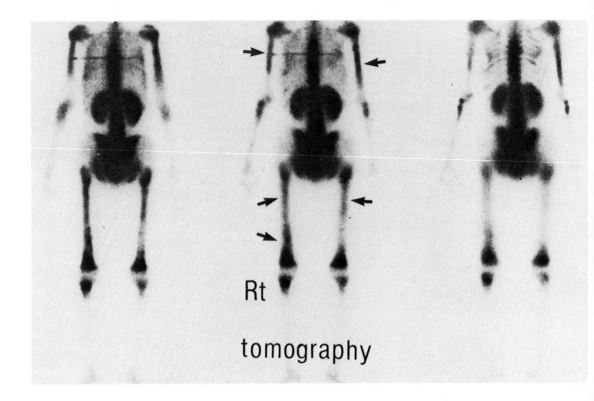

Rt

tomography

**Fig. 5:** Osteomyelitis. Multiple areas of increased uptake in the arms and legs (arrows) in a drug addict with multifocal osteomyelitis. Three tomographic sections.

### Osteochondromas

Bone scintigraphy is useful in evaluation of patients with hereditary multiple osteochondromas. The incidence of malignant degeneration of osteochondromas in these patients is about 20%. An osteochondroma will show avid accumulation of the isotope in its growing phase (Fig. 3). If, however, avid uptake is identified after the epiphysis has fused, that is, the quiescent phase, the physician should be alerted to the possibility of malignant degeneration. Two such cases have been reported. On biopsy one was a chondrosarcoma, the other an osteochondroma. It was concluded that the scintigraphy will not identify malignant degeneration but will distinguish active growing lesions from quiescent lesions. Again malignancy should be suspected if intense uptake is noted in an adult.[1]

### Fibrous Dysplasia

The lesions of fibrous dysplasia are hyperemic and consequently demonstrate intense uptake on delayed static images. Due to the intense uptake, however, this disease cannot readily be distinguished from a malignant disease process. Radiographs are necessary to make the proper diagnosis.

### Paget's Disease

Paget's disease occurs in about 3% of individuals over the age of 40. The scintigram demonstrates intense uptake, which is most likely related to the rich vascular supply within the bone. Due to

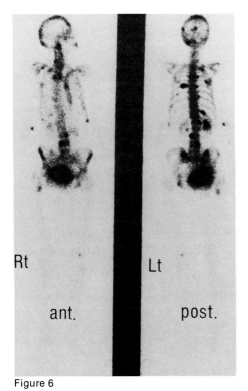

Rt

Lt

ant.

post.

Figure 6

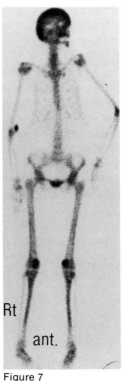

Rt

ant.

Figure 7

**Fig. 6:** Metastases. Numerous foci of increased uptake in the axial and appendicular skeleton in this patient are consistent with metastases.

**Fig. 7:** Hyperparathyroidism. Uniform increased uptake of the radionuclide results in a "superscan." Absence of kidney and bladder activity are clues indicating that there is abnormal bone uptake. Diffuse metastases can produce an identical appearance.

active bone remodeling the scans are positive in the early lytic phase of the disease as well as the late blastic stage (Fig. 4). However, the late so called "burn out" stage may produce a normal image. A correlation between radiographic and scintigraphic findings in 96 patients with Paget's disease has been reported. Of 316 lesions demonstrated in these patients, 60% were detected by both scintigraphy and radiographs, 27% were seen only by scintigraphy, and 13% were seen only on radiographs.[2]

In a long bone, the typical scintigraphic appearance is that of an area of increased uptake which corresponds to the outline of the bone and extends to the end of the bone. Although Paget's disease is often polyostotic, in its monostotic form, an area of increased uptake within the calvarium cannot be distinguished from metastatic disease and radiographic correlation is usually necessary. Scintigraphy has been reported to be superior to biochemical tests in assessing the extent of Paget's disease and in evaluating the response to calcitonin therapy.[3]

**Trauma**

Bone scintigraphy is useful in the detection of occult fractures occurring in the small bones of hands, feet, elbows, or other areas where there is a high clinical suspicion for fracture and the radiographs are normal.

It has been reported that scintigraphy may be positive as early as 7 hours after the trauma.[4] However, scintigraphy is most often positive between 24 and 48 hours after the trauma but may be delayed for days, especially in elderly patients. Activity peaks at 6 to 9 months. Uptake may persist for as long as 6 to 9 years.[5]

Numerous articles have been written evaluating the scintigraphic diagnosis of stress fractures.[6] Scintigraphy shows the earliest changes in patients with stress fractures. About two-thirds of stress fractures can be identified prior to the radiographic signs of fracture.[7] An average delay of 10.5 days between the positive radionuclide scan and the positive radiograph has been reported.[8] A patient whose bone scan is abnormal should be treated even in the absence of a positive radiograph in order to prevent long term disability or complete fracture of the affected bone.

**Inflammation**

The scintigraphic diagnosis of osteomyelitis can usually be made within 24 hours of the onset of symptoms, while radiographs are not positive for 7 to 10 days. The characteristic finding is a focal area of increased activity at the site of infection (Fig. 5). Hyperemia and associated bone resorption produce the avid uptake at the affected site. However, a rather high false negative rate in infants less than 3 months of age has been reported.[9]

In some patients the bone scan may be negative initially. If clinical suspicion is high, a gallium-67 citrate scan may be performed. The exact mechanism of gallium-67 localization in inflammatory disease is unknown. The labeling is mediated in some way through neutrophilic leukocytes.[10] Although the gallium scan is consistently abnormal in acute osteomyelitis, it produces a higher radiation dose to the patient and, therefore, the bone scan is preferred as the initial imaging modality.

In patients with chronic osteomyelitis it is not possible, by bone scintigraphy, to identify an acute process superimposed on the chronic process. Due to the active osteoblastic activity in chronic osteomyelitis, the bone scan will already be positive. However, gallium-67 has identified foci of acute infection superimposed on chronic osteomyelitis.[11] Gallium-67 is also the preferred agent for evaluating response to antibiotic therapy. As the patient responds to treatment, the scan ceases to be positive. In the same situation, however, the technetium scan continues to show accumulation at the affected site because of the reparative process within the bone.

**Metastatic Disease**

Scintigraphy is the most sensitive means for detecting osseous metastatic disease. There may be as long as an 18-month lag between the discovery of a metastatic lesion on a bone scan and its first appearance on a radiograph.[12] In evaluation of metastatic disease scintigraphy offers total body imaging on a single film (Fig. 6). Radiography is reserved for areas identified as abnormal by scanning.

In a patient with a known malignancy it must be remembered that benign causes of uptake such as degenerative change, trauma, Paget's disease, and other benign bone diseases may produce positive scans. In one series of patients with a known malignancy who had solitary areas of uptake, 36% had benign disease.[13]

Radiographic correlation is always necessary in this group of patients.

Occasionally, metastatic disease may present as focal areas of decreased uptake. These "cold spots" are commonly due to metastases from breast and lung carcinoma.[14] Radiation therapy has also been reputed to produce photopenic areas on bone scans 4 to 6 months after therapy.[15]

Metastatic disease may produce a "superscan" appearance. In this situation the axial and appendicular skeleton are seen exceptionally well. Decreased activity within the kidneys, bladder, and soft tissues indicate the presence of abnormal skeletal uptake. This pattern has been seen most often in patients with breast and prostate carcinoma. It can also be produced by metabolic bone disease (Fig. 7).

It should be remembered that scintigraphy can be normal in the presence of malignant bone disease. A false negative study is frequent in multiple myeloma and also occurs with metastatic

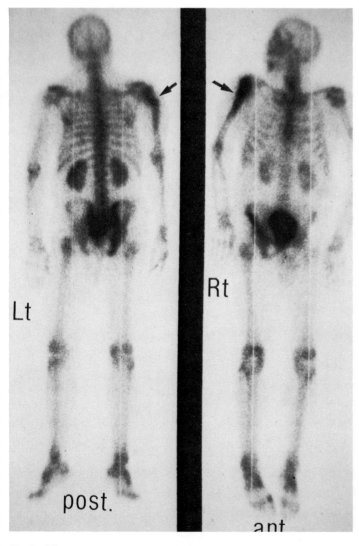

**Fig. 8:** Osteosarcoma. Increased uptake in the proximal right humerus. The finding is not specific. Other lesions have been excluded.

**Fig. 9A:** Avascular necrosis. Decreased uptake of technetium labeled MDP in right femoral head (arrows).

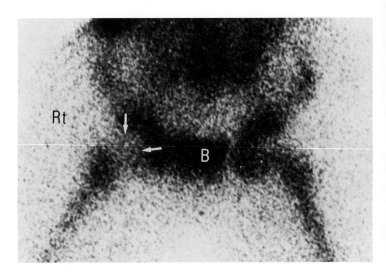

**Fig. 9B:** Radiograph shows sclerosis, fragmentation, and flattening of the femoral head.

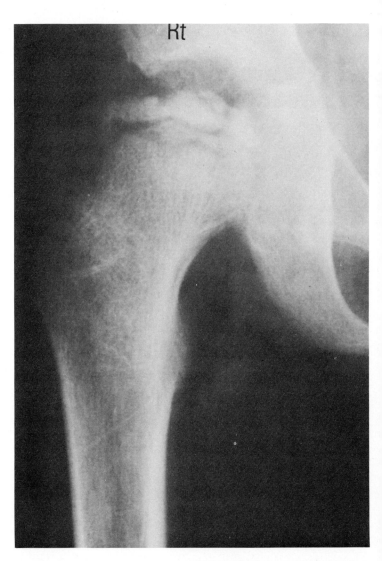

neuroblastoma. A small percentage of bone metastases in adults with positive radiographs are also missed. These are usually destructive lesion with little histologic osteoblastic activity.

## Primary Malignant Bone Neoplasms

Osteosarcomas have increased uptake on bone scintigraphy which is attributed to osteoblastic activity and extensive tumor vascularity. Mineralized metastatic lesions outside the skeletal system may also be identified. The uptake by a primary osteosarcoma is not specific (Fig. 8) and radiographs usually show a definite primary lesion at the time of initial study. In addition it should be remembered that the extent of abnormal radionuclide uptake may exceed the true extent of neoplasm in a long bone. The extent of neoplastic involvement is, however, rarely greater than the extent of increased uptake.

The widespread use of chemotherapy in the treatment of osteosarcoma has resulted in prolonged survival, and some patients will develop bone metastases prior to the development of lung metastases. These patients treated with chemotherapy can be easily followed by scintigraphy.

Malignant transformation in benign lesions such as enchondromas or osteochondromas can be excluded when scrintigraphy is normal or suspected when scintigraphy is positive in an adult. In addition, scintigraphy may identify multifocal lesions in a patient with multiple benign bone lesions or metastases who has symptoms and radiographs of a single site suggesting a primary bone tumor.

## Avascular Necrosis of the Hips

In early avascular necrosis, prior to the radiographic changes, scintigraphy will demonstrate decreased activity within the femoral head (Fig. 9). However, as the disease process continues and the reparative process begins, scintigraphy demonstrates increased uptake. This increased activity cannot be distinguished from inflammatory, traumatic, or degenerative disease.

Technetium labeled sulfur colloid, the agent commonly used for liver spleen scintigraphy, has proven to be extremely valuable. The isotope is taken up by functioning bone marrow. In normal patients marrow activity is identified within both femoral heads. In avascular necrosis decreased activity is identified in the abnormal hip.[16] We have found marrow imaging extremely useful (Fig. 10).

## Hip Prosthesis Imaging

There is controversy concerning the scintigraphic diagnosis of a loosened versus an infected prosthesis. It is generally agreed that 6 to 8 months after hip surgery there should be no significant uptake around the femoral or acetabular component of the hip prosthesis.[17] Focal areas of uptake at the end of the trochar in the femur is generally considered to be a sign of a loosened prosthesis (Fig. 11). Diffuse increased uptake around a prosthesis suggests inflammation. In many patients loosening and infection are not distinguishable, based on scintigraphic criteria alone.

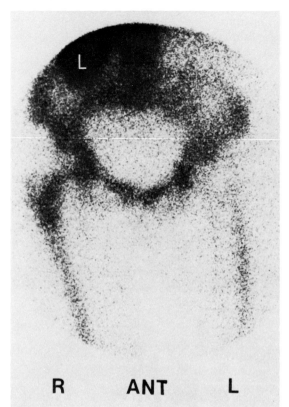

R ANT L

Figure 10

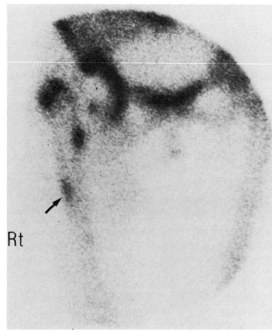

Rt

Figure 11

**Fig. 10:** Avascular necrosis. This technetium labeled sulfur colloid scan images the bone marrow. Absence of activity in the left proximal femur indicates avascularity. The hip was dislocated, but the bone was normal on radiographs.

**Fig. 11:** Loose prosthesis. Increased uptake at the tip of the trochar of the hip prosthesis (arrow) is consistent with loosening.

## Arthritis

Scintigraphy has limited usefulness in patient with arthritis. While it will demonstrate the extent of the disease, the type of arthritis cannot be determined. Additionally, there is normally uptake in the sacroiliac joints, shoulders, and wrists. Superimposed degenerative changes in these joints also cause diagnostic difficulty. Radiographs are necessary to arrive at a specific diagnosis.

## Metabolic Disease

Osteomalacia, hyperparathyroidism, hyperthyroidism, and renal osteodystrophy can all produce a "superscan" similar to diffuse bone metastases (Fig. 7). If multiple symmetric foci of activity corresponding to common sites for pseudofractures are identified, however, osteomalacia may be suggested as an etiology of the "superscan."

## Bone Density

Transmission scanning with a collimated I-125 beam has proven to be superior to radiographs in determining the bone density of the appendicular skeleton.[18] The axial skeleton cannot be evaluated by this technique. This is important since there may be statistically significant differences between the density of the axial and appendicular skeleton in some patients. Computed tomography can be used to determine accurately the density of the axial

Bone Radiology Case Studies

skeleton. A commercial CT scanner can make bone density determinations accurately and reproducibly by using special hardware and software in conjunction with a special calibration phantom.[19]

*— Richard Provus, MD*

# References

1. Epstein DA, Levin EJ: Bone scintigraphy in hereditary multiple exostoses. *Am J Rad* 1978; 130:331-333.
2. Wellman HN, Schauwecker D, Robb JA, et al: Skeletal scintimaging and radiography in the diagnosis and management of Paget's disease. *Clin Ortho Ped* 1977; 127:55-62.
3. Waxman AD, Drucker S, McKee D, et al: Evaluation of 99mTc-diphosphonate kinetics and bone scans in patients with Paget's disease before and after calcitonin treatment. *Radiology* 1977; 125:761-764.
4. Rosenthal L, Hill RO, Chuang S: Observations on the use of 99mTc-phosphate imaging in peripheral bone trauma. *Radiology* 1976; 119:637-641.
5. Fordham EW, Ramachandran PC: Radionuclide imaging of osseous trauma. *Seminar Nuclear Medicine* 1974; 4:411-429.
6. Wilcox JC, Jr. Monoit A, Green JP: Bone scanning in the evaluation of exercise related stress injuries. *Radiology* 1977; 123:699-703.
7. Geslien GE, Thrall SH, Espinosa SL, et al: Early detection of stress fractures using 99mTc-polyphosphate. *Radiology* 1976; 121:683-687.
8. Prather JL, Nusynowitz MC, Snowdy HA, et al: Scintigraphic findings in stress fractures. *J Bone Joint Surg* 1977; 59:869-874.
9. Ash JM, Gilday DL: The futility of bone scanning in neonatal osteomyelitis-concise communication. *J Nucl Med* 1980; 21:417-420.
10. Hoffner PB, Bekerman C, Henkin RE (eds.): *Gallium-67 Imaging.* John Wiley & Sons, 1978, pp 5-6.
11. Lisbona R, Rosenthall L: Observation on the sequential use of 99mTc-phosphate complex and gallium-67 imaging in osteomyelitis, cellulitis, and septic arthritis. *Radiology* 1977; 123:123-129.
12. Galesko CS: Skeletal metastases and mammary cancer. *Ann R Coll Surg Eng* 1972; 50:2-3.
13. Corcoran RJ, Thrall JH, Kyle RW, et al: Solitary abnormalities in bone scans of patients with extraosseus malignancies. *Radiology* 1976; 121:663-667.
14. Vieras F, Herzberg D: Focal decreased skeletal uptake secondary to metastatic disease. *Radiology* 1976; 118:121-122.
15. Hattner RS, Hartmeyer J, Wars WM: Characterization of radiation induced photopenic abnormalities on bone scans. *Radiology* 1982; 145:161-163.
16. Meyers MH, Downey JNT, Tillman MM: Determination of vascularity of the femoral head with technetium 99m-sulfur colloid. *J Bone Joint Surg* 1977; 59A:658-664.
17. Harris WH: Total joint replacement. *N Engl J Med* 1977; 247:650-651.
18. Cameron JR, Sorenson J: Measurement of bone mineral in-vivo: an improved method. *Science* 1963; 142:230-235.
19. Genant HK, Cann CE, Chafetz NI, et al: Advances in computed tomography of the musculoskeletal system. *Rad Clin of NA* 1981; 19:645-674.

# Study 39

This 42-year-old man was pulled into a machine by his arm. His right arm was amputated and his neck injured. The AP film demonstrates a fracture of the lateral mass of C7 (arrows). *How would you evaluate for other fractures, alignment of vertebra, and impingement by bone fragments on the spinal canal?*

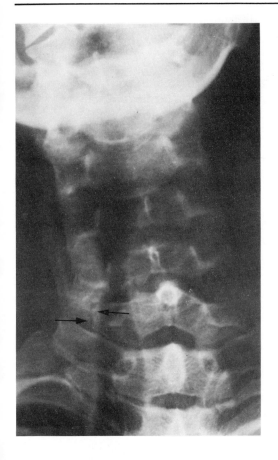

**Fig. 1A:** AP radiograph of the cervical spine.

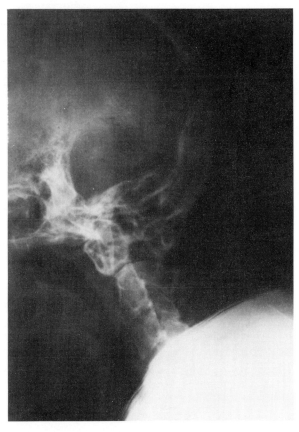

**Fig. 1B:** Attempted lateral radiograph of the cervical spine.

# Answer: Computed Tomography

Computed tomography (CT) was introduced by Hounsfield in 1972 and has revolutionized the radiographic evaluation of patients with suspected intracranial, thoracic, abdominal, retroperitoneal, and pelvic abnormalities. As clinical experience with CT has grown, so have the number of publications detailing its applicability and limitations in evaluating a variety of pathological conditions.

In 1979, Alfred[1] summarized specific indications for CT. These included many disease states solely or frequently encountered in orthopedic practice. Since then, the application of CT in orthopedics has continued to grow. The following cases illustrate some of the established indications for computed tomography in evaluating the musculoskeletal system.

## Axial Skeleton

Evaluation of the axial skeleton (spine and pelvis) with plain radiographs can be difficult. This is due in part to the complex anatomy and articulations of the spine, and to the complex three dimensional anatomy of the pelvis and sacrum. Multiple radiographs in a variety of projections are often necessary to evaluate a given area. Even utilizing complex motion tomography, complete evaluation, particularly of the thoracic spine and pelvis, can be difficult if not impossible. Nuclear medicine scans can document the presence of disease, but the pattern of uptake is often nonspecific. We have encountered a number of patients with abnormalities of the axial skeleton which were subtle or not perceptible on plain films but were obvious on CT images (Figs. 1-4).

CT, because of its cross sectional imaging format, is well suited to study the axial skeleton. An additional advantage is the ability to image the adjacent soft tissues and internal organs. This is particularly important in traumatized patients and patients with neoplastic disease. The cross sectional anatomy of both the spine and pelvis has been well described.[2-5]

In the traumatized patient, an additional advantage over conventional studies is that little patient movement is necessary. The uncooperative, semiconscious, or comatose patient often presents less of a problem with CT than with conventional radiographs.

Many studies have evaluated the clinical impact of CT on the diagnosis and management of patients with a variety of abnormalities of the spine and pelvis. Roub and Drayer[6] reported their experience in 188 patients with suspected spinal pathology. They found CT particular useful in evaluating the traumatized spine. In many cases it added important information about the integrity of the spinal cord and adjacent soft tissues which would not have been obtained by conventional, noninvasive studies. In all cases, CT identified the size and extent of bony injury unequivocally. Displacement of fragments and the presence of epidural

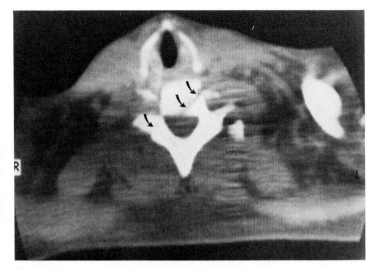

Figure 1C

**Fig.1C:** Transverse CT Scan. Fracture (arrows) involves the body and lateral mass of C7. The spinal canal is normal. On sagittal reconstruction the vertebrae were normally aligned.

**Fig. 2:** Fracture (arrows) of the C3 vertebral body which could not be identified on the plain radiographs.

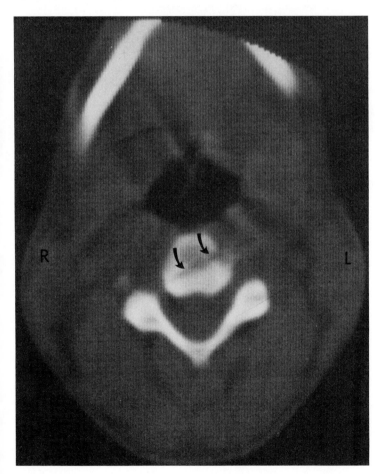

Figure 2

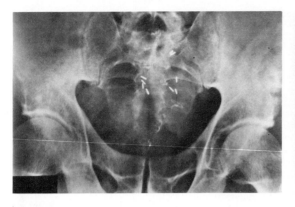

Figure 3A

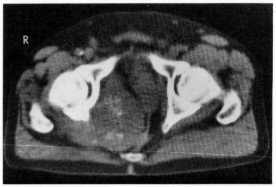

Figure 3B

**Fig. 3A:** The colon metastasis of the right pelvis is barely visible on this plain film.

**Fig. 3B:** The large calcified colon metastasis with bone erosion is obvious.

hematoma could clearly be seen. CT was also found to be valuable in evaluating neoplastic disease (Fig. 5), spinal dysraphism (Fig. 6), and in patients with prior spinal fusion (Fig. 7).

Gilula, et al[7] reported their experience with CT in pelvic pathology. They studied 43 patients with a number of pelvic abnormalities including benign and malignant neoplasms, trauma, and sacroiliitis. They found CT useful or definitive in 80% of all cases and in 96% of patients with neoplastic disease. CT accurately showed soft tissue extension of tumor and was judged invaluable in staging neoplastic disease, planning treatment, and posttherapy followup.

## Hip

Sauser, et al[8] and Shirkoda, et al[9] have described their experience with CT in hip trauma. A total of 23 cases were reported. Therapeutic planning was significantly affected in 10 of these patients because of the information obtained with CT. Two patients had acetabular fractures and nine patients had intra-articular fragments detected only with CT. In 14 of the 23 cases, the pathologic anatomy and extent of involvement of adjacent structures (ilium and sacroiliac joints) were more clearly appreciated on CT than on plain radiographs (Fig. 8).

Low back pain is a frequent presenting complaint in patients who are seen by orthopedic surgeons. Lumbar facet arthropathy (Fig. 9) and herniated discs (Fig. 10) are the major causes of sciatic and low back pain and may not be diagnosed or differentiated by pain radiographs, myelography, and even epidural venography. The CT appearance of both has been well described.[10-13]

CT can readily distinguish between disc and facet pathology.[11] Improved diagnosis has lead to improved surgical results in this group of patients. CT is also the most accurate means of diagnosing spinal stenosis (Fig. 11).[14]

## Sacroiliac Joints

CT has been used to evaluate the sacroiliac (SI) joints. Demonstration of the joints is uniformly better with CT than with either plain radiographs or plain tomography, but the role of CT in

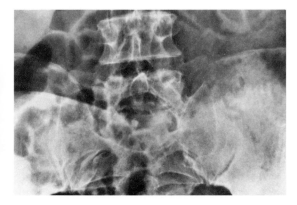

Figure 4A

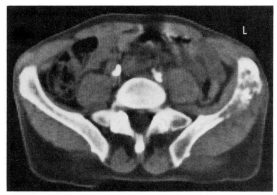

Figure 4B

evaluation is not established. Carrera, et al[15] found CT more sensitive than plain radiographs in detecting early changes of scaroiliitis. Borlaza, et al[16] found no significant difference between the two modalities when radiographs were interpreted by "experienced" radiologists. Radiation dosage with both modalities is similar.

**Fig. 4A:** Osteolytic thyroid metastasis of left iliac crest is subtle.

**Fig. 4B:** The metastasis is obvious. Note expansion of left iliac wing and soft tissue mass compared to right side.

## Extremities—Bones

CT clearly plays a secondary role in the radiographic evaluation of the bones of the extremities. The vast majority of traumatic, neoplastic, congenital, and metabolic osseous abnormalities can be identified and characterized with radiographs, conventional tomography, and nuclear medicine bone scans. In selected patients, however, CT can be invaluable.

Many studies have evaluated the role of CT in the identification, staging, therapy planning, and followup of patients with primary neoplasms of bone.[7,17–23] This material comprises over 200 individual cases from which the following conclusions can be drawn:

1. CT has detected subtle neoplasms not identified by other imaging modalities. Ginaldi and deSantos[22] described three cases of round cell tumors of bone detected only by CT. Radionuclide studies are useful in identifying a lesion. However, conventional radiography and tomography remain the principle means of identifiying and diagnosing osseous lesions except in areas which are difficult to image such as the sternal articulation of the clavicle.[18]
2. Neoplastic bone marrow involvement, adjacent soft tissue invasion, and neurovascular bundle invasion are most accurately defined by CT (Fig. 12).
3. CT is particularly useful in selecting patients for and planning of limb salvage procedures. It is also useful in selecting an optimal site for percutaneous biopsy.
4. CT is routinely used in radiation therapy planning and posttherapy followup.
5. CT can detect minimal changes in bone mineral content in the spine and has been used to follow patients being treated for

osteoporosis. In many patients there has been disparity between the mineral content of the spine as determined by CT and the mineral content of the extremities as determined by radionuclide photon emission.[24]

While metastatic disease has been clearly identified by CT when other studies were normal or equivocal the role of CT in routine evaluation is not yet defined.

## Extremities—Soft Tissue

CT is the imaging method of choice in identifying, characterizing, and staging soft tissue neoplasms of both the extremities and trunk (Figs. 12, 13).

The CT appearances of many other entities seen in orthopedic practice have been described. These include bursitis, Paget's disease (Fig. 14), osteomyelitis (Figs. 15, 16), Baker's cysts, congenital hip dislocations (Fig. 17) and many others (Fig. 18). In most instances, such entities can be adequately assessed using conventional radiographic methods. In problem cases, however, CT may add information useful in both diagnosis and management.

## Conclusion

The role of CT in evaluating disorders of the musculoskeletal system is still evolving. Neoplastic lesions of the spine and pelvis are best evaluated by CT. Equally established is evalution of trauma to the spine and pelvis. In a significant number of these cases, the information added by CT will greatly affect patient management.

CT can distinguish between the various causes of low back pain with sciatica and has already affected the surgical management of these patients. After radiography, it is becoming the imaging procedure of choice in this patient group because it is noninvasive and can be performed on an outpatient basis.

Bone density in the spine can be more accurately determined by CT than other methods.

In the extremities CT is valuable in the diagnosis and staging of soft tissue neoplasms. CT is valuable in determining the extent of bone neoplasms but plain films are still the best means of obtaining diagnostic information.

—*Michael Flisak, MD*

### References

1. Alfred RT: Special report: New indications for computerized body tomography. *AJR* 1979; 133:115-19.
2. Lee BCP, Kazam E, Newman AD: Computed tomography of the spine and spinal cord. *Radiology* 1978; 128:95-102.
3. Carrera GF, Haughton VM, Syvertsen A, et al: Computed tomography of the lumbar facet joints. *Radiology* 1980; 134:145-48.
4. Wyman AC, Lawson TL, Goodman LR: *Transverse Anatomy of the Human Thorax, Abdomen and Pelvis.* Boston, Little, 1978; pp 88-124.
5. Redman HC: Computed tomography of the pelvis. *Radiol Clin North Am* 1977; 15:441-448.
6. Roub LW, Drayer BP: Spinal computed tomography: Limitations and applications. *AJR* 1979; 133:267-273.

7. Gilula LA, Murphy WA, Tailor CC, et al: Computed tomography of the osseous pelvis. *Radiology* 1979; 132:107-114.

8. Sauser DD, Billimoria PE, Rowse GA, et al: Computed tomographic evaluation of hip trauma. *AJA* 1980; 135:269-274.

9. Shirkhoda A, Brashear R, Staab EV: Computed tomography of acetabular fractures. *Radiology* 1980; 134:683-688.

10. Williams AL, Haughton VM, Syvertsen A: Computed tomography in the diagnosis of herniated nucleus polposis. *Radiology* 1980; 135:95-99.

11. Carrera GF, Williams AL, Haughton VM: Computed tomography in sciatica. *Radiology* 1980; 134:137-143.

12. Carrera GF, Haughton VM, Syvertsen A, et al: Computed tomography of the lumbar facet joints. *Radiology* 1980; 134:145-148.

13. Mikhael MA, Ciric I, Tarkington JA, et al: Neuroradiological evaluation of lateral recess syndrome. *Radiology* 1981; 140:97-107.

14. Ulrich CG, Binet EF, Sanecki MG, et al: Quantitative assessment of the lumbar spinal canal by computed tomography. *Radiology* 1980; 134:137-143.

15. Carrera GF, Foley WD, Kozin F, et al: Computed tomography of sacroiliitis. *AJR* 1981; 136:41-46.

16. Borlaza GS, Seigel R, Kuhns LR, et al: Computed tomography in the evaluation of sacroiliac arthritis. *Radiology* 1981; 139:437-440.

17. Weis L, Heelan RT, Watson RC: Computed tomography of orthopedic tumors of the pelvis and lower extremities. *Clin Orthop* 1978; 130:254-259.

18. Berger PE, Kuhn JP: Computed tomography of tumors of the musculoskeletal system in children. *Radiology* 1978; 127:171-175.

19. Herman G, Rose JS: Computed tomography in bone and soft tissue pathology of the extremities. *J Comput Assist Tomogr* 1979; 3:58-66.

20. Levine E, Lee KR, Neff JR, et al: Comparison of computed tomography and other imaging modalities in the evaluation of musculoskeletal tumors. *Radiology* 1979; 131:431-437.

21. Destouet JM, Gilula LA, Murphy WA: Computed tomography of long-bone osteosarcoma. *Radiology* 1979; 131:439-445.

22. Ginaldi S, deSantos LA: Computed tomography in the evaluation of small round cell tumors of bone. *Radiology* 1980; 134:441-446.

23. Kenney PJ, Gilula LA, Murphy WA: The use of computed tomography to distinguish osteochondroma and chondrosarcoma. *Radiology* 1981; 139:129-137.

24. Cann EC, Genant HK: Precise measurement of vertebral mineral content using computed tomography. *J Comput Assist Tomogr* 1980; 4:493.

**Fig. 5A:** Non-Hodgkin's lymphoma. AP view of dorsal spine. There is subtle destruction of the right superolateral cortex of the T9 vertebral body (arrows).

**Fig. 5B:** CT scan at T9 level (same patient as 3A) clearly demonstrates a lytic lesion of the vertebral body (arrows). Pleural fibrosis (F) with focal calcifications in left pleural space.

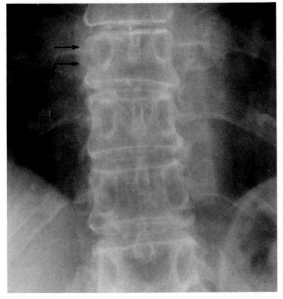

Figure 5A

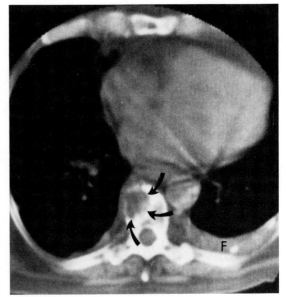

Figure 5B

Study 39

**Fig. 5C:** Lytic lesion of L3. Left paraspinal mass (arrows) resulted in lumbar plexopathy. Colon primary.

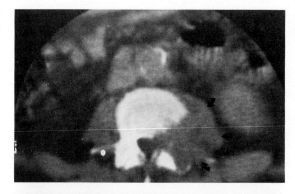

**Fig. 5D:** Two small blastic metastases (curved arrows) involving T11 vertebral body. Anterior osteophytes (straight arrows) are also present. Adenocarcinoma of prostate.

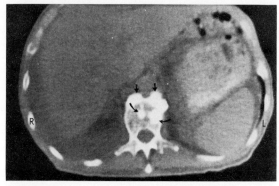

**Fig. 6:** Spina bifida with myelomeningocele at S1 level (arrows). Calcific densities within the meningocele represent residual myelographic contrast material.

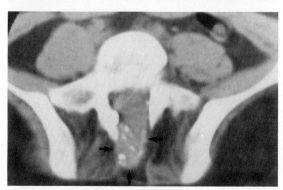

**Fig. 7:** Patient is post left hemilaminectomy and fusion at L5. Recurrent symptoms due to lateral recess stenosis (arrows) and overgrowth of scar tissue (arrow heads) through laminectomy defect.

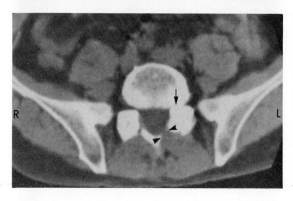

Bone Radiology Case Studies

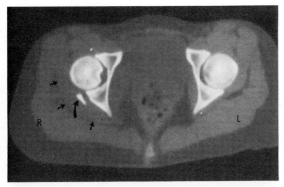

**Fig. 8A:** Fracture of posterior right acetabulum (curved arrow) with adjacent soft tissue swelling (straight arrows).

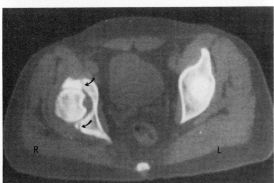

**Fig. 8B:** Fracture (arrows) of anterior and posterior portions of the right acetabulum.

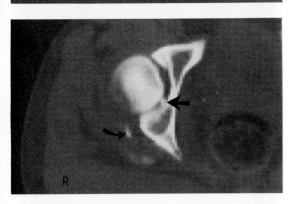

**Fig. 8C:** Small fracture fragment (curved arrow) from posterior right acetabulum. Intra-articular fragment (large arrow) is present.

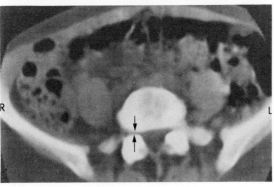

**Fig. 9:** Lumbar facet arthropathy. The facet joints are bilaterally obliterated. Bony overgrowth has caused narrowing of the right lateral recess (arrows).

**Fig. 10:** Herniated disc at L5-S1 causing characteristic obliteration of the ventral fat pad on the right side. Note normal appearing fat pad on left (arrows). Facet disease is also present.

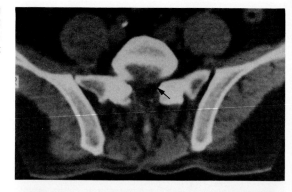

**Fig. 11:** Lumbar spinal stenosis. Both AP and transverse diameters are decreased. Bony canal has typical "Tri-Foil" appearance.

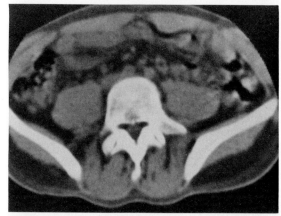

**Fig. 12:** Osteosarcoma of left femur. There is a soft tissue mass and increased density of the marrow cavity plus periosteal reaction (arrows).

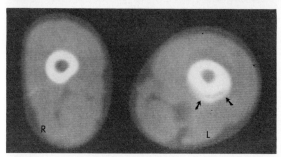

**Fig. 13A:** Rhabdomyosarcoma (arrows) of right buttock, apparently arising from gluteus medius.

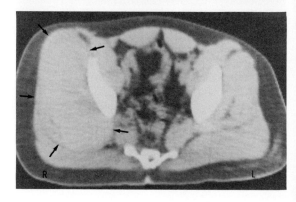

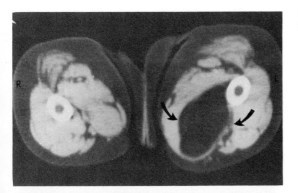

**Fig. 13B:** Large lipoma of left thigh (arrows).

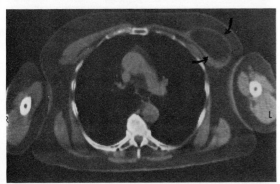

**Fig. 13C:** Lipoma of chest wall (arrows).

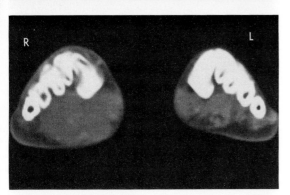

**Fig. 13D:** Fibromatosis of right foot. Homogenous soft tissue mass below metatarsals.

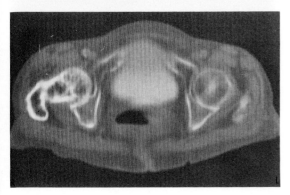

**Fig. 14:** Paget's disease involving right femur.

**Fig. 15:** Osteomyelitis of T12 vertebral body. Lytic lesions with cortical destruction (arrow) and subtle periosteal new bone (arrow heads). Left paraspinal soft tissue mass (curved arrows) is present.

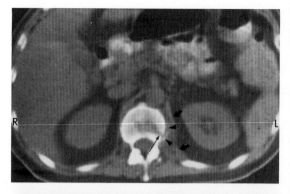

**Fig. 16:** Osteomyelitis right acromioclavicular joint. Section at level of upper clavicle demonstrates destruction of medial right clavicle (arrow) with adjacent soft tissue swelling (curved arrows). Lower section demonstrated destruction of lateral sternal manubrium.

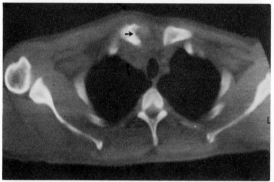

**Fig. 17:** Congenital dislocation of right hip. Femoral head is displaced superolaterally. Anterior acetabulum is poorly formed.

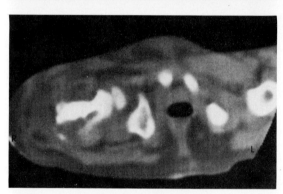

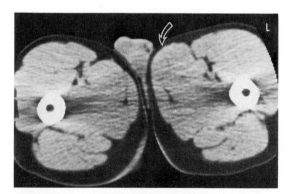

**Fig. 18A:** This 16-year-old boy has a palpable mass in the left upper thigh medially (arrow).

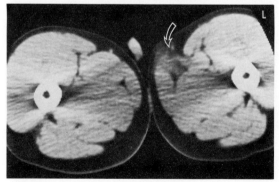

**Fig. 18B:** More distal section showing defect in adductor muscle (arrow). The adductor had torn and retracted upward, resulting in a palpable mass.

Bone Radiology Case Studies

# Appendix of Diagnoses

Section I: Radiographic Features of Bone and Joint Disease
    Turner's Syndrome


Section II: Size and Shape
    Congenital Tarsal Coalition
    Juvenile Chronic Arthritis
    Multiple Hereditary Exostosis with Madelung Deformity
    Rotational Subluxation of Navicular
    Sickle Cell Anemia (Anemias)
    Slipped Capital Femoral Epiphysis
    Traumatic (Plastic) Bowing Fracture


Section III: Density
    Acute Lymphocytic Leukemia (Lymphoreticular disorders)
    Benign Vertebral Sclerosis
    Osteoid Osteoma
    Rheumatoid Arthritis
    Skeletal Tuberculosis
    Solitary Plasmacytoma of Sternum
    Subacute Osteomyelitis


Section IV: Cortex and Trabeculae
    Congenital Absence of Vertebral Pedicle
    Fibrous Dysplasia
    Legg-Calvé-Perthes Disease
    Posterior Shoulder Dislocations
    Primary Lymphoma of Bone
    Radiation Bone Damage

Section V: Periosteum
   Neurofibromatosis
   Psoriatic Arthritis
   Sarcomatous Degeneration of an Enchondroma


Section IV: Soft Tissue
   Calcium Pyrophosphate Dihydrate (CPPD)
     Deposition Disease
   Diffuse Idiopathic Skeletal Hyperostosis
   Ewing's Sarcoma
   Gout
   Hemophilia (and Myeloproliferative disorders)
   Osteosarcoma
   Soft Tissue Fibrosarcoma


Section VII: Joints
   Galeazzi Fracture Dislocation
   Giant Synovial Cyst
   Isolated Traumatic Dislocation of Radial Head
   Osteochondral Fracture
   Partial Menisectomy with Torn Remnant (Arthrography)


Section VIII: Bone Imaging
   Computed Tomography
   Vertebral Column Osteoid Osteoma (Nuclear Medicine)
   Stress Fracture

Appendix of Diagnoses

# Index

Enchondromatosis 182, 183, 184, 203
    multiple 38, 182, 183
Endarteritis 150
Endocarditis
    subacute bacterial 102
Endocrinopathy 159
Ependymoma 176
Erosion 112, 114, 115, 175, 177, 191, 192, 193, 194, 195,
    196, 197, 198, 255
    articular 113
    asymmetric 115
    bone 23, 175, 254
    bony 112, 217, 255
    calcaneal 112, 194
    distal interphalangeal 198
        joint 192
    odontoid 24
    osseous 113, 114
    vertebral artery 146
Erthroleukemia 242
Erythema 106
Erythematosis
    systemic lupus 102, 106
Erythroblastosis 47
    fetalis 42, 48
Erythrocyte 242
Erythropoiesis 46
Exophthalmos 176, 177
Exostosis
    multiple 39
        hereditary 37-39, 291, 308

**F**
Fabry's disease 140
Fibroblast 202, 216
Fibroma
    chondromyxoid 78, 85, 184
Fibromatosis 329
    benign juvenile 219
Fibrosarcoma 153, 205, 206, 216, 217, 218, 219
    soft tissue 215-219
Fibrosis 23, 242
    annulus 98, 228, 230, 238
    interstitial
        diffuse 105
        pulmonary 179
    pleural 326
    pulmonary 190
Flat foot 44, 58, 67
    hypermobile 61
    peroneal 59
    spastic 59
        peroneal 59
Fluorosis 72, 231
Forestier's disease 229, 232
Fracture 25, 26, 48, 128, 150, 153, 160, 162, 175, 183,
    184, 242, 258, 264, 292, 321, 326
    acute 146
    angulated 31, 34
    avulsion 294
    Bankart's 137
    bowing 30, 34

traumatic (plastic) 29-35
    Chauffeur's 296
    Colles' 294, 296
    complete 30
    Darrach-Hughston-Milch 294
    Dorsal Barton's 294
    Essex-Lopresti's 296
    fatigue 301
    femoral neck 140, 153
    Galeazzi 293-296
    greenstick 30, 32, 33, 34, 35
    impacted 11, 128
    impaction 131, 132, 135, 136
    incomplete 11, 30, 128
    insufficiency 301
    isolated ulnar 296
    Monteggia's 290
    multiple oblique 30
    osteochondral 59, 283-287
    pathologic 44, 159
    Piedmont 294
    reverse Hill-Sachs 136
    reverse Monteggia 294
    Smith's 294, 296
    spontaneous 174
    stress 30, 210, 299-304, 308, 312
    subcortical 141
    tibial 34
    torus 30
    trochanter 137
    Volar Barton's 294
Fungal disease 74
Fusion 58, 62, 145, 174
    apophyseal 198
    calcaneo-navicular 61
    cartilagenous 61, 62
    fibrous 61, 62
    joint 62
    non-bony 60
    premature 80
    spinal 322
    talo-calcaneal 61, 62
    tarsal
        arthritic 58
        infectious 58
        traumatic 58

**G**
Gallstones
    pigmented 48
Gangrene
    gas 200
Gaucher's disease 53, 140
Glioma 176
    optic 175, 176, 178, 179
Globin 51
    abnormal 42
        synthesis 43, 51
Gout 114, 190, 238, 244, 245, 251-256, 262
Granulation tissue 104
Granulocyte 242, 244
Granulocytopenia 50, 244

Granuloma
    eosinophilic 85, 166, 210, 211, 222
Granulomatosis 26
Granulomatous disease 91
Granulomatous tissue 84

**H**
Hand-foot syndrome 53
Hamartoma 176
    cartilagenous 182
Heart disease
    congenital 50
    valvular 105
Heavy chain disease 120
Hemangioma 13, 182, 183
    joint 19
        knee 24
    synovial 242
Hemangiopericytoma 216
Hemarthrosis 53, 118, 242
Hematogenous spread 89
Hematologic disease 6, 72
Hematoma 9, 131, 172, 241, 244, 322
Hematopoiesis 243
    extramedullary 42, 248
Hemi-hypertrophy 172
Hemimelia 58, 291
Hemiplegia 108
Hemochromatosis 231, 238
Hemoglobin 43, 51, 52
    abnormal 51
Hemoglobin C 53
Hemoglobin S 48, 53, 54
Hemoglobinopathy 51
    sickle 140, 253
Hemoglobinuria 46, 50
    paroxysmal nocturnal 42, 50
Hemolysis 43, 46, 50, 51, 52
Hemolytic disease
    isoimmune 42, 48
Hemophilia 19, 24, 42, 90, 238, 241-249
Hemorrhage 204, 242, 270
    intravascular 242
    subperiosteal 172, 173, 175, 242
Hemosiderin deposition 242
Henoch-Schonlein disease 19
Hepatosplenomegaly 21, 50, 118, 123, 243, 244, 245
Heterozygous form 48
Heterozygous S 51
Histiocytoma
    malignant 78
        fibrous 206, 216
Histiocytosis X 90
Hodgkin's disease 120, 122
Holt-Oram syndrome 44
Homocystinuria 53
Homozygous S disease 51
Hurler's disease 38
Hyaline membrane disease 50
Hydrocephalus 176
    obstructive 176
Hydropneumothorax 208

Hyperbilirubinemia
    indirect 48
Hypercalcemia 72, 120
Hyperemia 72, 90, 108, 312
Hyperlipidemia 140
Hyperostosis 229, 231
    ankylosing 228, 229
    cervical 228
    diffuse idiopathic skeletal 227-233
    infantile cortical 12
    spiculated 232
    spinal 229
Hyperostotica
    spondylosis 228
Hyperparathyroidism 6, 8, 10-11, 70, 72, 159, 181, 238, 239, 258, 316
Hyperphosphatasia 162
Hyperplasia
    marrow 46, 47, 48, 51, 52, 53
        exuberant 46
Hypertension 176
    portal 243
Hyperthyroidism 159, 316
Hypertrophy 70, 103, 172, 173, 242
Hyperuricemia 140, 253
Hypogammaglobulinemia 19
Hypogonadism 159
Hypoparathyroidism 231
Hypophosphatasia 162, 231, 238
Hypoplasia 44, 61
    phalangeal 46
    radial element 44
Hypotension 245
Hypothyroidism 70, 238
Hypoxia
    tissue 44

**I**
Ileostomy 150
Infarct 6, 48, 50, 51, 51, 53, 72, 104, 107, 184, 185, 203, 210, 301
Infarction
    myocardial 238
Infection 6, 16, 19, 20, 38, 44, 46, 51, 52, 53, 58, 84, 88, 89, 90, 91, 93, 96, 98, 99, 120, 128, 153, 166, 223, 244, 262, 306, 315
Inflammation 150, 254, 258, 312, 315
    acute 237
    arthritic 58
    chronic 104
    synovial 242
Inflammatory disease 74, 315
Iridocyclitis
    acute 22
    chronic 22
Iron deficiency 42, 50
Ischemia 53, 142, 150

**J**
Jaundice 50
Joint damage
    progressive 254

Joint destruction 72
  disabling 22
  peripheral 22
  severe 24
Joint disease 109
  degenerative 71, 72, 258, 281
  interphalangeal 191
  space 242

## K

Keratoconjunctivitis sica 105
Ketosis 253
Klinefelter's syndrome 70, 291
Kyphoscoliosis 173, 174
Kyphosis 153

## L

Lead poisoning 9, 253
Legg-Calvé-Perthes disease 139-142
Leiomyosarcoma 216
Lesion 4, 21, 38, 39, 62, 74, 76, 78, 84, 104, 107, 120, 122,
  123, 126, 156, 157, 160, 161, 162, 166, 174, 175, 176,
  182, 183, 184, 191, 202, 203, 204, 207, 209, 210, 211,
  212, 213, 218, 226, 269, 306, 310, 311, 313, 323
  aggressive 72, 170
  articular 90
  bilateral symmetric 84
  bone 5, 11, 88, 122, 156, 159, 166, 209, 212
    benign 315
    fibrous 159
    lytic 207
  bony 159
  cardiovascular 176
  congenital 217, 290
  cystic 110
    intraosseous 173, 175, 177
  destructive 89, 92, 315
  epiphyseal 84
  expansile rib 159
  extrameniscal 264, 268-270
  homogenous 160
  intra-articular 79
  intraosseous 175
  lucent 96, 162
  lytic 10-11, 87, 88, 118, 120, 122, 123, 125, 126, 202,
    203, 242, 244, 245, 326, 330-331
    geographic metaphyseal-diaphyseal 183
    multiple coalescent 118
    rib 120, 223
  malignant 167, 213
  meniscal 264, 267-268
  metaphyseal 225
  metastatic 315
  mixed 118
  monostotic 160
  nail 190
  neoplastic 324
  osseous 323
  psoriatic 190
  sclerotic 121, 122, 203, 245
  skeletal 76, 172
    tuberculous 88

skin 159, 172, 190, 199, 245
skull 122
spine 90
sternal 74
subperiosteal 79, 80
Leukemia 19, 47, 50, 166, 222, 244, 245
  acute 119, 120, 121, 244
  Burkitt's 118
  childhood 118
  granulocytic
    acute 242, 244
    chronic 42, 242, 243, 244-245
  lymphocytic 118
    acute 42, 117-126
  myelogenous 118
    acute 42, 118
    chronic 42
Leukocyte 21, 84, 103, 237, 253, 254, 312
Leukocytosis 21, 22, 23
Ligamentosa
  spondylitis ossificans 228
Lipoma 329
Liposarcoma 206, 216, 217
Lupus erythematosus
  systemic 19
Lymphadenopathy 22, 118, 245
  generalized 21
Lymphoblast 167
Lymphocyte 102, 103, 104, 118, 120, 167
Lymphoma 74, 98, 118, 166, 216
  bone 165-168
  disseminated 166
  histiocytic 78, 123, 166, 222
  Hodgkins 42, 118, 166
  lymphocytic 124
  metastatic 8, 222
  non-Hodgkins 42, 118, 166
  primary 22
Lymphoproliferative disease 253

## M

Macrocephaly 175
Macrocranium 173
Macroglobulinemia 123
  Waldenstrom's 120, 123
Maffucci's syndrome 182, 183
Marfanoid habitus 179
Marfan's disease 175
Mastectomy
  radical 152
Mastocytosis 42
  systemic 245, 249
Mediterranean fever
  familial 19
Melanoma 75
  malignant 125, 173
  metastatic 206
Meningioma 176
Meningocele 174, 176, 179, 326
Meniscectomy
  partial 264-282
Mental retardation 44, 176

malignant 173
Sclerosis 6, 12, 48, 49, 50, 53, 60, 61, 71, 72, 79, 80, 84, 85,
    86, 90, 96, 97, 98, 108, 109, 115, 118, 119, 122, 123,
    124, 141, 145, 150, 151, 152, 156, 160, 162, 168, 175,
    184, 185, 192, 193, 197, 198, 225, 226, 230, 236, 243,
    246, 247, 249, 255, 302, 303
    benign 95-99
        vertebral 95-99
    bone 4, 91
    circumscribed 96
    discogenic 97
    focal 72
    iliac 195
    juxta-articular 115
    noninfectious 96
    non-neoplastic segmental 96
    reparative 30
    sacral 195
    segmental anterior 99
    tuberous 172, 245
    vertebral 96, 97
Scoliosis 153, 173, 174, 179, 308
    cervical 174
    idiopathic 174
    lumbar 151, 174
Serum sickness 19
Sequestration 48, 51, 52, 84, 225
Short status syndrome 16
    congenital 16
Sickle cell disease 6, 42, 45, 245
    hemoglobin C 51
Sickle cell-thalassemia 51, 54
Sickling disease 42
Silver's syndrome 291
Sinusitis 157
    chronic 157
Sjogren's syndrome 105
Skeletal disease 5
Slipped epiphysis
    femoral 19
        capital 69-71, 140, 153
Spherocytosis 53
    hereditary 42, 48
Spina bifida 145, 326
Spina ventosa 91, 93
Splenomegaly 22, 48
    massive 46
Spondylitis 191
    ankylosing 22, 98, 115, 195, 198, 229, 230, 231, 232
Spondylolisthesis 97
Spondylolysis 145, 147, 306, 308
Spondylosis
    cervical 229
    deformans 230, 231
Stasis
    vascular 51
Stenosis
    artery 176
        renal 176
    aqueductal 176
    pulmonic valve 176
    recess 327

spinal 322
    lumbar 328
Still's disease 18
Sturge-Weber syndrome 172
Subluxation 27, 104, 107, 109, 112, 115, 141, 145, 192,
    194, 198
    atlantoaxial 24, 115
    hip 142
    humeral 193
    irreversible 106
    rotational, of navicular 25-28
    rotatory 192
    volar 106
Surgery 26, 61, 62, 76, 80, 82, 85, 89, 162, 167, 168, 175,
    212, 216, 218, 237, 238, 242, 254, 263, 269, 274, 285,
    291, 301, 315, 322, 324
Symphalangism 58
Synchondrosis 58
    neurocentral 145, 146
Syndesmosis 58
Syndesmophyte 195, 198
    spinal 199
Synostosis 58, 61, 66, 146
    familial carpal 291
    familial tarsal 291
    local anterior 67
    talo-navicular 60
    tibiofibular 291
Synovectomy 23
Synovial cyst 260
    giant 259-262
Synovioma 166
Synovitis 19, 22, 108, 110, 112, 270
    acute 141
    chronic 115
    diffuse proliferative 103
    nonspecific 19
    villonodular 262
        pigmented 270
Syphilis
    congenital 47, 91
    infantile 50
Syringomyelia 176

**T**
Talar beak 61, 63
Thalassemia 42, 45, 46, 48, 51, 53, 54, 128
    beta 54
        major 52
    major 45, 46, 47
    minor 46
Thrombocythemia 242, 243
Thrombocytopenia 42, 50, 118, 244
    congenital hypomegakaryocytic 45
    with absent radii syndrome 42, 44, 45
Thrombophlebitis 107, 260, 268, 277
Thrombosis 44, 107
    cerebral 238
    venous 50
Thrombus 104
Trauma 19, 26, 38, 58, 89, 96, 97, 98, 104, 130, 140, 146,
    153, 155, 171, 172, 175, 183, 200, 237, 242, 254, 258,